ALLE·ZEIT·WACH
1842

M. Middeke · H. Holzgreve (Eds.)

New Aspects in Hypertension

Adrenoceptors

With the Assistance of B. Riepl

With 76 Figures and 18 Tables

Springer-Verlag Berlin Heidelberg New York
London Paris Tokyo

Dr. Martin Middeke

Professor Dr. Heinrich Holzgreve

Medizinische Poliklinik
der Ludwig-Maximilians-Universität München
Pettenkoferstr. 8 a
8000 München 2

"New Aspects in Hypertension - Adrenoceptors" Symposium
November 1985, Munich

ISBN-13:978-3-642-71420-7 e-ISBN-13:978-3-642-71418-4
DOI: 10.1007/978-3-642-71418-4

Library of Congress Cataloging-in-Publication Data

New aspects in hypertension.
1. Hypertension - Etiology. 2. Adrenergic receptors. I. Middeke, M. (Martin), 1948-
II. Holzgreve, Heinrich. III. Riepl, B. [DNLM: 1. Hypertension - physiopathology.
2. Receptors, Adrenergic - physiology. WG340 N532]
RC685.H8N48 1986 616.1'32071 86-17782
ISBN-13:978-3-642-71420-7

Softcover reprint of the hardcover 1st edition 1986

2127/3145-5 4 3 2 1 0

Preface

This book reports on the current state of knowledge about adrenoceptors and their involvement in the pathogenesis and treatment of high blood pressure. This is a relatively recent and extremely exciting addition to the field of hypertension research. The development of new analytical procedures, such as radioligand-binding methods, has made it possible to identify and quantify the adrenoceptors in different tissues and in circulating blood cells. As a consequence, much new and valuable information has been obtained. An understanding of the role of the β-adrenoceptor-adenylatecyclase-cAMP system in hypertension is one such product of this new approach.

Both review articles and new experimental and clinical data are included in this volume. New aspects of the distribution, identification and regulation, and the chronopharmacology of adrenoceptors, as well as beta blockade, will be highlighted.

The clinical contributions concern the normal regulation of the β-adrenoceptor-adenylatecyclase-cAMP system, and how it is altered in hypertensives as a possible mechanism in the pathogenesis and maintenance of essential hypertension. With this knowledge it is becoming easier to explain the molecular and cellular action behind the familiar role of the sympathico-adrenergic system in the development of hypertension and the mechanism of beta blockade. The vast majority of the data available in this field is confined to peripheral mechanisms, owing to the limited possibilities for investigating the central nervous system under clinical conditions. The presentations and discussions show the direction that future experimental and clinical research will have to take to obtain a universal picture of the central and peripheral sympathico-adrenergic mechanisms involved in the development of hypertension.

We would very much like to thank all contributors to this book for their willingness to make their research available to the public and for the speedy submission of their contributions.

Neither the symposium itself nor the publication of the contributions would have been possible had it not been for the generous support of ICI Germany.

Munich, June 1986 *M. Middeke and H. Holzgreve*

Table of Contents

List of Contributors

S. Bauer
Pharmakologisches Institut der Universität Heidelberg
Im Neuenheimer Feld 366, 6900 Heidelberg, Federal Republic of Germany

L. H. Block
Kantonsspital Basel, Dept. für Innere Medizin
Petersgraben 4, 4031 Basel, Switzerland

F. Bompart
Department of Clinical Pharmacology, University College London and The Middlesex Hospital Medical School, The Rayne Institute
5 University Street, London WC1E 6JJ, England

U. Borchard
Institut für Pharmakologie der Universität Düsseldorf
Moorenstraße 5, 4000 Düsseldorf 1, Federal Republic of Germany

A. Borghetti
Istituto di Clinica Medica e Nefrologia, Università di Parma
Via Gramsci 14, 43100 Parma, Italy

O. E. Brodde
Universitätsklinikum Essen, Biochem. Forschungslabor der Medizinischen Klinik und Poliklinik, Abteilung für Nieren- und Hochdruckkranke, Hufelandstraße 55, 4300 Essen 1, Federal Republic of Germany

G. Bruschi
Istituto di Clinica Medica e Nefrologia, Università di Parma
Via Gramsci 14, 43100 Parma, Italy

M. E. Bruschi
Istituto di Clinica Medica e Nefrologia, Università di Parma
Via Gramsci 14, 43100 Parma, Italy

A. Cavatorta
Istituto di Clinica Medica e Nefrologia, Università di Parma
Via Gramsci 14, 43100 Parma, Italy

J. M. Cruickshank
ICI plc Pharmaceuticals Division
Mereside, Alderley Park, Macclesfield, Cheshire SK10 4TH, England

A. Daul
Universitätsklinikum Essen, Biochem. Forschungslabor der Medizinischen Klinik und Poliklinik, Abteilung für Nieren- und Hochdruckkranke, Hufelandstraße 55, 4300 Essen 1, Federal Republic of Germany

A. Distler
Universitätsklinikum Steglitz, Medizinische Klinik und Poliklinik, Abt. für allg. Innere Medizin und Nephrologie
Hindenburgdamm 30, 1000 Berlin 45, Federal Republic of Germany

E. Fritschka
Universitätsklinikum Steglitz, Medizinische Klinik und Poliklinik, Abt. für allg. Innere Medizin und Nephrologie
Hindenburgdamm 30, 1000 Berlin 45, Federal Republic of Germany

M. Göthert
Institut für Pharmakologie und Toxikologie, Universität Bonn
Reuterstraße 2b, 5300 Bonn, Federal Republic of Germany

R. Grandt
Pharmakologisches Institut der Universität Heidelberg
Im Neuenheimer Feld 366, 6900 Heidelberg, Federal Republic of Germany

C. Greiner
Pharmakologisches Institut der Universität Heidelberg
Im Neuenheimer Feld 366, 6900 Heidelberg, Federal Republic of Germany

D. Hafner
Institut für Pharmakologie der Universität Düsseldorf
Moorenstraße 5, 4000 Düsseldorf 1, Federal Republic of Germany

H. Haller
Universitätsklinikum Steglitz, Abteilung für Innere Medizin
Hindenburgdamm 30, 1000 Berlin 45, Federal Republic of Germany

S. Harwig
Universitätsklinikum Steglitz, Abteilung für Innere Medizin
Hindenburgdamm 30, 1000 Berlin 45, Federal Republic of Germany

H. Holzgreve
Medizinische Poliklinik, Universität München
Pettenkoferstraße 8a, 8000 München 2, Federal Republic of Germany

K. H. Jakobs
Pharmakologisches Institut der Universität Heidelberg
Im Neuenheimer Feld 366, 6900 Heidelberg, Federal Republic of Germany

W. P. Koella
4104 Oberwil/Basel, Switzerland

W. Krawietz
Medizinische Klinik I, Zentralklinikum Augsburg, Lehrkrankenhaus der Ludwig-Maximilians-Universität München
8900 Augsburg, Federal Republic of Germany

A. Kribben
Universitätsklinikum Steglitz, Abteilung für Innere Medizin
Hindenburgdamm 30, 1000 Berlin 45, Federal Republic of Germany

P.-H. Lang
Klinikum der Johann-Wolfgang-Goethe-Universität, Zentrum der Pharmakologie, Theodor-Stern-Kai 7, 6000 Frankfurt 70, Federal Republic of Germany

B. Lemmer
Klinikum der Johann-Wolfgang-Goethe-Universität, Zentrum der Pharmakologie, Theodor-Stern-Kai 7, 6000 Frankfurt 70, Federal Republic of Germany

T. Lenz
Universitätsklinikum Steglitz, Abteilung für Innere Medizin
Hindenburgdamm 30, 1000 Berlin 45, Federal Republic of Germany

X. Liang Wang
Universitätsklinikum Essen, Biochem. Forschungslabor der Medizinischen Klinik und Poliklinik, Abteilung für Nieren- und Hochdruckkranke, Hufelandstraße 55, 4300 Essen 1, Federal Republic of Germany

M. Luedersdorf
Universitätsklinikum Steglitz, Abteilung für Innere Medizin
Hindenburgdamm 30, 1000 Berlin 45, Federal Republic of Germany

M. Middeke
Medizinische Poliklinik der Ludwig-Maximilians-Universität
Pettenkoferstraße 8 a, 8000 München 2, Federal Republic of Germany

M. Minuth
Pharmakologisches Institut der Universität Heidelberg
Im Neuenheimer Feld 366, 6900 Heidelberg, Federal Republic of Germany

N. O'Hara
Universitätsklinikum Essen, Biochem. Forschungslabor der Medizinischen Klinik und Poliklinik, Abteilung für Nieren- und Hochdruckkranke, Hufelandstraße 55, 4300 Essen 1, Federal Republic of Germany

D. Palm
Zentrum der Pharmakologie, Klinikum der J. W. Goethe Universität, Theodor-Stern-Kai 7, 6000 Frankfurt/Main, Federal Republic of Germany

Th. Philipp
Universitätsklinikum Steglitz, Medizinische Klinik und Poliklinik Hindenburgdamm 30, 1000 Berlin 45, Federal Republic of Germany

B. N. C. Prichard
Department of Clinical Pharmacology, University College London and The Middlesex Hospital Medical School, The Rayne Institute 5 University Street, London WC1E 6JJ, England

J. Schloos
Zentrum der Pharmakologie, Klinikum der J. W. Goethe Universität, Theodor-Stern-Kai 7, 6000 Frankfurt/Main, Federal Republic of Germany

D. Schütz
Institut für Pharmakologie der Universität Düsseldorf Moorenstraße 5, 4000 Düsseldorf 1, Federal Republic of Germany

H. M. Thiede
Universitätsklinikum Steglitz, Abteilung für Innere Medizin Hindenburgdamm 30, 1000 Berlin 45, Federal Republic of Germany

A. Wellstein
Zentrum der Pharmakologie, Klinikum der J. W. Goethe Universität, Theodor-Stern-Kai 7, 6000 Frankfurt/Main, Federal Republic of Germany

P. Zubin
Pharmakologisches Institut der Universität Heidelberg Im Neuenheimer Feld 366, 6900 Heidelberg, Federal Republic of Germany

Central Nervous Noradrenergic and Adrenergic Systems and their Functions

W. P. KOELLA
4104 Oberwil/Basel, Switzerland

Introduction

It is not unusual to hear or read that the therapeutic effects of beta-adrenoceptive blocking agents (BABAs) upon a variety of cardiovascular disorders - including hypertension - are satisfactorily explained by a preferentially, if not exclusively, peripheral locus of action of these drugs. In other words, one tends to assume that BABAs correct, for example, an abnormally elevated blood pressure by interfering with signal transmission at a variety of peripheral, post- and presynaptically located beta-adrenergic receptor sites. Van Zwieten and Timmermans [63], on the basis of their results obtained with atenolol and metoprolol, were ready to conclude that "a central mechanism (does not) underly the antihypertensive activity of beta-blockers."

Yet, closer scrutiny of a vast variety of effects induced by adrenergically active substances clearly indicates that the situation is by no means that simple. In the first place, one has to be aware that the net effect upon, for instance, the blood pressure, of a BABA that supposedly acts solely in the periphery a priori includes an indirect central component: information about the drop in blood pressure, as induced through the pharmacological action upon the vascular musculature and the heart muscle, is signalled back via sinoaortic receptors and pathways to the CNS. The latter, in turn, initiates countermeasures and thus reduces to some extent the pharmacologically induced change in the periphery.

Furthermore, a good many of the BABAs, in particular those of a more lipophilic nature, *do* penetrate the blood-brain barrier to reach the brain tissue proper. Experiments in animals and observations in human volunteers and patients have shown that such penetrating beta-blockers *are* capable of producing typically central effects [4, 5, 10, 16, 20, 25, 30, 45]. Furthermore, beta-blockers have been used successfully to treat a variety of "central" afflictions, in particular anxiety [18, 23, 26, 30, 31, 47, 50]. Thus, it seems that the possibility of a central component of action of lipophilic BABAs - in the sense of a directly, i.e., pharmacologically, induced change in activity of some "strategic" central structure with an autonomic output to the periphery - contributing to such typically vegetative-autonomic effects as lowering of the blood pressure (as well as of more somatic effects) should not be too lightheartedly dismissed. As recently outlined [30], one can contemplate indeed that the lipophilic BABAs bind to beta-receptors situated on neurons of adrenergically innervated and autonomically (as well as somatically) active central nervous networks.

New Aspects in Hypertension: Adrenoceptors
M. Middeke and H. Holzgreve (Eds.)
Springer-Verlag Berlin Heidelberg New York 1986

Moreover, BABAs may act via their affinity to a variety of *non*adrenergic receptors (e.g., of the 5-HT variety) and/or via their "unspecific" membrane-stabilizing effects.

Even if, for the sake of simplicity, a specific and truly (beta-)adrenergic mode of central action of BABAs, and of adrenergic agents in general is considered, proper understanding of these mechanisms and their functional consequences still requires adequate knowledge of the location of the central-nervous adrenoceptors and, even more, of their "downstream" functional connections, *together* with their "input" in terms of various ascending and descending noradrenergic and adrenergic fiber systems that project to these receptor areas.

It is the aim of the present paper to supply, although in somewhat cursory manner, this information. Readers interested in considerably more detail are kindly referred to the papers and book chapters which are mentioned in the text and which, in fact, have been used extensively for the "education" of this writer. The very same and additional references can be consulted for information about a variety of other - nonadrenergic - "wet" neurotransmission systems.

Anatomy of the Central Noradrenergic and Adrenergic Systems

Noradrenergic, truly adrenergic, and dopaminergic fiber systems constitute but three of a vast variety of virtually ubiquitous aminergic, aminoacidergic, or polypeptidergic neurohumoral transmission instruments that handle information transfer through, and to some extent into, as well as out of, the central nervous system. The unifying feature of all these transmission systems is that they transmit information electrically along the axons of their neurons and then across the synaptic cleft or across the space surrounding extrasynaptic receptors by means of a transmitting substance. The latter then binds to specialized receptors situated on both the post- and presynaptic membrane and thus leads to activation of the receptor and then to activation of one of a variety of postreceptor, or second messenger mechanisms.

Noradrenergic and, to some extent, adrenergic neurons have been detected and followed to their usually widely divergent projection sites by means of the fluorescence technique of Falck and co-workers [13] and, later, by means of the methods of imunofluorescence as well as, in part, by biochemical methods [24]. From the early work of Dahlström and Fuxe [11], Andén and co-workers [1], Ungerstedt [61], supplemented by more recent studies of Livett [35], Maeda and collaborators [38], Pickel and co-workers [51], Swanson and Hartman [57], Commissiong and co-workers [8], Loewy and collaborators [37], and many others - performed mostly on the rat, but also in a number of other species - we have now come to possess ample and unequivocal evidence that noradrenergic (NA), adrenergic (A), and dopaminergic (DA) nerve fibers emerge from a series of catecholaminergic cell-body agglomerations in the brain stem: the various "Ai" nuclei. These cells, with their emerging axons, give rise to ascending and descending fiber tracts which project to different areas of the forebrain, the length of the brain stem (including the diencephalon), the cerebellum, and the spinal cord.

Fibers emerging from A6, in the locus coeruleus, and A7, part of the subcoeruleus nucleus (both located in the upper pontine area and both mainly noradrenergic in nature), form what is usually referred to as the dorsal ascending noradrenergic fasciculus. It runs through the lateral hypothalamus (the medial forebrain bundle) and innervates virtually the entire neocortex, the cingular cortex, the hippocampus, the amygdala, the subiculum, the septum, and the piriform cortex. A descending portion of the dorsal bundle, also originating in A6 and A7, projects to the cerebellar cortex and to the spinal cord. In the latter it terminates mainly in the ventral horn region [9]. The adrenergic nucleus A1, the noradrenergic A2 and A4 (in the medul-

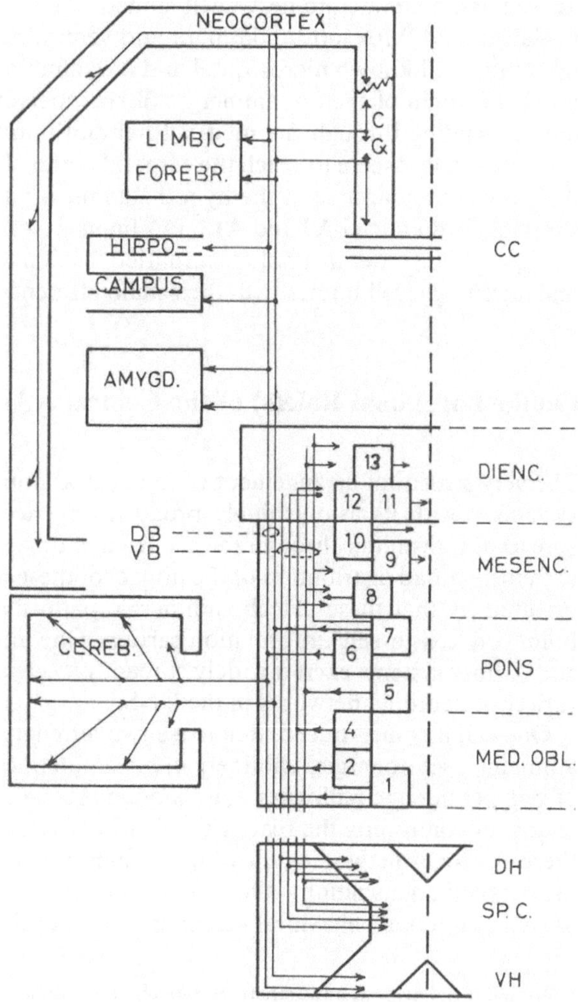

Fig. 1. Schematic representation of the various adrenergic and noradrenergic nuclei *[1–7 (8)]* with their most important projections to the various structures and networks of the CNS. The projections of the exclusively, or quasi-exclusively dopaminergic nuclei *(9–13)* are not shown. *CC*, corpus callosum; *CCx*, cingular cortex; DB, VB, dorsal and ventral noradrenergic bundles; *DH, VH*, dorsal and ventral horns of the spinal cord gray matter *(SP.C.)*; *CEREB*, cerebellum; *DIENC.*, diencephalon; *MESENC.*, mesencephalon. (Adapted in part from Andén et al. [1])

la), A5, and (part of) A7 (in the pons) give rise to the ventral ascending bundle which innervates the various parts of the brain stem, including some of the (serotonergic) raphé nuclei and, rather densely, the hypothalamus. From A1, A2, and A5 arise descending fibers which reach the intermedio-lateral cell column of the thoracic and upper lumber spinal cord. These are the loci that contain the somata of the cholinergic preganglionic efferent sympathetic fibers. In addition, the three A-nuclei just mentioned also innervate the dorsal horn. Of interest also is the observation that A1 projects to the nucleus motorius of the vagal nerve and to the nucleus of the solitary tract [61].

A8 in the rostral midbrain is clearly a "mixed" nucleus, containing noradrenergic as well as dopaminergic nerve cell somata. The almost exclusively dopaminergic nuclei A9 and A10 (substantia nigra and ventral tegmental area, respectively) give rise to the well-known nigrostriatal and mesolimbic pathways. A12 and A13 are the points of origin of the dopaminergic fibers innervating the median eminence and, after ascending through the medial forebrain bundle, higher forebrain structures. The latter in fact seem to reach the cerebral cortex. Finally, A11, which is situated in the paraventricular area of the hypothalamus, is mainly dopaminergic in nature; it supplies, as do nuclei A9 and A13, DA fibers descending into the spinal cord.

Figure 1 illustrates in a rather simplified fashion the location of the noradrenergic and adrenergic cell bodies with their main efferent connections.

On the Functional Role(s) of the Central NA- and A-Systems

The very structural arrangement of the central noradrenergic and adrenergic fiber systems - with its astonishingly broad divergence, together with the even wider spread of transmitter through release from extrasynaptic varicosities, and, thus the extremely broad distribution of the impact of these neurohormones - makes it a priori unlikely that these catecholaminergic pathways subserve a role as "point-to-point" or "cell-to-cell" information carriers. One must rather postulate that the NA- and A-fiber systems exert a widely spread, yet selective, modulatory influence on a variety of neuronal networks in the CNS.

One can assume, indeed, that these two adrenergic systems - together with dopaminergic, serotonergic, cholinergic, histaminergic, trace-aminergic, and a variety of polypeptidergic pathways - are among the main central nervous instruments in charge of controlling the reactivity of those networks. One can assume further that these neuronal networks (allowing, though, for overlap and interaction) subserve the detailed organization - the actual "making" - of the vast variety of extroversive as well as internal behavioral activities[1]. Thus it follows that these aminergic as well

[1] We define behavior as any activity initiated by the animal organism which ensures survival of the individual and of the species and, true mainly for higher species, provides enjoyment of the good things of life. With this broad definition, one a priori must distinguish - while allowing for overlap, coexistence, cooperation, and interaction - between extroversive, i.e., overt, and internal, i.e., covert, behaviors. The former comprise mainly (skeleto-)motor activities of various complexities (posturing, locomotion, respiration, fighting, flight, searching and ingestion of food, playing, vocalization, writing, etc.), but also a variety of vegetative-autonomic activities that can be observed from

as peptidergic fiber systems are the prime controllers of *vigilance*, i. e., the level of responsiveness to internal and external stimuli, in the various behavioral systems.

In the following section we shall make an attempt towards an interpretation of the functional role(s) of the central nervous noradrenergic and adrenergic fiber systems in terms of a recently developed novel concept of vigilance; for details on this general theory of vigilance, the reader is referred to more detailed treatments [27, 28, 29].

As to the ascending noradrenergic fiber systems, there can be little doubt that they exert a mainly activating, i. e., reactivity-enhancing, influence on the networks of the anterior brain stem and the forebrain. A few examples may underline this statement. Electrical stimulation of the locus coeruleus of the cat is followed by an electroencephalographic, behavioral, and autonomic arousal pattern not unlike the one produced by the "classical" reticular stimulation. The electrocortical effect is reduced, in a dose-dependent fashion, by local application of beta-adrenergic antagonists [26]. Redmond and coworkers [52] noted that electrical stimulation of the locus coeruleus produces marked alerting responses in macaques. According to Tanaka and collaborators [59], electrical stimulation of the locus coeruleus drives release of NA from the cerebral cortex. Poisoning of the ascending NA pathways by local (intracerebral) application of 6-hydroxydopamine (6-OHDA) in rats leads to selective slowing of the cortical EEG without affecting to any marked degree the motor activity of the animals [33, 43].

Reduction of the release of NA by activation of the (preferably) presynaptic $alpha_2$-receptors with, for example, clonidine is followed by deactivation and sedation in rats and cats [22, 32]. Mason and Iversen [41] showed that lesions of the coeruleo-cortical NA fiber systems elevates resistance to extinction. According to the same authors [42] NA systems are involved in the control of attentional behavior (the "classical" vigilance indicator). Mason and Fibiger [40] have demonstrated that depletion of brain NA through infusion of 6-OHDA into the dorsal bundle of rats leads to impairment of the animals' ability to ignore irrelevant stimuli, i. e., impairment of an "attentional filtering process." Anlezark and co-workers [2] were able on the basis of their experiments to state that coeruleocortical NA fibers are involved in the reinforcement of the process of learning; rats with lesions in these fiber systems are slowed down in the process of acquisition. Lesions in the locus coeruleus have been found to impair intracranial self-stimulation [17]. In turn, electrostimulation of the coeruleus yields excellent self-stimulation behavior. Margules [39] has noted that the performance-impairing effect of painful stimuli on conditioned behavior is supported by beta-adrenergic, yet antagonized by alpha-adrenergic, mechanisms in the amygdala. Jaekel (cited in Koella [26]) has shown that treatment of monkeys (in an ethological setting) with propranolol or oxprenolol is followed by signs of tranquilization and anxiolysis, by lowered aggressiveness, and an increase in social contacts.

---

the outside and may at times assume the function of language (blushing, paling, sweating, miosis, mydriasis, defecation, micturition, etc.). The latter comprise all activities that take place on the inside of the organism and are not directly observable from the outside. In this class of behaviors one can include the vast variety of vegetative-autonomic and endocrine activities (e. g., circulation, excretion, digestion, and uptake of foodstuffs, variations in, and maintenance of, body temperature, particular patterns of endocrine output, etc.), but also mental or psychic activities (such higher functions as perception, recognition, association, learning, feelings, moods, drives, etc.).

Evidently, ascending noradrenergic fiber tracts appear to be clearly and positively involved in the elevation of vigilance in a variety of higher function behavioral systems. It is thus not surprising if one notes that there is rather high central NA activity during waking [53] as well as during REM sleep, i. e., when, during the dreams, higher functions - or at least what in animals may be referred to as higher functions - perform quite well, although in a somewhat "dereistic" fashion.

Adrenergic receptors, supposedly residing in the diencephalon, are assumed to play a role in the regulation of body temperature. Feldberg and Myers [14] have shown that the injection of noradrenaline into the rostral ventricular space of cats (and a variety of other species) induces hypothermia. When injected into the cat's anterior hypothalamus, adrenaline and noradrenaline were found to be more potent as hypothermic agents than isoproterenol [54]. Burks [6] has demonstrated that intraventricularly administered phentolamine, but not practolol, propranolol, or sotalol, antagonized the hypothermic response to (intraventricularly administered) noradrenaline (100 μg in 100 μl saline). Clonidine and a number of other still more selective alpha$_2$-receptor agonists (given i. p.) produced hypothermia in mice and rats, respectively [46, 62]. Such experiments suggest the conclusion that alpha$_2$-adrenergic receptors are involved in the initiation of all peripheral autonomic activities that lead to a drop in body temperature, i. e., an increased heat loss. While the intimate details about this adrenergic response, such as the controversy as to whether these effects are due to the activation of pre- or postsynaptic receptors, are not known, one can at least postulate that ascending noradrenergic or adrenergic fibers arising from one or more of the A-nuclei project to receptor sites in the anterior hypothalamus, which in turn are functionally connected to networks that control the hypothermic mechanisms.

The functional role of the adrenergic innervation of the cerebellum - mainly supplied by the locus coeruleus - is not well understood, simply because we still do not well understand the role played by the cerebellum in the organization and regulation of biomotor activity. Still, there is good evidence about the intimate mechanisms that come into play at the cellular level. Thus, it is well established that the noradrenergic fibers project, among a variety of other sites, to the cerebellar Purkinje cells, where they exert a beta-receptor-mediated inhibitory effect [21]. According to Moises and coworkers [48], noradrenaline, while reducing the spontaneous discharge rate of the Purkinje cells, enhances their reactivity to other (e. g., aminoacidergic) inputs and thus elevates their signal-to-noise ratio. The thought is not too far-fetched that this NA input facilitates the coactivation of cerebellar networks involved in the organization of motor activity; but just how these networks affect motor activity is not yet well understood.

Of the various noradrenergic and adrenergic fiber tracts that descend into the spinal cord, one, originating in A6 (the locus coeruleus), innervates the ventral horn, i. e., the site of the alpha- and gamma-motoneuron somata, as well as some interneurons. Activation of descending NA fibers through (local) application of cyclobenzaprine to the locus coeruleus leads to a marked attenuation of the EMG of the gastrocnemius muscle, for example [7]; i. e., an inhibition of the respective alpha-motoneurons. Incidentally, according to the same author, the intravenous injection of L-DOPA leads - probably via newly synthesized DA - to the activation of gamma-motoneurons. This effect varies in dependence on whether 5-HT is present (both alpha- and gamma-motoneurons are activated) or partially depleted (only gamma-motoneurons are activated). Regardless of such complications, it appears likely that the activation of a descending NA fiber tract may be instrumental for the establishment of the alpha-motoneuron "paralysis" typically observed during REM sleep. That is to say, enhanced activity of ascending and descending NA fibers could explain two of the characteristic features of REM sleep: high vigilance in the higher function systems and low vigilance in the motor systems.

The descending noradrenergic projections to the spinal cord dorsal horn clearly relate to the "endogenous analgesic mechanisms." After the discovery of the analgesic effect of electrical brain stimulation in the periaqueductal gray [34, 44] and of the endogenous opioids and their respective receptors [55], it has been shown that descending monoaminergic - in particular NA and 5-HT - pathways are intimately involved in the establishment of such "endogenous" analgesia. Fields and Basbaum [15] have shown that electrical stimulation of the locus coeruleus of the rat induces analgesia not unlike that produced by electrical stimulation of the periaqueductal gray. According to Takagi [58], one must assume that the analgesic effect elicited through microinjection of morphine into the paragigantocellular reticular nucleus is also mediated through descending noradrenergic pathways. The activation of dorsal horn neurons induced through peripheral (nociceptive) application of heat or bradykinin is counteracted by local (i.e., intraspinal) application of noradrenaline (and serotonin) [3, 12]. In the rat, the analgesic effect of morphine applied into the periaqueductal gray is antagonized by the topical (i.e., segmental) application of phentolamine (and methysergide) [66, 67]. Finally, electrical (nociceptive) stimulation of spinal afferent fibers elicits an enhanced release of noradrenaline (and serotonin) from the spinal cord, an effect which is eliminated after severance of the spinal cord [67]. The available evidence allows the conclusion that this analgesic or at least "proanalgesic" influence of descending noradrenergic (and possibly adrenergic) pathways is mediated preferably through alpha-adrenergic receptors, whereas beta-adrenergic receptors seem to mediate rather antianalgesic effects [56].

Of special interest in connection with the main topic of this symposium are the descending noradrenergic and adrenergic projections to the intermedio-lateral column of the thoracic and upper lumbar spinal cord, i.e., the sites of the perikarya of the preganglionic (cholinergic) efferent sympathetic fibers. It is already known that A1 nuclei (mainly adrenergic in nature) and A2, A5, A6, and A7 nuclei (all mainly noradrenergic) send their descending axons to this typically autonomic-vegetative area of the spinal cord gray matter. According to Loewy and Neil [36], electrical stimulation of, for instance, the nucleus A5 elicits a pressure response. Yet, chemical stimulation of the same area by iontophoretic application of glutamate rather yields depressor responses. Loewy and Neil are inclined to explain this apparent discrepancy by assuming that glutamate may in fact inhibit the A5 cells via an activation of some (more sensitive) local inhibitory interneurons. Neumayr and co-workers [49] found that electrical stimulation of the region of the A1 nucleus brings about excitation (i.e., actually facilitation) of the preganglionic sympathetic fibers. Ward and Gunn [64] observed marked blood pressure increases and an inhibition of the depressor effect (elicited by aortic nerve stimulation) in response to electrical stimulation of the subcoeruleus region (A7). According to Guyenet and Cabot [19], locally applied clonidine is more effective than adrenaline and noradrenaline, inhibiting

Table 1. Schematic listing of various functional roles of the ascending and descending noradrenergic and adrenergic pathways. Arranged spatially to coincide with the quasi-anatomical map shown in Fig. 1.

Higher functions	
Cortical arousal ↑	
Orienting response ↑	
Attention ↑	
Learning ↑	
Extinction ↑	
Read-out ↑	
Cognitive functions ↑	
Recognition ↑	
Intracerebral self-stimulation ↑	
Anxiety-fear ↑↓	
Drives ↓↑	*Temperature regulation*
	Heat loss ↑
Motor functions	
Regulation of motor activity ↑↓	
	Autonomic regulation
	Higher centers of regulation:
	Circulation ↑↓
	Respiration ↑↓
	Metabolism ↑↓
	Digestion ↓
	Sensory gating
	Internal analgesia ↑
	Sympathetic output
	Regulation of sympathetic tone ↑(↓)
	Circulation
	Respiration (bronch.)
	Temperature regulation metabolism
	Motor excitability
	Excitability of
	Alpha-motoneurons ↓
	Gamma-motoneurons ↓↑

cell firing in the intermedio-lateral column of the pigeon. This effect is antagonized by the local application of the alpha$_2$-blockers yohimbin and piperoxan, but not by the alpha$_1$-blocker prazosin or by the beta-antagonist sotalol. Loewy and Neil [36] are ready to assume that such results "suggest the existence of an alpha$_2$-receptor on, or near, the sympathetic preganglionic neurons." In favor of an excitatory influence of descending NA and A fibers on the sympathetic preganglionic neurons are the experimental results of Taylor and Brody [60]. They stimulated in spinal cats the lateral columns (the site of the descending NA neurons) and elicited thus a pressure response which could be attenuated by infusion of alpha-antagonists into the spinal subarachnoid space.

In Table 1 we have attempted to summarize in an integrated fashion the various functions of the central NA and A systems. Like all summaries, this compilation of functions is incomplete, yet it may emphasize the diversity of functions of the two catecholaminergic transmitter systems.

Epilogue

This short discussion of the central noradrenergic and adrenergic fiber systems has, we hope, revealed that these "wet" neurotransmission instruments subserve a variety of functions. Or, to put it more concisely, they exert a rather uniform, at most a binary, influence on a variety of functional (i.e., in fact, behavioral) systems: an up- and/or down-modulation or control of reactivity of neuronal networks involved in the "making" of a vast variety of extroversive and internal behaviors. The central noradrenergic and adrenergic fiber systems affect the reactivity of the networks of higher function (perception, cognition, sensation, memory), motor, nociception, and vegetative-autonomic (temperature regulation, circulation, respiration, etc.) systems.

Concerning the higher functions, there is ample evidence that the effect of the ascending, mainly noradrenergic, pathways is "facilitatory" in nature; they almost uniformly elevate the level of responsiveness - i.e., the vigilance - in those systems. And there is good evidence that this noradrenergic vigilance-enhancing effect (supported and supplemented by activity in ascending cholinergic pathways, see Koella [27]) is mediated largely by beta-adrenergic mechanisms.

Concerning the motor, sensory, and vegetative functions the situation is less clear, with respect to both the direction of the modulatory effect (up and/or down) and the detailed transmission mechanism. Still, the bulk of the evidence suggests that central noradrenergic and, in part, adrenergic pathways actively support hypothermia (i.e., counteract hyperthermia), induce a loss of tonus in the (spinal) alpha-motoneurons, lead to analgesia, and enhance the sympathetic tone in the peripheral vegetative sphere. Yet for some of these "systems" there remains the not inconsiderable uncertainty about the involvement within the central domain of any particular receptor type in the making of those modulatory effects.

The feelings of uncertainty are further intensified by the very fact that the effects of central noradrenergic and adrenergic mechanisms are in part supplemented and in part counteracted (in the sense of an antagonistic innervation) by other wet, e.g., serotonergic, cholinergic, dopaminergic, and polypeptidergic, mechanisms. This multitude of inputs makes analysis of the actual effect of a given single channel on a particular network rather difficult; in many cases a good deal of additional experimental work is necessary to clarify the situation, with respect not only to the effects of the catecholamines, but also to those of the other neurohumors. We hope indeed that this attempt towards an integrative view of the functions of the central noradrenergic and adrenergic systems may help to define the direction of future research.

References

1. Andén NE, Dahlström A, Fuxe K, Larsson K, Olson L, Ungerstedt U (1966) Ascending monoamine neurons to the telencephalon. Acta Physiol Scand 67: 313-326
2. Anlezark GM, Crow TJ, Greenway AP (1973) Impaired learning and decreased cortical norepinephrine after bilateral locus coeruleus lesions. Science 181: 682-684
3. Belcher G (1977) Correlation between effects of brain stem stimulation and effects of 5-hy-

droxytryptamine and noradrenaline on non-nociceptive and nociceptive spinal interneurons. Br J Pharmacol 61: 149P-150P
4. Betts TA, Alford C (1985) Beta-blockers and sleep. Eur J Clin Pharmacol 28 [Suppl]: 65-68
5. Betts TA, Knight R, Crowe A, Blake A, Harvey P, Mortiboy D (1985) Effect of beta-blockers on psychomotor performance in normal volunteers. Eur J Clin Pharmacol 28 [Suppl]: 39-49
6. Burks TF (1972) Central alpha adrenergic receptors in thermoregulation. Neuropharmacology 11: 615-624
7. Commissiong JW (1981) Spinal monoaminergic systems: an aspect of somatic motor function. Fed Proc 40: 2771-2777
8. Commissiong JW, Galli CL, Neff NH (1978) Differentiation of dopaminergic and noradrenergic neurons in rat spinal cord. J Neurochem 30: 1095-1099
9. Commissiong JW, Gentleman S, Neff NH (1979) Spinal cord dopaminergic neurons: evidence for an increased nigrospinal pathway. Neuropharmacology 18: 565-568
10. Cove-Smith JR, Kirk CA (1985) CNS-related side-effects with metoprolol and atenolol. Eur J Clin Pharmacol 28 [Suppl]: 69-72
11. Dahlström A, Fuxe K (1964) Evidence for the existence of monoamine-containing neurons in the central nervous system: I. Demonstration of monoamines in the cell bodies of brain stem neurons. Acta Physiol Scand 62 [Suppl 232]: 1-55
12. Duggan AW, Headley PM (1977) The effects of noradrenaline and 5-hydroxytryptamine on the responses of dorsal horn neurons to noxious and innocuous skin stimuli. Br J Pharmacol 61: 149P
13. Falck B, Hillarp NA, Thieme G, Torp H (1962) Fluorescence of catecholamines and related compounds condensed with formaldehyde. J Histochem Cytochem 10: 348-354
14. Feldberg W, Myers RD (1964) Effects on temperature of amines injected into the cerebral ventricles. A new concept of temperature regulation. J Physiol (Lond) 173: 226-237
15. Fields HL, Basbaum AI (1978) Brain stem control of spinal pain-transmission neurons. Annu Rev Physiol 40: 217-248
16. Foerster EC, Greminger P, Siegenthaler W, Vetter H, Vetter W (1985) Atenolol versus Pindolol: side effects in hypertension. Eur J Clin Pharmacol 28 [Suppl]: 89-91
17. German DC, Bowden DM (1974) Catecholamine system as the neural substrate for intracranial self-stimulation: a hypothesis. Brain Res 73: 381-419
18. Gosling RH (1977) Clinical experience with oxprenolol in the treatment of anxiety in the United Kingdom. In: Kielholz P (ed) Beta-blockers and the central nervous system. Huber, Bern, pp 125-130
19. Guyenet PG, Cabot JB (1981) Inhibition of sympathetic preganglionic neurons by catecholamines and clonidine: mediation by an alpha-adrenergic receptor. J Neurosci 1: 908-917
20. Harms D (1985) Visual reaction times may be improved by certain beta-blockers. Eur J Clin Pharmacol 28 [Suppl]: 51-54
21. Hoffer BJ, Siggins GR, Oliver AP, Bloom FE (1973) Activation of the pathway from locus coeruleus to rat cerebellar Purkinje neurons: pharmacological evidence of noradrenergic central inhibition. J Pharmacol Exp Ther 184: 553-569
22. Kleinlogel H, Scholtysik O, Sayers AC (1975) Effects of clonidine and BS 100-151 on the EEG sleep pattern in rats. Eur J Pharmacol 33: 159-163
23. Kielholz P (ed) (1978) A therapeutic approach to the psyche via the beta-adrenergic system. Huber, Bern
24. Kobayashi RM, Palkovits M, Jabobowitz DM, Kopin IJ (1975) Biochemical mapping of the noradrenergic projection from the locus coeruleus. Neurology 25: 223-233
25. Koella WP (1977) Anatomical, physiological, and pharmacological findings relevant to the central nervous effects of the beta-blockers. In: Kielholz P (ed) Beta-blockers and the central nervous system. Huber, Bern, pp 21-34
26. Koella WP (1978) Central effects of beta-adrenergic blocking agents: mode and mechanisms of action. In: Kielholz P (ed) A therapeutic approach to the psyche via the beta-adrenergic system. Huber, Bern, pp 11-29
27. Koella WP (1982) A modern neurobiological concept of vigilance. Experientia 38: 1426-1437
28. Koella WP (1984) The organization and regulation of sleep; a review of the experimental evidence and a novel integrated model of the organizing and regulating apparatus. Experientia 40: 309-338

29. Koella WP (1984) Vigilance - local vigilance - the vigilance profile. A new concept and its application in neurobiology and biological psychiatry. Acta Neurol Scand 69 [Suppl 99]: 35-41
30. Koella WP (1985) CNS-related (side-)effects of beta-blockers with special reference to mechanisms of action. Eur J Clin Pharmacol 28 [Suppl]: 55-63
31. Lader M (1974) The peripheral and central role of the catecholamines in the mechanisms of anxiety. Int Pharmacopsychiatry 9: 125-137
32. Leppävuori A, Putkonen PTS (1980) Alpha-adrenoceptive influences on the control of the sleep-waking cycle in the cat. Brain Res 193: 95-115
33. Lidbrink P (1974) The effect of lesions of the ascending noradrenaline pathway on sleep and waking in the rat. Brain Res 74: 19-40
34. Liebeskind JG, Guilbaud G, Besson JM, Oliveras JL (1973) Analgesia from electrical stimulation of the periaqueductal gray matter in the cat; behavioral observations and inhibitory effects on spinal cord interneurons. Brain Res 50: 441-446
35. Livett BG (1973) Histochemical visualization of peripheral and central adrenergic neurones. Br Med Bull 29: 93-103
36. Loewy AD, Neil JJ (1981) The role of descending monoaminergic systems in central control of blood pressure. Fed Proc 40: 2778-2785
37. Loewy AD, McKellar S, Saper CF (1979) Direct projection from the A5 catecholamine cell group to the intermedio-lateral cell column. Brain Res 174: 309-314
38. Maeda T, Pin C, Salvert D, Ligier M, Jouvet M (1973) Les neurones contenant des catécholamines du tegmentum pontique et leurs voies de projection chez le chat. Brain Res 57: 119-152
39. Margules DL (1971) Alpha- and beta-adrenergic receptors in amygdala: reciprocal inhibitors and facilitators of punished operant behaviour. Eur J Pharmacol 16: 21-26
40. Mason ST, Fibiger HC (1979) Noradrenaline and selective attention. Life Sci 25: 1949-1956
41. Mason ST, Iversen SD (1975) Learning in the absence of forebrain noradrenaline. Nature 258: 422-424
42. Mason ST, Iversen SD (1979) Theories of the dorsal bundle extinction effect. Brain Res Rev 1: 107-137
43. Matsuyama S, Coinet J, Mouret J (1975) 6-hydroxydopamine intracysternale et sommeil chez le rat. Brain Res 57: 85-95
44. Mayer DJ, Wolfle TL, Akil H, Carder B, Liebeskind JC (1971) Analgesia from electrical stimulation in the brain stem of the rat. Science 174: 1351-1354
45. McDevitt DG (1985) Beta-blockers and psychometric performance: studies in normal volunteers. Eur J Clin Pharmacol 28 [Suppl]: 35-38
46. McLennan PL (1981) The hypothermic effect of clonidine and other imidazolines in relation to their ability to enter the central nervous system in mice. Eur J Pharmacol 69: 477
47. Middlemiss DN, Buxton DA, Greenwood DT (1981) Betaadrenoceptor antagonists in psychiatry and neurology. Pharmacol Ther 12: 419-437
48. Moises HC, Woodward DJ, Hoffer BJ, Freedman R (1979) Interactions of norepinephrine with Purkinje cell responses to putative aminoacid neurotransmitters applied by microiontophoresis. Exp Neurol 64: 493-515
49. Neumayr RJ, Hare RD, Franz DN (1974) Evidence for bulbospinal control of sympathetic preganglionic neurons by monoaminergic pathways. Life Sci 14: 793-806
50. Noyes R (1982) Beta-blocking drugs and anxiety. Psychosomatics 23: 155-170
51. Pickel VM, Segal M, Bloom FE (1974) A radioautographic study of the efferent pathways of the nucleus locus coeruleus. J Comp Neurol 155: 15-41
52. Redmond DE, Huang YH, Snyder DR (1976) Behavioral effects of stimulation of the nucleus locus coeruleus in the stump-tailed monkey, macaca arctoides. Brain Res 116: 502-510
53. Reis DJ, Weinbren M, Corvelli A (1968) A circadian rhythm of norepinephrine regionally in the cat brain: its relationship to environmental lighting and to regional diurnal variations in brain serotonin. J Pharmacol Exp Ther 164: 135-146
54. Rudy TA, Wolf HH (1969) Receptor selectivity of the hypothermic response to intracerebrally injected catecholamines in cats. Fed Proc 28: 443
55. Snyder SH (1977) Opiate receptors and internal opiates. Sci Am 236: 44-56
56. Spencer PSJ (1976) Some aspects of the pharmacology of analgesia. J Int Med Res 4 [Suppl 2]: 1-14
57. Swanson LW, Hartman BK (1975) The central adrenergic system. An immunofluorescence

study of the location of cell bodies and their efferent connections in the rat utilizing dopamine-β-hydroxylase as a marker. J Comp Neurol 163: 467–506
58. Takagi H (1980) The nucleus reticularis paragigantocellularis as a site of analgesic action of morphine and enkephalin. Trends Pharmacol Sci 1: 182–184
59. Tanaka C, Inagaki C, Fujiwara H (1976) Labeled noradrenaline release from rat cerebral cortex following electrical stimulation of locus coeruleus. Brain Res 106: 384–389
60. Taylor DG, Brody MJ (1976) Spinal adrenergic mechanism regulating sympathetic outflow to blood vessels. Circ Res 38 [Suppl 2]: 10–20
61. Ungerstedt U (1971) Stereotaxic mapping of the monoamine pathways in the rat brain. Acta Physiol Scand [Suppl] 367: 1–29
62. Van der Laan JW, van Veenendaal W, Voorthuis P, Weick G, Hillen FC (1985) The effects of centrally acting adrenergic agonists on temperature and on explorative and motor behaviour. Relation with effects on quasi-morphine withdrawal behaviour. Eur J Pharmacol 107: 367–373
63. Van Zwieten PA, Timmermans PBMWM (1985) Brain levels and acute antihypertensive activity of beta-blockers. Eur J Clin Pharmacol 28 [Suppl]: 13–19
64. Ward DG, Gunn CG (1976) Locus coeruleus complex: differential modulation of depressor mechanisms. Brain Res 107: 407–411
65. Westerlund A (1985) Central nervous system side-effects with hydrophilic and lipophilic beta-blockers. Eur J Clin Pharmacol 28 [Suppl]: 73–76
66. Yaksh TL (1978) Direct evidence that spinal serotonin and noradrenaline terminals mediate the spinal antinociceptive effects of morphine in the periaqueductal gray. Brain Res 160: 180–185
67. Yaksh TL, Hammond DL, Tyce GM (1981) Functional aspects of bulbospinal monoaminergic projections in modulating processing of somatosensory information. Fed Proc 40: 2786–2794

Discussion

Göthert: You showed this remarkable divergence of noradrenergic neurons in the central nervous system very nicely and the relation 1:1000000. Basically, that is only one facet of the overall picture when you consider that in the cortex, for example, hardly any of the noradrenergic neurons form true synapses and that norepinephrine exerts a relatively diffuse influence over relatively large neuronal territories.

Koella: Yes, you could almost put it that way. When a pronounced noradrenergic release occurs, the entire cortex is flooded, as it were, with norepinephrine. This substance is released not only directly into the subsynaptic cleft but, as you mentioned, into tissue, so that the cells are exposed to relatively high concentrations of norepinephrine as well as epinephrine. The same applies to serotonin, dopamine, and so forth.

Borchert: I have a question concerning species variability. If I am correctly informed, most studies have been carried out in the rat. Are there very great differences among warm-blooded species in terms of the transmitters dopamine and, above all, norepinephrine?

Koella: Yes, of course there are. You have correctly noted that many studies have been carried out in rats. Many studies, particularly those conducted in our laboratories, have used cats. We are aware of differences between individual species, chiefly of a quantitative nature. But in essence the findings are very similar when you consider the entire range of the continuum – I would not venture to say from mouse to man, but at least to monkeys. Generally speaking the relations are similar. From species to species, however, there are quantitative differences as well as differences in distribution, the influence on various cortical areas, and so forth. Doubtless there are also organizational differences in terms of spinal projections of autonomous activities. I'm glad you mentioned that, because we do wish, after all, to apply the findings to homo sapiens.

Peripheral Sympathoadrenal System: Transmitter Release and Distribution of Adrenoceptors

M. GÖTHERT

Institut für Pharmakologie und Toxikologie der Medizinischen Fakultät
der Rheinischen-Friedrichs-Wilhelms-Universität, Reuterstraße 2b, 5300 Bonn 1, FRG

Introduction

In a brief report on the peripheral sympathoadrenal system, few aspects of this vast field can be discussed. Accordingly, this paper will focus on three main topics. In the first section, effects of hormones released under stress conditions and of co-transmitters, released together with noradrenaline (NA) on NA release will be described. The second part is a report on the differentiation and distribution of adrenoceptors mediating effects in sympathetically innervated tissues. The final section will be devoted to adrenoceptors in human blood vessels.

Effects of Cotransmitters and of Hormones Released During Stress on Noradrenaline Release

Activation of the sympathoadrenal system, for instance during dynamic exercise or stress, leads to the release of noradrenaline from the varicosities of the terminal postganglionic sympathetic nerve fibres and of adrenaline (as well as small amounts of noradrenaline) from the chromaffin cells of the adrenal medulla. Adrenaline release will be dealt with only in the context of the possibility that adrenaline may influence noradrenaline release from the varicosities.

The principle of Dale, namely that one neuron can store and release only one neurotransmitter, is no longer valid [16]. Thus, the storage vesicles of sympathetic nerve fibres contain not only NA but also ATP. When action potentials invade the varicosities and lead to its depolarization, ATP is coreleased together with NA. ATP and its degradation product adenosine are capable of activating P_2 and P_1 purinoceptors in vascular smooth muscle, respectively; these receptors mediate relaxation [4]. In addition, adenosine stimulates presynaptic P_1 purinoceptors, which in turn mediate an inhibition of further release of NA and ATP [32]. In this way, adenosine formed from released ATP may play a role in fine regulation of transmitter release.

Neuropeptide Y, composed of 36 amino acids, is another cotransmitter released together with NA from the varicosities of the terminal sympathetic nerve fibres (Fig. 1). This peptide, which produces a powerful vasoconstriction, inhibits the stimulation-evoked release of noradrenaline [5, 20] and of neuropeptide Y [1] in isolated

New Aspects in Hypertension: Adrenoceptors
M. Middeke and H. Holzgreve (Eds.)
Springer-Verlag Berlin Heidelberg New York 1986

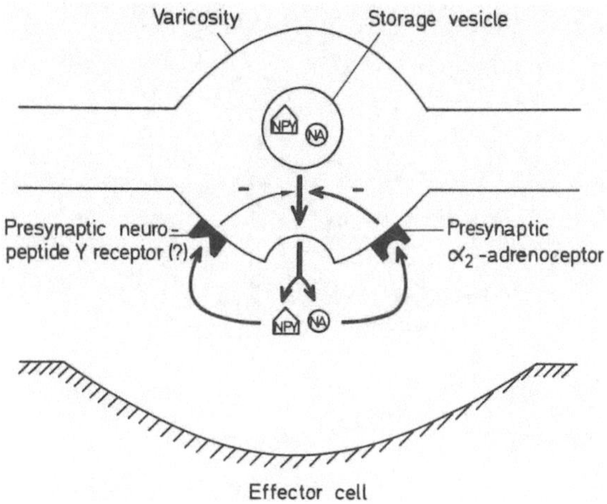

Fig. 1. Autoinhibition of noradrenaline *(NA)* and neuropeptide Y *(NPY)* release from sympathetic nerves via negative feedback loops mediated by presynaptic α_2-adrenoceptors and, probably, presynaptic NPY receptors. –, inhibition of release

cardiovascular tissue, probably by activiting inhibitory presynaptic neuropeptide Y receptors (Fig. 1). Hence, transmitter release appears to be controlled by this short negative feedback loop.

Facilitatory β_2-adrenoceptors on the postganglionic sympathetic nerve terminals of heart and blood vessels may play a role in the development of essential hypertension [21]. Under stress conditions, enhanced levels of adrenaline, released at increased rate from the adrenal medulla, are present in the synaptic cleft between noradrenergic varicosities and effector cells, from where adrenaline is taken up by the amine "pumps" into the varicosities and, finally, its storage vesicles (Fig. 2). This adrenaline can be released together with NA and activate the presynaptic β_2-adrenoceptors, thus increasing further transmitter release via a positive feedback loop (Fig. 2). There is experimental evidence that this mechanism is involved in the development of increased blood pressure in spontaneously hypertensive rats [2].

Stress induces not only an activation of the sympathoadrenal system but also an increased release of adrenocorticotropic hormone (ACTH) from the hypophysis. As shown in rabbit pulmonary arteries, the electrically evoked noradrenaline release is increased by $ACTH_{1-24}$. $ACTH_{7-38}$, an ACTH receptor antagonist, abolishes the facilitatory effect of $ACTH_{1-24}$, but the latter is not affected by saralasin [8]. α-MSH, which represents the amino acid sequence 1-13 of the ACTH molecule, and the full amino acid sequence of porcine ACTH, also facilitate the evoked release, but $ACTH_{4-10}$ is ineffective [9]. These results correspond to the relative potencies of the peptides at activating ACTH receptors in the adrenal cortex. In conclusion, ACTH and related peptides appear to increase the action-potential-induced NA release by activating facilitatory presynaptic ACTH receptors. It is not yet clear whether these ACTH receptors on the postganglionic sympathetic nerve terminals can be activated by blood-borne ACTH under stress conditions, since the EC_{50} for the facilitatory

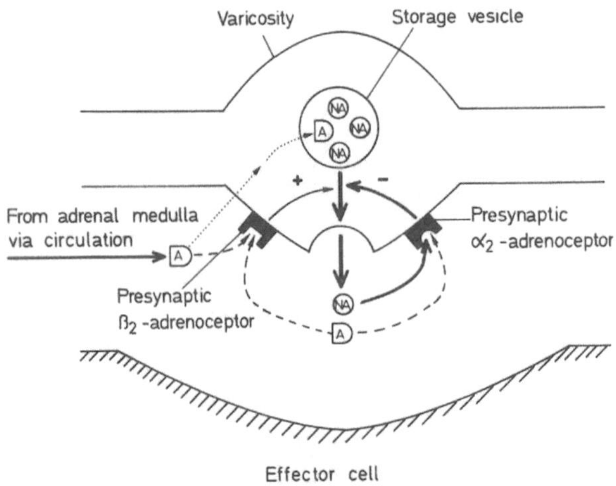

Fig. 2. Autoinhibition of noradrenaline *(NA)* release from sympathetic nerves via a negative feedback loop mediated by presynaptic α_2-adrenoceptors, and an autofacilitatory feedback loop triggered by adrenaline *(A)* acting on presynaptic β_2-adrenoceptors. A, originally released from the adrenal medulla and taken up into the sympathetic neuron, is released from the varicosity with NA. +, facilitation of release; −, inhibition of release; *dotted arrows,* neuronal and vesicular uptake of A [10]

effect of ACTH in the rabbit pulmonary artery is about 40 times higher than the ACTH concentration in human blood during stress. However, preliminary experiments in the human pulmonary artery (Göthert and Hentrich, unpublished) revealed that $ACTH_{1-24}$ is more potent in this species than in rabbits. Furthermore, it is conceivable that the sensitivity of ACTH receptors may be increased in arterial hypertension of the systemic or pulmonary circulation.

Differentiation and Distribution of Adrenoceptors

Adrenoceptors in sympathetically innervated tissues are differentiated according to their pharmacological properties into the α_1-, α_2-, β_1- and β_2-receptor subtypes. With respect to their localization "before" or "behind" the synaptic cleft (i.e., on the noradrenergic nerve terminal or the effector cell, pre- and postsynaptic adrenoceptors can be distinguished (see above).

Although considerable progress toward elucidating the chemical structure of adrenoceptors has been made in the past 5 years [25], the classification of the adrenoceptors is at present mainly based on determinations of the potencies or affinities of adrenoceptor agonists and antagonists. Such experiments have been carried out both in functional investigations on isolated tissues or intact organisms and in radioligand-binding studies on intact cells or fragments of the cell membrane. The development of agonists and antagonists with a marked preference for one of the adrenoceptor subtypes was a prerequisite for a more clear-cut differentiation of the various receptor subtypes. Some of these compounds are listed in Table 1; the selec-

Table 1. Agonists and antagonists acting preferentially on a certain adrenoceptor subtype

Adrenoceptor subtypes	Agonists	Antagonists
α_1	Cirazoline Phenylephrine Methoxamine	Prazosin Terazosin BE 2254
α_2	B-HT 920 B-HT 933 Guanfacine	Rauwolscine Yohimbine BDF 6143
β_1	Prenalterol	Atenolol
β_2	Procaterol Salbutamol	ICI 118-551

Table 2. Distribution and function of peripheral α-adrenoceptors

Localization	Subtype	Function
Presynaptic		
Noradrenergic nerve fibres	α_2	Inhibition of noradrenaline release
Cholinergic nerve fibres	α_2	Inhibition of acetylcholine release
Postsynaptic		
Heart	α_1	Positive inotropic effect
Blood vessels	α_1, α_2	Contraction of smooth muscle
Liver	α_1	Glycogenolysis
Fat cells	α_2	Inhibition of lipolysis
Pancreas	α_2	Inhibition of insulin release
Thrombocytes	α_2	Aggregation

tion of drugs was mainly guided by the application of drugs in the investigations quoted below, i.e., in the last section of this report.

Within the last decade, distribution and function of pre- and postsynaptic adrenoceptor subtypes have been extensively investigated. Some of the results are listed in Table 2 (α-adrenoceptors) and Table 3 (β-adrenoceptors) and will not be discussed in detail, since they are generally well known. Only few points will be briefly touched upon.

Presynaptic α_2-adrenoceptors mediating inhibition of transmitter release occur both on noradrenergic ("autoreceptors"; Fig. 2, Table 2;) [10, 18, 26, 27] and cholinergic nerve fibres ("heteroceptors"; Table 2;) [24]. The α_2-adrenoceptors on the cholinergic neurons play a role for instance in the emergence of the gastrointestinal side effects of clonidine, which inhibits acetylcholine release by activating these receptors, thus leading to constipation. In the medial layer of blood vessels, α_1- and α_2-adrenoceptors may coexist, both of which mediate vasoconstriction (Table 2). It has been suggested that these two receptor populations may have different anatomical locations in relation to the sympathetic nerve terminals. Thus, α_1-adrenoceptors appear to be innervated and, hence, are probably localized intrasynaptically, where-

Table 3. Distribution and function of peripheral β-adrenoceptors

Localization	Subtype	Function
Presynaptic		
Noradrenergic nerve fibres	β_2	Increase in noradrenaline release
Postsynaptic		
Heart	β_1, $(\beta_2)^a$	Positive inotropic, chronotropic, bathmotropic, and dromotropic effects
Blood vessels[b]	β_2	Relaxation of smooth muscle
Bronchial system	β_2, $(\beta_1)^a$	Relaxation of smooth muscle
Uterus	β_2	Relaxation of smooth muscle
Gastrointestinal tract	β_1	Relaxation of smooth muscle
Liver	β_2	Glycogenolysis
Fat cells	β_1	Lipolysis

[a] Minor percentage (about 10%–25%) of the total β-adrenoceptor population in a tissue, in which both subtypes coexist.
[b] Human cerebral blood vessels: β_1 [6]

as α_2-adrenoceptors may predominantly be localized extrasynaptically [19]. However, this hypothesis is still a matter of debate [28].

As outlined in Table 3, both β-adrenoceptor subtypes can coexist in the same tissue, e.g., in the heart [3, 30] or bronchial system [22]. Therefore, it can be concluded that the development of agonists or antagonists which selectively act on β-adrenoceptors in only one of these tissues will probably not be possible; even a drug with an extremely high selectivity for one of the β-adrenoceptor subtypes will interact at least with a minor population of the β-adrenoceptors present in any of these tissues.

Whereas in most blood vessels of various animal species vasodilatation is mediated via postsynaptic β_2-adrenoceptors, the β_1-receptor subtype appears to be involved in the dilator response of human cerebral blood vessels (Table 3). In view of this rather unexpected result, it is evident that only investigations in human tissues will provide a reliable link between experimental pharmacology in animals and clinical pharmacology.

Adrenoceptors in Human Blood Vessels

In the last decade a large number of studies on adrenoceptors has been carried out in human blood vessels, removed by biopsy or necropsy. Postsynaptic α-adrenoceptors have been characterized extensively in femoral arteries and veins [7] and in mesenteric arteries and veins of humans [33]. Femoral arteries were less sensitive to NA than femoral veins. Among the agonists investigated (NA, guanfacine, phenylephrine), NA was most potent in both types of femoral blood vessels. In arteries the α_1-adrenoceptor agonist phenylephrine had a higher intrinsic activity than the preferential α_2-adrenoceptor agonist guanfacine, whereas in veins the reverse order was observed with respect to both intrinsic activity and potency. The α_2-preferential antagonists rauwolscine and yohimbine were less potent against NA in arteries than in veins. In arteries the selective α_1-adrenoceptor antagonist prazosin was a potent competitive antagonist, but in veins this drug was a weak noncompetitive antagonist [7]. These findings obtained in human femoral blood vessels suggest that arterial smooth muscle contains more α_1- than α_2-adrenoceptors, whereas the reverse holds true for venous smooth muscle. Similarly, Törnebrandt et al. [33] observed that human mesenteric arteries are primarily endowed with postsynaptic α_1-adrenoceptors, whereas the mesenteric veins are mainly equipped with α_2-adrenoceptors. Thus, it is conceivable that drugs which preferentially act on adrenoceptors in resistance or capacitance vessels can be developed.

Postsynaptic β-adrenoceptors in human blood vessels have been less well investigated than α-adrenoceptors. In human mesenteric arteries and veins contracted with prostaglandin $F_{2\alpha}$, no vasodilatory effect of isoprenaline or terbutaline was detectable [33]. In contrast, isoprenaline was found to produce a relaxation of strips of human saphenous veins contracted with noradrenaline, suggesting that postsynaptic vasodilatory β-adrenoceptors appear to be present in this blood vessel. As outlined above (Table 3), such receptors were identified in human cerebral blood vessels and probably belong to the β_1-receptor subtype [6].

It has been shown recently that the sympathetic nerves of the human saphenous vein [13, 17] and pulmonary artery [15] are endowed with inhibitory α_2-autoreceptors. In these blood vessels, NA and the preferential α_2-adrenoceptor agonists α-methyl-NA and B-HT 920 inhibited the electrically evoked ^{3}H-noradrenaline release, whereas the α_1-adrenoceptor agonist methoxamine was ineffective. α_2-Adrenoceptor antagonists, such as rauwolscine and BDF 6143, increased NA release by preventing endogenous NA from activating the inhibitory autoreceptors (see Fig. 2). Prazosin was ineffective in this respect. The concentration-response curve of B-HT 920 for its inhibitory effect on NA release was shifted to the right by rauwolscine.

Presynaptic facilitatory β_2-adrenoceptors (Fig. 2), which may play an important role in the development of hypertension (see above, section on NA release), were also identified on the sympathetic nerves of various human blood vessels, including omental arteries and veins [31], digital arteries [29], metatarsal veins [23], saphenous veins [12, 34], and pulmonary arteries [11]. It was shown in these blood vessels that isoprenaline, adrenaline (in the presence of rauwolscine), and preferential β_2-adrenoceptor agonists such as salbutamol and procaterol increased the action-potential-induced NA release, whereas the β_1-preferential agonists NA (in the presence of rauwolscine) and prenalterol were ineffective. The concentration-response curve of procaterol was shifted to the right by the preferential β_2-adrenoceptor antagonist ICI 118-551, but was not affected by the β_1-preferential antagonist atenolol; the latter also did not produce a shift to the right of the concentration-response curve of isoprenaline. Experiments in the human pulmonary artery support the assumption that an adenylate cyclase is involved in the β_2-adrenoceptor-mediated facilitation of NA release, since forskolin produced a potentiation of the response to isoprenaline [14].

The complex interplay of the various adrenoceptors present in one synapse was examined in the human saphenous vein by Verbeuren et al. [34]. Transmural electrical stimulation of the sympathetic nerves produced a contraction of the vascular strips; this effect was caused by an activation of the postsynaptic α-adrenoceptors by released NA. When isoprenaline was administered an increase in evoked ^{3}H-NA release and in contractile response to nerve stimulation was observed. The increased contraction occurred in spite of the relaxing effect of isoprenaline mediated by postsynaptic β-adrenoceptors, and is obviously due to the increased concentration of endogenous NA at the postsynaptic α-adrenoceptors. Hence, at least in the human saphenous vein, the functional importance of the presynaptic β_2-adrenoceptors prevails over that of the postsynaptic β-adrenoceptors.

Summary

Activation of the sympathoadrenal system, for instance during stress, results in release of NA from the varicosities of the terminal postganglionic sympathetic nerve fibres and of adrenaline (as well as smaller amounts of NA) from the chromaffin cells of the adrenal medulla. In addition to the main transmitter NA, a variety of other compounds (e.g., ATP, adrenaline, and neuropeptide Y) coexist in the sympathetic nerve terminals, are coreleased upon action potentials invading the varicosities, and activate pre- and postsynaptic adrenoceptors, purinoceptors, and neuropeptide Y receptors; the latter mediate inhibition of NA release and powerful vasoconstriction. Under stress conditions there is also an increased release of ACTH, which in turn may facilitate NA release by activating presynaptic ACTH receptors.

The peripheral pre- and postsynaptic adrenoceptors are differentiated according to their pharmacological properties into α_1-, α_2-, β_1-, and β_2-adrenoceptors. The differentiation was based on experiments with newly developed drugs with high selectivity for one of the receptor subtypes. The various adrenoceptors play an important role in the regulation of cardiovascular and other vegetative functions.

In several tissues different adrenoceptors coexist. For instance, on the myocardial cell β_1-receptors prevail, but 10%–25% of the β-adrenoceptors belong to the β_2-subtype. These receptors mediate modifications of heart rate, of contractility, and of the electrophysiological properties. A positive inotropic effect is also mediated via α_1-adrenoceptors. α_2- and β_2-adrenoceptors mediating inhibition and facilitation of noradrenaline release, respectively, are present on the sympathetic nerves of the heart and of blood vessels of various species of animals and humans. Postsynaptically, activation of α_1- and α_2-adrenoceptors causes vasoconstriction; stimulation of β_2-adrenoceptors produces vasodilatation.

References

1. Archelos J, Reinecke M, Lang RE (1985) Neuropeptide Y is a transmitter in cardiac sympathetic nerves. Naunyn-Schmiedebergs Arch Pharmacol [Suppl] 329: R 88
2. Borkowski KR, Quinn P (1985) Adrenaline and the development of spontaneous hypertension in rats. J Auton Pharmacol 5: 89-100
3. Brodde OE, Karad K, Zerkowski HR, Rohm N, Reidemeister JC (1983) Coexistence of β_1- and β_2-adrenoceptors in human right atrium. Direct identification by ($\pm$)-[^{125}J]iodocyanpindolol binding. Circ Res 53: 752-758
4. Burnstock G (1985) Neurohumoral control of blood vessels: some future directions. J Cardiovasc Pharmacol 7: S 137-S 146
5. Dahlöf C, Dahlöf P, Tatemoto K, Lundberg JM (1985) Neuropeptide Y (NPY) reduces field stimulation-evoked release of noradrenaline and enhances force of contraction in rat portal vein. Naunyn-Schmiedebergs Arch Pharmacol 328: 327-330
6. Edvinsson L, Owman C, Sjöberg NO (1976) Autonomic nerves, mast cells, and amine receptors in human brain vessels. A histochemical and pharmacological study. Brain Res 115: 377-393
7. Glusa E, Markwardt F (1983) Characterization of postjunctional α-adrenoceptors in isolated human femoral veins and arteries. Naunyn-Schmiedebergs Arch Pharmacol 323: 101-105
8. Göthert M (1981) $ACTH_{1-24}$ increases stimulation-evoked noradrenaline release from sympathetic nerves by acting on presynaptic ACTH-receptors. Eur J Pharmacol 76: 295-296
9. Göthert M (1984) Facilitatory effect of adrenocorticotropic hormone and related peptides on Ca^{2+}-dependent noradrenaline release from sympathetic nerves. Neuroscience 11: 1001-1009
10. Göthert M (1985) Role of autoreceptors in the function of the peripheral and central nervous system. Arzneimittelforschung Drug Research 35 (II): 1909-1916
11. Göthert M, Hentrich F (1985) Identification of presynaptic β_2-adrenoceptors on the sympathetic nerve fibres of the human pulmonary artery. Br J Pharmacol 85: 933-941
12. Göthert M, Hentrich F (1986) Presynaptic β-adrenoceptors in human blood vessels and their possible relationship to adenylate cyclase. In: Grobecker H, Philippu A, Starke K (eds) New aspects of the role of adrenoceptors in the cardiovascular system. Springer, Berlin Heidelberg New York
13. Göthert M, Schlicker E, Hentrich F, Rohm N, Zerkowski HR (1984) Modulation of noradrenaline release in human saphenous vein via presynaptic α_2-adrenoceptors. Eur J Pharmacol 102: 261-267
14. Hentrich F, Göthert M, Greschuchna D (1985) Involvement of cAMP in modulation of noradrenaline release in the human pulmonary artery. Naunyn-Schmiedebergs Arch Pharmacol 330: 245-247
15. Hentrich F, Göthert M, Greschuchna D (1986) Noradrenaline release in the human pulmonary artery is modulated by presynaptic α_2-adrenoceptors. J Cardiovasc Pharmacol 8: 539-544
16. Hökfelt T, Johansson O, Ljungdahl Å, Lundberg JM, Schultzberg M (1980) Peptidergic neurones. Nature 284: 515-521
17. Janssens W, Verhaeghe R (1983) Modulation of the concentration of noradrenaline at the neuroeffector junction in human saphenous vein. Br J Pharmacol 79: 577-585
18. Langer SZ (1980) Presynaptic regulation of the release of catecholamines. Pharmacol Rev 32: 337-363
19. Langer SZ, Shepperson NB (1982) Recent developments in vascular smooth muscle pharmacology: the postsynaptic α_2-adrenoceptor. Trends Pharmacol Sci 3: 440-444
20. Lundberg JM, Stjärne L (1984) Neuropeptide Y (NPY) depresses the secretion of ^{3}H-noradrenaline and the contractile response evoked by field stimulation in rat vas deferens. Acta Physiol Scand 120: 477-479
21. Majewski H, Rand MJ (1984) Prejunctional β-adrenoceptors and hypertension: a hypothesis revisited. Trends Pharmacol Sci 5: 500-502
22. Minneman KP, Hegstrand LR, Molinoff PB (1979) Simultaneous determination of $beta_1$- and $beta_2$-adrenergic receptors in tissues containing both receptor subtypes. Mol Pharmacol 16: 34-46
23. Moulds RFW, Stevens MJ (1983) Facilitatory prejunctional β-adrenoceptors in human arteries and veins. Gen Pharmacol 14: 81-83

24. Muscholl E (1980) Peripheral muscarinic control of norepinephrine release in the cardiovascular system. Am J Physiol 239: H 713–H 720
25. Shreeve SM, Fraser CM, Venter JC (1985) Adrenergic and cholinergic neurotransmitter receptor structure. In: Bevan JA, Godfraind T, Maxwell RA, Stoclet JC, Worcel M (eds) Vascular neuroeffector mechanisms. Elsevier, Amsterdam, pp 77–82
26. Starke K (1977) Regulation of noradrenaline release by presynaptic receptor systems. Rev Physiol Biochem Pharmacol 77: 1–124
27. Starke K (1981) Presynaptic receptors. Ann Rev Pharmacol Toxicol 21: 7–30
28. Stevens MJ, Moulds RFW (1985) Neuronally released norepinephrine does not preferentially activate postjunctional α_1-adrenoceptors in human blood vessels in vitro. Circ Res 57: 399–405
29. Stevens MJ, Rittinghausen RE, Medcalf RL, Moulds RFW (1982) Prejunctional β-adrenoceptors in human digital arteries. Eur J Pharmacol 83: 263–270
30. Stiles GL, Taylor S, Lefkowitz RJ (1983) Human cardiac beta-adrenergic receptors: subtype heterogeneity delineated by direct radioligand binding. Life Sci 33: 467–473
31. Stjärne L, Brundin J (1976) β_2-Adrenoceptors facilitating noradrenaline secretion from human vasoconstrictor nerves. Acta Physiol Scand 97: 88–93
32. Su C (1983) Purinergic neurotransmission and neuromodulation. Ann Rev Pharmacol Toxicol 23: 397–411
33. Törnebrandt K, Nobin A, Owman C (1985) Pharmacological characterization of alpha-adrenergic receptor subtypes mediating contraction in human mesenteric arteries and veins. Blood Vessels 22: 179–195
34. Verbeuren TJ, Lorenz RR, Aarhus LL, Shepherd JT, Vanhoutte PM (1983) Prejunctional beta-adrenoceptors in human and canine saphenous veins. J Auton Nerv Syst 8: 261–271

Discussion

Werdan: Can one estimate what percentage of alpha and beta receptors are saturated with epinephrine and norepinephrine under physiological conditions?

Göthert: Needless to say, that is very difficult under physiological conditions if you mean conditions at rest.

Werdan: Conditions at rest, yes.

Göthert: I would say a certain impulse frequency is always present, which is transmitted via the sympathetic nerve endings. But under conditions of rest a very partial saturation occurs – I would say in the order of less than 20%. Under conditions of stress, of course, the system can be powerfully activated by endogenous catecholamines.

Koella: I am very interested in the picture in which you showed the influence of ACTH in response to various frequencies. Interestingly, at low frequencies of 0.66 ACTH was highly effective. When you moved up to 2 or 6 there was no effect.

Göthert: I wouldn't say no effect. After all, there was an increase by 30%–50%.

Koella: But that reminds me somewhat of experiments we performed with Schaeppi some time back, in which we clearly demonstrated on pupillary muscles that the relative occupation of and binding to beta receptors and alpha receptors are largely frequency-dependent. Maybe there is some common ground there.

Göthert: I agree, but I'd like to add the comment that all presynaptic receptor mechanisms are strongly frequency-dependent, and showing this frequency dependence is a major part of demonstrating presynaptic receptor-mediated effects. Release evoked by low frequencies is always more strongly influenced by presynaptic receptors than that by higher frequencies. On the other hand, I should also like to emphasize that ACTH remains bound to its receptor for a relatively long time. Even when stress is long ago passed and the sympathetic system is no longer strongly activated, ACTH is still present at the noradrenergic nerve endings and is still able to activate these receptors, even in case of low impulse frequency. In this way large quantities of norepinephrine may still be released. I should perhaps also add that we have meanwhile been able to identify these ACTH receptors in the human vascular system. They are therefore not restricted to rabbits.

Unidentified: A short question on this point. What is one to imagine about the in vivo situation when it is stated that a receptor can be especially well demonstrated in the presence of particularly low stimulus frequencies? The reason I ask is - you know the story with the cardiac $alpha_1$ receptors - there it was the same thing. They can be well demonstrated with especially low frequencies, but functionally they are of no relevance whatsoever.

Göthert: I'd say the functional relevance of the presynaptic adrenoceptors, which we are chiefly concerned with in this context...

Unidentified: I was speaking of ACTH.

Göthert: Good. As far as the adrenoceptors are concerned it has been conclusively demonstrated by the group headed by Starke, who performed these in vivo experiments in rabbits. With the ACTH receptors the whole thing is still more or less in the rudimentary phase. I published the first paper as a 'rapid communication' in the *European Journal of Pharmacology* four years ago, and last year the main report appeared. In fact, though, I would just like to repeat what I said in conclusion: The physiologic significance could lie in the fact that these receptors can be stimulated at a time when the molecule is still bound to the receptor, so that the stimulus frequency is again relatively low. When stress is passed we can still release a large quantity of norepinephrine. On the other hand, I must comment on this aspect from another point of view as well. In rabbits we needed relatively high concentrations of ACTH in order to increase the release; in humans the receptor is more sensitive. Indeed, we come into a range that is relevant and corresponds to ACTH release under conditions of stress.

Borchert: I wanted to return briefly to the presynaptic beta receptors. It is always surmised that beta receptor blockers play a role, at least therapeutically. I find it difficult to understand why. If only $beta_2$ receptors are present, how are the $beta_1$-selective substances comparable in efficacy to nonselective blockers?

Göthert: I'd first like to emphasize one thing: you are just as aware as I am that purely selective substances do not exist. And in antihypertensive therapy we should not forget that the beta-receptor blockers are administered in substantially higher doses than in other indications. At the moment, however, this is a very hypothetical opinion: the dosage is even sufficient to produce a blockade of $beta_2$ receptors. But I should like to emphasize a point that will also be underscored by the Rand group: The maintenance of hypertension by these receptors is probably influenced less than the development of the hypertension. This was recently shown extraordinarily well by Bokowsky and Quinn, who published a paper this year in the *Journal of Autonomic Pharmacology* in which they showed the development of hypertension in SH rats. In fact, the process is slowed down when the animals are adrenalectomized. The development of spontaneous hypertension can also be delayed by the administration of the $beta_2$ blocker ICI-118-551. There is some evidence indicating that $alpha_2$ receptors play a role in the development of hypertension, but certainly not exclusively. Even in these demedullated animals hypertension still develops, though it is much less pronounced than in non-demedullated animals.

Von Eiff: Norepinephrine release on termination of stress in humans differs according to which parameters one looks at. The question is whether it occurs as a result of inhibiting mechanisms influencing ACTH release via coping mechanisms. Do you regard that as possible?

Göthert: I could only speculate on that. I'd say that although the findings have been validated, they are experimental and still too preliminary for one to venture a detailed conclusion for humans with all its consequences. But I certainly do regard it as possible.

Neyses: Is it known which receptors are responsible for protein synthesis leading to vascular hypertrophy, and might the ACTH receptors play a much greater role in the long-term development of hypertension than short-term changes in contractility?

Göthert: I'd like to deal with the second part of the question first. Again I must pass. With the ACTH receptors we are only at the stage where we can demonstrate them in vitro; of course it is important to note that we have demonstrated them not only in animals but also in humans. We simply haven't published those findings yet. As for the first part of your question, I would say that basically no other receptors could be responsible than those which also mediate the other effects.

Characterization of Adrenoceptors: Receptor-Binding Studies and Agonist-Antagonist Interaction*

A. Wellstein

Zentrum der Pharmakologie, Klinikum der J. W. Goethe-Universität, T. Stern-Kai 7, 6000 Frankfurt 70, FRG

Introduction

In the last decade receptor-binding studies have received ever increasing attention. Especially in adrenergic pharmacology, they have proved to be very powerful and reliable tools in many respects, as outlined in the different articles of the present volume and in the literature [2, 7, 11, 12, 17, 20]. However, it must be pointed out that despite such numerous reports, there are still some contradictions and especially confusion about when acceptable proof has been obtained that a radioligand under investigation has indeed bound at receptors [8, 20]. In the present paper, we discuss aspects and prerequisites of the receptor binding approach and how this could provide a better understanding of the action of the classical β-adrenoceptor antagonist, propranolol.

Methods

Receptor Binding Studies

Membranes containing β-adrenoceptors were prepared from rat salivary glands or rat reticulocytes as described by Wellstein et al. [18]. In brief, salivary glands were removed, homogenized in 310 mosmol/liter sodium phosphate buffer (pH 7.4), and washed thrice in this buffer by centrifugation (20000 *g*; 15 min). Of the final suspension of 1 g gland per 10 ml buffer, 100 µl was used in the assay. Reticulocyte-rich blood was obtained from rats on the 7th day after a 3-day treatment with 40 mg/kg 1-acetyl-2-phenylhydrazide daily (Schuchardt, Munich, FRG; [5]). Cells were washed in the above buffer, lysed in hypotonic buffer (17 mosmol/liter), and membranes were washed free of hemoglobin as described by Wiemer et al. [19]. Of the final suspension of membranes in the original volume of blood, 50 µl was used in the assay. The incubation volume of 300 µl contained membranes (50 or 100 µl), 20 µl of the radioligand ^{3}H-CGP 12177 (Amersham-Buchler; Braunschweig, FRG;

* The support of the *Deutsche Forschungsgemeinschaft*, the provision of a 9836 Hewlett-Packard computer and a liquid scintillation counter by the *Dr. Robert-Pfleger-Stiftung*, and the provision of a multifold filtration device by the *Paul- and Cilli-Weill-Stiftung* are gratefully acknowledged

New Aspects in Hypertension: Adrenoceptors
M. Middeke and H. Holzgreve (Eds.)
Springer-Verlag, Berlin Heidelberg New York 1986

30–40 Ci/mmol; [15]) in the concentrations indicated in the figures, 30 µl of competing ligand or buffer, and additional buffer or plasma to fill up the volume. All drugs were dissolved in the 310 mosmol/liter sodium phosphate buffer. After 60 min incubation at 25 °C, the whole volume was passed through glass fiber filters (AP 15 Millipore; Dreieich, FRG) using a multifold filtration device. Retained radioactivity on the filters was detected in a liquid scintillation counter.

Investigation in Volunteers

Six healthy male volunteers received placebo or 240 mg (±)-propranolol (3 × 80 mg of Dociton; ICI, Plankstadt, FRG) orally in a double-blind fashion; exercise heart rate and plasma concentrations of the drug were monitored thereafter, as described in detail elsewhere [18].

Calculations

Estimation of parameters was performed by the GIP program [16, 19] for nonlinear, least-square curve fitting [6] using the following equation for competitive antagonists (Eq. 1) [4, 18]:

$$B = B_{max} \times L/(L + K_D \times (1 + i/K_i)) + nsb \times L$$

where B is bound radioligand at the respective concentration L with a maximal binding capacity B_{max}, an equilibrium dissociation constant K_D, and nonspecific binding nsb. i is the concentration of inhibitory (nonlabelled) ligand – if present – with the respective equilibrium dissociation constant K_i.

In addition, the following extension of the above equation by the Hill slope n was used (Eq. 2):

$$B = B_{max}/(1 + (K_D/L)^n) + nsb \times L$$

In the case of multiple saturable binding sites, Eq. 1 was extended by additional terms as described by Wiemer et al. [19].

Results

As shown in Fig. 1 A, the radioligand ^{3}H-CGP 12177 binds at rat salivary gland membranes in a saturable fashion with a B_{max} value of 240 fmol/mg protein and a K_D value of 0.8 nmol/liter. Nonspecific binding is neglectably small (about 1% at K_D of the radioligand). The binding parameters of the radioligand can either be esti-

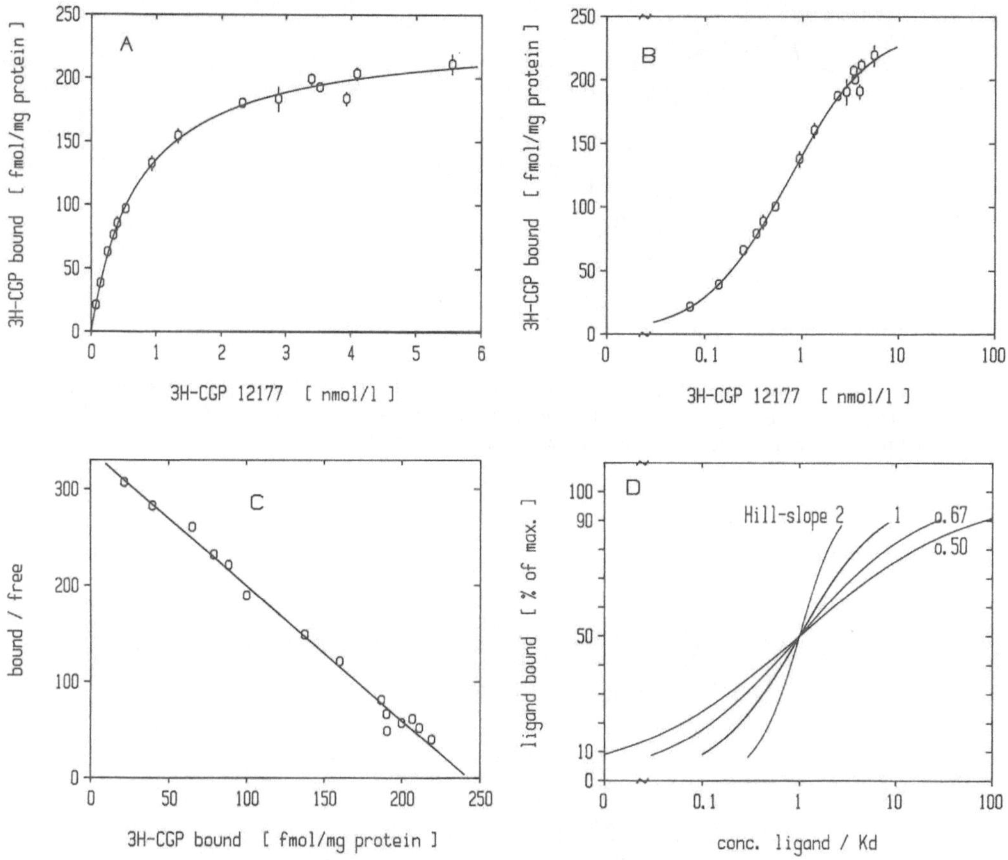

Fig. 1. Binding of the radioligand ^{3}H-CGP 12177 at rat salivary gland membranes. **A,** linear-linear plot; **B,** log-linear plot; **C,** Scatchard transformation; **D,** functions with different Hill slopes. *Abscissa,* multiples of K_D; *ordinate,* percentages of maximum; B_{max}, 240 fmol/mg protein; K_D, 0.8 nmol/liter; nonspecific binding at K_D: 1% of total binding

mated by a nonlinear procedure, fitting Eq. 1 to the data or by a linear regression analysis after a linearizing Scatchard transformation [14] as shown in Fig. 1 c. Binding of ^{3}H-CGP 12177 at salivary gland membranes increases within 2 decades of radioligand concentration around the K_D value from 9% to 91% of the maximum as can be seen both in panel A and B of Fig. 1. This finding is *always* associated with a straight line in the Scatchard transformation and a Hill slope of unity. If Hill slopes of 2, 0.67, or 0.5 become apparent - as shown in the simulated functions in panel D of Fig. 1 (Eq. 2) - the curve moves from 9% to 91% of maximum within 0.5, 1.5, or 2 log units around its EC_{50} or K_D (or IC_{50}) concentration. In general, the Hill slope can be estimated as: 2/log (concentrations of ligand which induce an increase on the ordinate from 9% to 91% of maximum).

The results of the competition experiments of catecholamines for binding of the radioligand depicted in Fig. 2 prove that this radioligand labels β-adrenoceptors: (−)-Isoprenaline is the most potent of the three catecholamines [1]. The relative

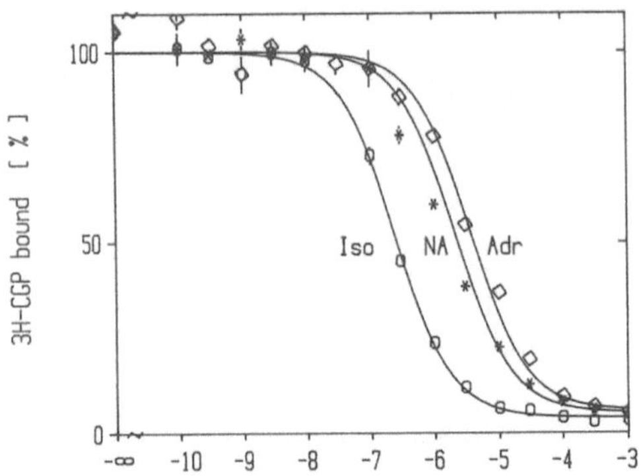

Fig. 2. Competition of catecholamines for the binding of ^{3}H-CGP 12177 at rat salivary gland membranes. The rank order of potency (−)-isoprenaline (*Iso*) > (−)-noradrenaline (*NA*) ⩾ (−)-adrenaline *(Adr)* indicates that the radioligand labels β_1-adrenoceptors

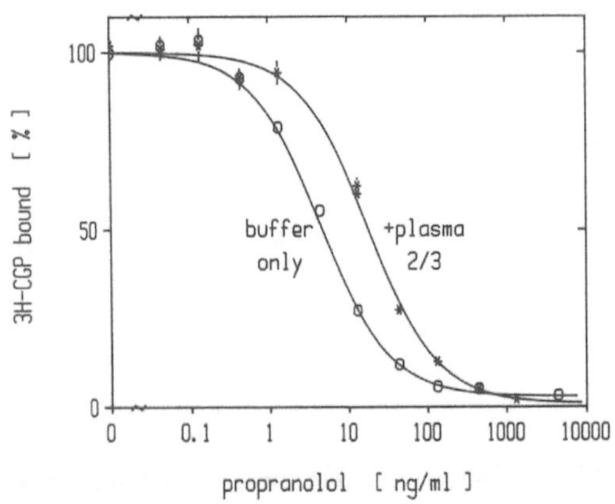

Fig. 3. Competition of (±)-propranolol for the binding of ^{3}H-CGP 12177 at rat reticulocyte membranes in the absence and presence of human plasma

potency of (−)-noradrenaline ⩾ (−)-adrenaline indicates that β_1-subtypes are labelled [9, 10].

The competition of (±)-propranolol for the radioligand binding at rat reticulocyte membranes gives a K_i value around 3 nmol/liter in the presence of buffer. This finding is also indicative of β-adrenoceptors as the binding site of the radioligand [7]. In the presence of human plasma, however, (2/3 v/v) this K_i value is shifted by about 1 log unit to the right due to protein binding of the lipophilic (±)-propranolol. Receptor binding of the hydrophilic radioligand is not affected by inclusion of plasma in the assay [17].

The relevance of these binding experiments is finally shown in Fig. 4: Exercise tachycardia is inhibited by propranolol present in the extracellular plasma compartment at concentrations which are in agreement with the inhibitory effects at β-adrenoceptors in receptor binding studies in vitro (c.f. IC_{50} values in Figs. 3 and 4 in the presence of plasma.

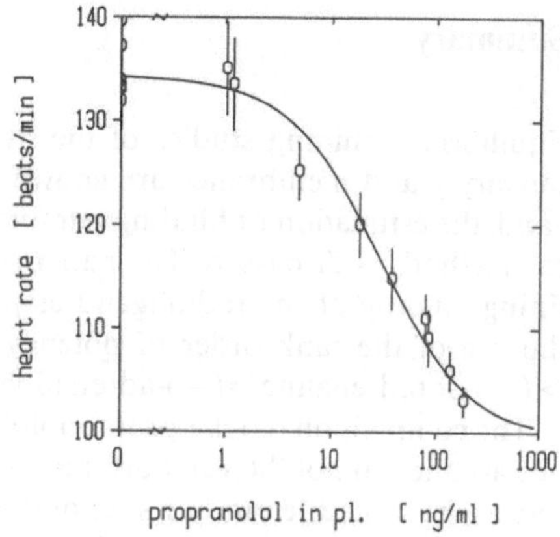

Fig. 4. Inhibition of exercise tachycardia in man by propranolol. *Ordinate,* heart rate after 4-min exercise (75% of maximum); *abscissa,* plasma concentrations of propranolol

Discussion

Receptor binding studies have allowed direct labelling of receptors. Certain principles must, however, be kept in mind. Saturable binding alone does not prove labelling of a drug receptor but might also speak in favor of a drug acceptor site. The proof of drug receptors as the site of binding of a radioligand stems from the use of classical pharmacological tools, such as the rank order of potency of well-defined ligands [3, 4]. If the potency of antagonist drugs is well established (i.e., their K_D or their K_i values; [7]), they may also serve to define the binding site as a drug receptor of a certain type. This is exemplified for propranolol in the example presented here where propranolol shows K_i values in agreement with those of a β-adrenoceptor interaction.

Finally one should always try to correlate receptor-mediated effects with those observed via the receptor binding approach. In the case of β-adrenoceptors, this may be the cAMP synthesis at the biochemical level [5, 7, 11], in vitro experiments with intact human tissue [7], or even effects in man like the inhibition of exercise tachycardia presented here [18]. In the latter case, it can be shown by this approach that antagonist present in plasma is in fact in a rapid equilibrium with the concentration at β-adrenoceptors in man. One can thus extrapolate from the in vitro findings the antagonistic effects in man if the respective plasma concentrations of the active compound are known. Thus, in vitro receptor interaction is a good measure for the prediction of clinical effects of β-adrenoceptor antagonists and perhaps other classes of drugs [13].

If receptor binding studies are used in this sense, they prove to be valuable tools for a better understanding of drug-induced, pathophysiological, or other regulatory events as reviewed by Motulsky and Insel [12]. They may furthermore increase our understanding of drug action and support a rational discussion of the potential use of new approaches to drug therapy [13].

Summary

Equilibrium binding studies of the hydrophilic radioligand ^{3}H-CGP 12177 at rat salivary gland membranes are shown. Using saturation isotherms of this radioligand, the estimation of binding parameters by linearization procedures and nonlinear methods is discussed. The paper shows which criteria are prerequisites for defining binding of the radioligand as β-adrenoceptor binding at the β_1-subtype by the use of the rank order of potency of well-defined agonists: (−)-isoprenaline > (−)-noradrenaline ⩾ (−)-adrenaline.

The competition of (±)-propranolol for binding of this radioligand shows K_i values around 3 nmol/liter in buffer medium and is thus also a proof of β-adrenoceptors as the saturable binding sites of the radioligand. In the presence of human plasma, an apparent reduction of the potency of (±)-propranolol in the competition for the radioligand binding is observed, which is due to plasma protein binding of (±)-propranolol. Finally, it is shown that IC_{50} values calculated from the inhibition of exercise tachycardia in man dependent on plasma concentrations of (±)-propranolol are in agreement with the in vitro β-adrenoceptor interaction of (±)-propranolol in the presence of human plasma. Thus, it is concluded that under appropriate conditions, receptor binding studies are a valuable tool for the understanding of the mechanisms underlying drug-receptor interaction.

Abbreviations:
K_D: equilibrium dissociation constant of radioligand; K_i: equilibrium dissociation constant of inhibitory ligand; IC_{50}: half-maximally inhibitory concentration; B_{max}: maximal capacity of receptor binding.

References

1. Ahlquist RP (1948) A study of adrenotropic receptors. Am J Physiol 153: 586–600
2. Brodde OE, Engel G, Hoyer D, Bock KD, Weber F (1981) The β-adrenergic receptor in human lymphocytes: Subclassification by the use of a new radio-ligand, $(+/-)^{125}$-iodocyanopindolol. Life Sci 29: 2189–2198
3. Furchgott RF (1972) The classification of adrenoceptors (adrenergic receptors). An evaluation from the standpoint of receptor theory. In: Blaschko H, Muscholl E (eds) Catecholamines. Springer, Berlin Heidelberg New York, pp 283–335, Handbook of experimental pharmacology, vol 33
4. Gaddum JH (1957) Theories of drug antagonism. Pharmacol Rev 9: 211–218
5. Gauger D, Kaiser G, Quiring K, Palm D (1975) The β-adrenergic receptor adenyl cyclase-system of rat reticulocytes. Naunyn-Schmiedebergs Arch Pharmacol 289: 379–389
6. Gauss CF (1809) Theoria motus corporum coelestium in sectionibus conicis solem ambientium. Lib II, Sect III, Hamburgi Sumtibus, Frid Perthes et IH Besser
7. Gille E, Lemoine H, Ehle B, Kaumann AJ (1985) The affinity of (−)-propranolol for β_1- and β_2-adrenoceptors of human heart. Differential antagonism of the positive inotropic effects and adenylate cyclase stimulation by (−)-noradrenaline and (−)-adrenaline. Naunyn-Schmiedebergs Arch Pharmacol 331: 60–70
8. Laduron PM (1984) Criteria for receptor sites in binding studies. Biochem Pharmacol 33: 833–839

9. Lands AM, Arnold A, McAuliff JP, Luduena FP, Brown TG (1967 a) Differentiation of receptor systems activated by sympathomimetic amines. Nature 214: 597-598
10. Lands AM, Luduena FP, Buzzo HJ (1967 b) Differentiation of receptors responsive to isoproterenol. Life Sci 6: 2241-2249
11. Lefkowitz RJ, Stadel JM, Caron MG (1983) Adenylate cyclase-coupled beta-adrenergic receptors: structure and mechanisms of activation and desensitization. Annu Rev Biochem 52: 159-186
12. Motulsky HJ, Insel PA (1982) Adrenergic receptors in man. Direct identification, physiologic regulation, and clinical alterations. N Engl J Med 307: 18-29
13. Palm D, Wellstein A (1985) Multipotente Arzneistoffe - Hybride und Pseudohybride. In: Holzgreve H (ed) Kombinierte Alpha- und Beta-Adrenozeptorenblockade mit symbiontischen Molekülen. Ein neues Therapiekonzept bei Hypertonie und koronarer Herzkrankheit. MMW Medizin Verlag, München, pp 28-56
14. Scatchard G (1949) The attraction of proteins for small molecules and ions. Ann NY Acad Sci 51: 660-672
15. Staehelin M, Simons P, Jaeggi K, Wigger N (1983) CGP12177. A hydrophilic β-adrenergic receptor radioligand reveals high affinity binding of agonists to intact cells. J Biol Chem 258: 3496-3502
16. Von Hattingberg HM, Brockmeier D, Kreuter G (1977) A rotating iterative procedure (RIP) for estimating hybrid constants. Eur J Clin Pharmacol 11: 381-388
17. Wellstein A, Palm D, Wiemer G, Schäfer-Korting M, Mutschler E (1984) Simple and reliable radioreceptor assay for β-adrenoceptor antagonists and active metabolites in native human plasma. Eur J Clin Pharmacol 27: 545-553
18. Wellstein A, Palm D, Belz GG, Pitschner HF (1985) Receptor binding of propranolol is the missing link between plasma concentration kinetics and effect time course in man. Eur J Clin Pharmacol 29: 131-147
19. Wiemer G, Wellstein A, Palm D, von Hattingberg HM, Brockmeier D (1982) Properties of agonist binding at the β-adrenoceptor of the rat reticulocyte. Naunyn-Schmiedebergs Arch Pharmacol 321: 11-19
20. Williams LT, Lefkowitz RJ (1978) Receptor binding in adrenergic pharmacology. Raven, New York

Discussion

Skrabal: Binding studies yield information on two basic points: binding affinity and capacity. Theoretically it is conceivable that in physiological regulation of the receptors the binding affinity and the capacity are changed in direct or inverse relationship to each other. Is it possible to predict the in vivo action from the relationship of affinity and binding capacity? The second question in this context is: Are there any underlying physiological laws? For example, when the binding capacity increases, how does the affinity change?

Wellstein: Affinity and capacity are two quantities that are independent of each other, in the sense that capacity is more or less the quantity given by the body and affinity the quantity given by the pharmacologists or the people who synthesize drugs. With beta blockers, for example, we have affinities in the picomolar to micromolar range. If you take pindolol on the one hand and atenolol on the other, you have such a wide range that the affinity and the capacity are again independent of each other. As to the question of regulation and what can change: For the agonist norepinephrine, for example, this is very difficult to demonstrate. In humans receptor occupation does not necessarily parallel the effect of the agonist. When you take an agonist, you often have the full effect with very low receptor occupation. Pharmacologists speak of 'spare receptors,' meaning that you only need a very small proportion of the receptors to achieve the full effect. It is certainly conceivable that you have 100% capacity of the receptors but only 10% of them are required. In this case you could have small changes in this portion of spare receptors or in the coupling of receptors without seeing any difference in the total capacity. You would observe it, for example, as a left or right shift in the agonist dose-effect curves in humans.

Brodde: May I add something to that, Dr. Skrabal? You also asked whether an upregulation always has a large effect or not. It must be stated clearly that changes in the number of receptors per se have no effect at all. They can vary directly with the receptor responsiveness or inversely. A small example: In advanced age the number of beta receptors is elevated. However, the responsiveness, i.e., the synthesis of cAMP, is depressed. In other words, if you were to measure only beta receptors you would say: "aha, in elderly people the responsiveness of beta receptors is markedly higher than in young people," whereas precisely the opposite is the case. When you measure receptor binding, you should also measure some functional response, in the case of beta receptors cAMP.

Wellstein: You will have noticed that our instruments are predominantly antagonists, propranolol, for example. You have these problems to a lesser degree because you simply see to what extent you can inhibit effects that are already present. With agonists it is very, very complicated because you have at least one parameter to change.

Agonist Interaction with α_2-Adrenoceptors of Human Platelets*

J. SCHLOOS and D. PALM

Zentrum der Pharmakologie, Klinikum der J. W. Goethe Universität, Theodor-Stern-Kai 7, 6000 Frankfurt/Main 70, FRG

Introduction

The development of radioligand binding technique during the past decade has led to increased understanding of the cascade of events in hormone-receptor coupling and receptor-mediated signal-transducing processes [14].

Investigations of ligand-receptor interaction in human tissues were facilitated by the demonstration that circulating blood cells, e.g., lymphocytes which possess β_2-adrenoceptors [1, 8] or platelets where α_2-adrenoceptors are located [18], are conveniently available for the study of receptors in man.

Several groups have applied radioligand binding methods in studies focused on alterations in platelet α_2-adrenoceptor density and binding affinity in a variety of pathological or altered physiological states, i.e., hypertension [19], asthma [23], major depressive illness [6], clonidine medication [2], variations in plasma levels of catecholamines [12, 22], menstrual cycle [27], and age [3, 36] (for review see: [17]).

In studies of radioligand binding to α_2-adrenoceptors, the selective antagonist ^{3}H-yohimbine [18] is commonly used as a radioligand. In such binding experiments, receptor occupancy by agonists, but not antagonists, promotes or stabilizes a high-affinity, guanine-nucleotide-sensitive state of the receptor [25, 33]. Guanine nucleotides have also been shown to regulate the functions of adenylate-cyclase-coupled receptors by decreasing high-affinity binding for hormones or agonist drugs [28]. Jakobs and coworkers [13] have shown that agonist-induced α-adrenergic inhibition of platelet adenylate cyclase is dependent on the presence of GTP. Thus, with antagonist radioligands, agonist-receptor interactions and the sensitivity to GTP or stable analogues can only be studied by indirect approaches, i.e., by competition experiments. In order to circumvent this shortcoming of studies conducted with antagonist radioligands we have investigated labeling of α_2-adrenoceptors with agonist radioligands. The most potent α-adrenoceptor agonists are (−)adrenaline and the new arylimidazoline derivative UK-14304. The latter has previously been described acting as a selective full agonist at α_2-adrenoceptors in physiological and biochemical studies [5, 9, 15, 31]. As it is available now as a radioligand, we examined the binding properties at human platelet membranes of the tritiated compound UK-

* This work was supported by a grant from the *Deutsche Forschungsgemeinschaft*. We are indebted to the *Robert-Pfleger-Stiftung* for generous gift of the Packard Tri-Carb and the Hewlett-Packard computer and to the *Paul-* and *Cilli-Weill-Stiftung* for the filtration device.

New Aspects in Hypertension: Adrenoceptors
M. Middeke and H. Holzgreve (Eds.)
Springer-Verlag Berlin Heidelberg New York 1986

14304 in comparison to ^{3}H-yohimbine. The present study was undertaken in an attempt to investigate coupling of the hormone-receptor complex to the effector system via the regulatory GTP-binding subunit by examining agonist-receptor interactions directly. This approach should provide a better insight into this first step in activation or inhibition of adenylate cyclase by catecholamines and may lead to a better understanding of the functional changes of adrenoceptor mediated effects.

Methods

Platelet membranes were prepared by a method according to Newman et al. [20] with slight modifications. In brief, platelet rich plasma obtained from the local blood bank was centrifuged (17500 *g*, 15 min, 25 °C), and the resulting pellet was washed in Tris buffer A (50 mmol/liter TrisHCl, 20 mmol/liter EDTA, 150 mmol/liter NaCl; pH=7.4), resuspended in an ice-cold hypotonic buffer B (5 mmol/liter TrisHCl, 5 mmol/liter EDTA; pH=7.4), and homogenized with an Ultra-Turrax (Janke & Kunkel, Staufen, FRG). After centrifugation (35000 *g*, 15 min, 4 °C), the membrane pellet was washed in ice-cold Tris buffer C (50 mmol/liter Tris HCl, 0.8 mmol/liter EDTA; pH=7.4), resuspended in the same buffer, and stored at −20 °C until use. At the day of assay, membrane pellets were washed three times in ice-cold buffer C and centrifuged (35000 *g*, 15 min, 4 °C) after each wash, and resuspended in the assay buffer (50 mmol/liter TrisHCl, 0.8 mmol/liter EDTA, 0.8 mmol/liter ascorbic acid, 0.3 mmol/liter catechol, 0.3 mmol/liter dithiothreitol, 10 mmol/liter $MgCl_2$; pH=7.4). Platelet membranes were adjusted to a final concentration of 0.8–1.0 mg of protein/ml in the assays which were performed in a total volume of 250 μl/assay cup.

After incubation at 25 °C for 60 min, bound and free radioligand were separated by rapid filtration under reduced pressure over glass-fibre filters (Whatman GF/C) using a 12-well cell harvester device (Skatron, Düsseldorf, FRG). Each filter was rinsed immediately with 10 ml ice-cold buffer C, and retained radioactivity was detected in a scintillation cocktail (Opti-Fluor, Packard Instruments, Frankfurt, FRG) by liquid scintillation spectrometry (Tri-Carb 4450, Packard Instruments, Frankfurt, FRG) at 46% efficiency. All assays were performed in triplicate and repeated as indicated in the text.

Data Analysis

Using a Hewlett-Packard 9836 desk computer, data were analysed by a nonlinear least-squares curve-fitting procedure applied to a model for ligand-receptor interactions. This generalized model is based on the equations according to Feldman [7]. The interactive computer program written in HP language was developed by D. Brockmeier and H. M. von Hattingberg [32, 33]. A two-tailed *t*-test was used to examine differences, $p < 0.05$ being set as significant. Experimental data presented in the text and figures are mean values ± SEM.

Drugs

Yohimbine, (methyl-^{3}H)- (spec. act. 75.0–85.8 Ci/mmol) and UK-14304, (imidazolyl-4,5-^{3}H)- (spec. act. 77.0–88.0 Ci/mmol) were purchased from New England Nuclear, Dreieich, FRG. The following drugs were kindly donated by the indicated companies: UK-14304 (5-bromo-6-(2-imidazoline-2-ylamino)-quinoxaline) tartrate (Pfizer Central Research, Sandwich/Kent, England); (−)adrenaline bitartrate (Sterling-Winthrop Research Institute, New York, USA); phentolamine methansulfonate (Ciba-Geigy, Wehr/Baden, FRG). Other reagents were obtained from the pharmaceutical company of origin or commercial sources.

Results

Binding of the radioligand ^{3}H-UK-14304 (^{3}H-UK) at 25 °C was rapid, with a association rate constant *(k_1)* of 3.7×10^7 M^{-1} min^{-1} calculated from kinetic experiments. Dissociation of the ligand showed a first-order process with a $t_{½}$ of 15.4 min (not depicted). This indicates that binding of ^{3}H-UK to human platelet membranes is reversible, reaching equilibrium at 25 °C during the 60-min incubation period.

Since specific binding of ^{3}H-UK was enhanced in the presence of $MgCl_2$, all binding assays were performed with a maximal effective concentration of 10 mmol/liter $MgCl_2$, which did not alter binding of ^{3}H-yohimbine (^{3}H-YOH) [24].

Saturation isotherms of specific binding of the antagonist ^{3}H-YOH and the agonist ^{3}H-UK to α_2-adrenoceptors of human platelet membranes are shown in Fig. 1. For ^{3}H-YOH saturations, no influence of 0.1 mmol/liter of the nonhydrolyzable GTP analogue Gpp(NH)p on the binding parameters was observed. In the absence of Gpp(NH)p the calculated K_D value was 6.18 ± 0.36 nmol/liter and the B_{max} value was 198 ± 8 fmol/mg protein (n=3), similar to that reported previously [25]. Addition of 0.1 mmol/liter Gpp(NH)p did not affect binding capacity (B_{max}= 185 ± 22 fmol/mg protein) or affinity (K_D=6.11 ± 0.46 nmol/liter) of the radioligand.

In contrast to antagonist binding, saturation experiments of ^{3}H-UK binding revealed a smaller portion of binding sites, with a B_{max} value of 107 ± 6 fmol/mg protein (n=6), i.e., 54% of ^{3}H-YOH-labeled sites in the mean. Binding of this agonist radioligand was of high affinity (K_D= 1.51 ± 0.13 nmol/liter; n=6) and addition of 0.1 mmol/liter Gpp(NH)p almost abolished specific binding of ^{3}H-UK over the concentration range of 0.2–50 nmol/liter used in this study. In both radioligand assays, nonspecific binding was determined in the presence of 10 μmol/liter phentolamine, a nonselective α-antagonist, revealing an amount of ~10% of total binding at the respective K_D concentration of the radioligands.

The effect of 0.1 mmol/liter Gpp(NH)p on competition of the agonist (−)adrenaline with ^{3}H-YOH for binding is depicted in Fig. 2A. The shallow competition curves derived in the absence of Gpp(NH)p are well described by a two-site model reflecting binding of (−)adrenaline to a high-affinity binding state with a calculated K_i of 15.3 ± 2.8 nmol/liter and a B_{max} of 56% ± 2% (n=7) of ^{3}H-YOH-labeled sites. The K_i value of the low-affinity binding of (−)adrenaline (K_i= 829 ± 190 nmol/

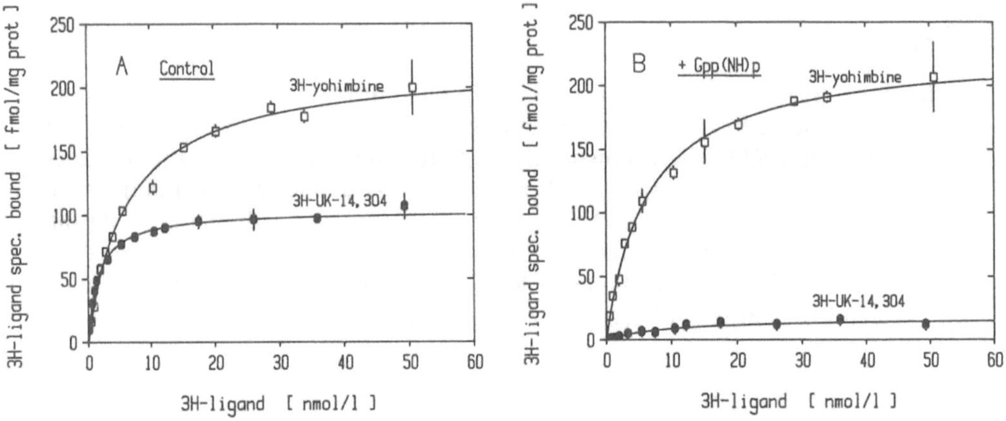

Fig. 1. Equilibrium binding of ^{3}H-yohimbine and ^{3}H-UK-14304 in the absence **(A)** and presence **(B)** of 0.1 mmol/liter Gpp(NH)p. Membranes (0.2 mg protein) were incubated with various concentrations (0.2–50 nmol/liter) of the respective radioligand for 60 min at 25 °C. Nonspecific binding for ^{3}H-YOH and ^{3}H-UK (13% and 8% of total binding at the respective K_D concentration) was determined in the presence of 10 μmol/liter phentolamine in parallel incubations and subtracted from total binding. Data *points* ± SEM are from a representative experiment performed in triplicate. Parameters of specific binding were calculated by a computer-assisted nonlinear least-squares fitting procedure using a model for one specific and a nonspecific class of binding sites. ^{3}H-YOH (control): K_D=5.89 nmol/liter, B_{max}=214.1 fmol/mg protein; in the presence of 0.1 mmol/liter Gpp(NH)p: K_D=5.70 nmol/liter, B_{max}=222.4 fmol/mg protein; ^{3}H-UK (control): K_D=1.57 nmol/liter, B_{max}=104.1 fmol/mg protein; in the presence of 0.1 mmol/liter Gpp(NH)p no reliable binding parameters can be calculated

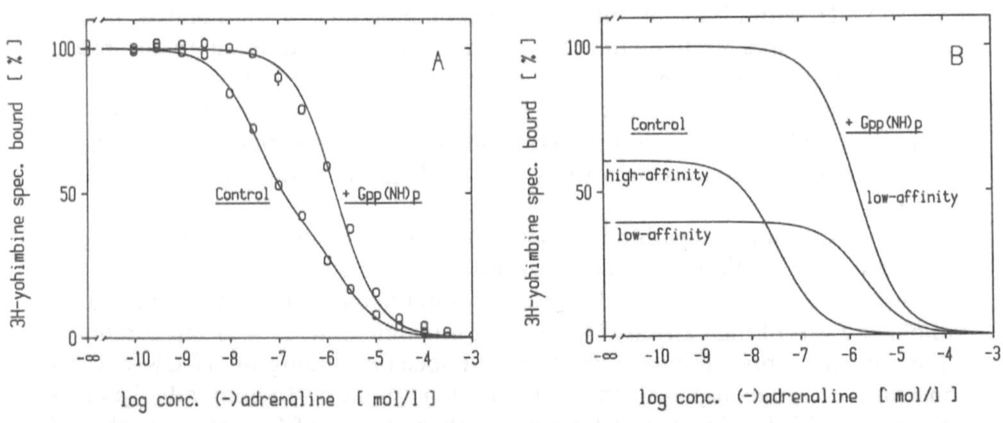

Fig. 2. A Competition isotherms of (−)adrenaline vs ^{3}H-yohimbine (7.2 nmol/liter) in the absence and presence of 0.1 mmol/liter Gpp(NH)p. In the absence of Gpp(NH)p, the shallow competition curve can be resolved into two components of different affinity and capacity (K_{iH}=11.5 nmol/liter, K_{iL}=662.0 nmol/liter; B_{maxH}=60.6%, and B_{maxL}=39.4% of total B_{max}). In the presence of 0.1 mmol/liter Gpp(NH)p, the data are well described by a model of homogeneous binding sites where adrenaline binds with low affinity (K_{iL}=503.9 nmol/liter).

In **B** functions of the two binding components from shallow control competition curve analysis are depicted separately (high-affinity and low-affinity component). Note that the IC_{50} value of the low affinity component is in close agreement with the IC_{50} value of the function obtained by analysis of the competition curve measured in the presence of Gpp(NH)p

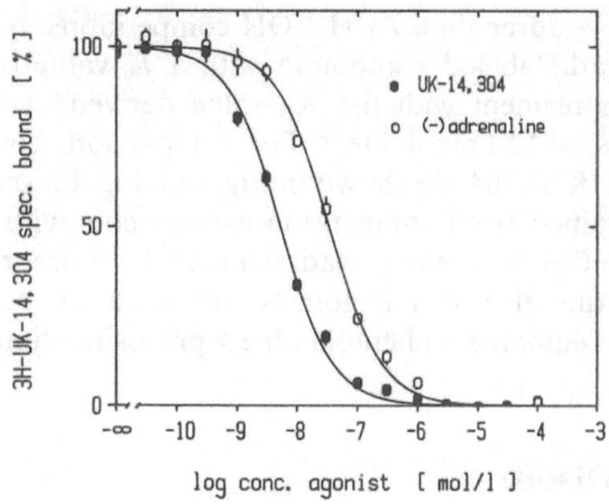

Fig. 3. Competition isotherms of UK-14304 (●) and (−)adrenaline (○) vs ^{3}H-UK-14304 (3.7 nmol/liter). The K_i values calculated from the monophasic competition curves are 1.42 nmol/liter for UK-14304 and 9.87 nmol/liter for (−)adrenaline

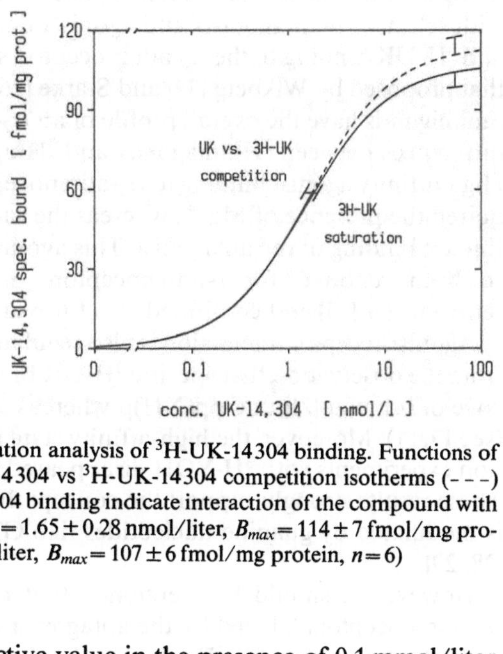

Fig. 4. Comparison of competition and saturation analysis of ^{3}H-UK-14304 binding. Functions of the mean values derived by analysis of UK-14304 vs ^{3}H-UK-14304 competition isotherms (- - -) and saturation isotherms (——) of ^{3}H-UK-14304 binding indicate interaction of the compound with a single class of binding sites (competition: $K_i = 1.65 \pm 0.28$ nmol/liter, $B_{max} = 114 \pm 7$ fmol/mg protein, $n = 3$; saturation: $K_D = 1.51 \pm 0.13$ nmol/liter, $B_{max} = 107 \pm 6$ fmol/mg protein, $n = 6$)

liter) is in the same range as the respective value in the presence of 0.1 mmol/liter Gpp(NH)p ($K_i = 639 \pm 98$ nmol/liter).

The functions of the separated high- and low-affinity components from the shallow competition isotherms and the function of the monophasic competition isotherm in the presence of Gpp(NH)p are depicted in Fig. 2B. In comparison to agonist vs ^{3}H-YOH experiments, competition curves of UK-14304 and (−)adrenaline vs ^{3}H-UK are monophasic representing a single site-to-site interaction (Fig. 3). The affinity of (−)adrenaline ($K_i = 9.6 \pm 0.5$ nmol/liter; $n = 3$) calculated from competition with ^{3}H-UK agrees with the K_i value of the high-affinity binding derived from

(−)adrenaline vs ^{3}H-YOH competitions. Nonlabeled UK-14304 competes for the radiolabeled compound with a K_i value of 1.65 ± 0.28 nmol/liter and is thus in agreement with the K_D value derived by ^{3}H-UK saturation experiments (mean $K_D = 1.51$ nmol/liter). For comparison, competition and saturation functions of UK-14304 are shown in Fig. 4 on log/lin scales. The potency order of agonists obtained from competition experiments with ^{3}H-UK is identical to that when ^{3}H-YOH is used: (−)adrenaline > (−)noradrenaline ≫ (−)isoprenaline. This holds true also if antagonists are used as competitors vs ^{3}H-UK and ^{3}H-YOH: yohimbine > phentolamine ≫ prazosin > timolol (data not depicted).

Discussion

The binding characteristics of ^{3}H-yohimbine (^{3}H-YOH) and ^{3}H-UK-14304 (^{3}H-UK) to human platelet membranes both satisfy criteria [35] which are required for identification of a pharmacological or physiological receptor, i. e., binding of the radioligands was saturable, reversible, and of high affinity. Competition experiments with selective α-antagonists and agonists demonstrated the specificity of ^{3}H-YOH and ^{3}H-UK binding to the α_2-adrenoceptor, since the rank order of potency obeyed that proposed by Wikberg [34] and Starke [26]. Although the sites labeled with both radioligands have the overall profile of an α_2-adrenoceptor, a number of significant differences between ^{3}H-antagonist and ^{3}H-agonist binding should be emphasized. High-affinity agonist binding to α_2-adrenoceptors of human platelet membranes required the presence of Mg^{2+}, whereas the same conditions did not significantly influence binding of the antagonist. This agonist-selective sensitivity for Mg^{2+} has also been reported for β-adrenoceptors in rat lung membranes [10] and rat reticulocytes [33] and confirmed also for platelet α_2-adrenoceptors [4].

Agonist-receptor interaction is also regulated by Gpp(NH)p, as can be concluded from the observation that specific ^{3}H-UK binding was almost abolished in the presence of 0.1 mmol/liter Gpp(NH)p whereas ^{3}H-YOH binding remained unaffected (see Fig. 1). Moreover, the high-affinity state induced by (−)adrenaline in competition experiments with ^{3}H-YOH disappeared under the same conditions (see Fig. 2). These results strongly support the concept that agonist, but not antagonist, binding is modulated by guanine nucleotides like GTP or the stable analogue Gpp(NH)p [28, 29].

However, it should be mentioned that obviously only a portion of the total α_2-adrenoceptors labeled by the antagonist can be transferred into a high-affinity agonist binding state (see Fig. 1). This has been demonstrated also for ^{3}H-noradrenaline [16] and ^{3}H-adrenaline binding [11] to α-adrenoceptors. The use of ^{3}H-(−)adrenaline as the physiological ligand is biased by the lower affinity and much higher amount of nonspecific binding (~50% at K_D concentration) of ^{3}H-(−)adrenaline binding to platelet membranes [24], reported also for rat brain α_2-adrenoceptors [30]. These disadvantages can be overcome by the use of ^{3}H-UK, which is more suitable for direct agonist binding studies due to lower nonspecific binding (~10% at K_D concentration) and higher affinity.

The labeling of the agonist UK-14304 obviously does not influence its interaction with α_2-adrenoceptors, for nonlabeled UK-14304 exhibits the same binding characteristics as are revealed by ^{3}H-UK saturation and competition experiments (see Fig. 4). An isotope effect based on radiolabeling of UK-14304 can thus be excluded. That ^{3}H-UK labels exclusively the high-affinity binding state can be deduced from the finding that (−)adrenaline competes with ^{3}H-UK with K_i values equal to those calculated for binding to the high-affinity state in ^{3}H-YOH competitions (see Fig. 2 and 3). Monophasic competition for ^{3}H-agonist labeled receptors have also been described for bovine cerebral cortex membranes by Perry and U'Prichard [21].

From these observations, it can be concluded that ^{3}H-UK binds to the agonist-induced or -stabilized high-affinity state of the platelet α_2-adrenoceptor.

The unique characteristics of direct labeling of agonist high-affinity binding state might be exploited as follows: Recent evidence shows that variations in plasma catecholamine concentrations modulate the affinity of human platelet α_2-adrenoceptors for agonists, whereas the total number of α_2-adrenoceptors and the affinity for antagonists remain unchanged [12, 22]. At present, it is not clear whether a variety of pathological or altered physiological states produce changes in total adrenoceptor density, as suggested by antagonist radioligand binding, or whether coupling of the receptor with the GTP-binding regulatory subunit is affected in a more pronounced manner. To evaluate this first step in α_2-adrenoceptor-mediated physiological events, ^{3}H-UK is proposed as a valuable tool for studying direct agonist binding to α_2-adrenoceptors of human platelets.

Summary

Differences between agonist and antagonist interactions with α_2-adrenoceptors of human platelet membranes were studied comparing binding properties of the radioligands ^{3}H-UK-14304 (^{3}H-UK) (an agonist) and ^{3}H-yohimbine (^{3}H-YOH) (an antagonist).

Binding of ^{3}H-UK revealed single site-to-site interaction with an equilibrium dissociation constant (K_D) of 1.51 ± 0.13 nmol/liter at 25 °C and a capacity (B_{max}) of 107 ± 6 fmol/mg of protein (n=6). The binding sites showed the characteristics of an α_2-adrenoceptor with respect to the potency order of agonists and antagonists.

In comparison with ^{3}H-YOH binding (K_D=6.18 ± 0.36 nmol/liter; B_{max}=198 ± 8 fmol/mg of protein; n=3) about 54% of the antagonist sites were labeled by ^{3}H-UK. Guanylylimidodiphosphate [Gpp(NH)p], a nonhydrolyzable GTP analogue, reduced binding of ^{3}H-UK to a hardly detectable amount at a concentration of 0.1 mmol/liter without altering binding parameters of ^{3}H-YOH.

Competition experiments carried out with (−)adrenaline vs ^{3}H-YOH revealed a two-site interaction for (−)adrenaline with high affinity (K_i=15.3 ± 2.8 nmol/liter) for 56% ± 2% and low affinity (K_i=829 ± 190 nmol/liter) for 44% ± 2% of the ^{3}H-YOH labeled sites (n=7). Gpp(NH)p (0.1 mmol/liter) diminished the number of high-affinity sites by transition into the low-affinity state. In competition experiments using (−)adrenaline vs ^{3}H-UK a single dissociation constant for (−)adrenaline (K_i=9.6 ± 0.5 nmol/liter; n=3) can be calculated from the monophasic competition curves. This indicates single site-to-site interaction for (−)adrenaline with the

Gpp(NH)p-sensitive high-affinity binding state labeled by ^{3}H-UK. The differences between antagonist and agonist binding noted support the concept of high-affinity and low-affinity states of the α_2-adrenoceptor for agonists.

Therefore, ^{3}H-UK should prove to be a valuable tool for agonist interaction in studies of physiological or pathophysiological alterations of α_2-adrenoceptors in tissues and blood cells with respect to the GTP-sensitive binding state of agonists.

References

1. Brodde OE, Engel G, Hoyer D, Bock KD, Weber F (1981) The β-adrenergic receptor in human lymphocytes: Subclassification by the use of a new radioligand, (±)-^{125}Iodocyanopindolol. Life Sci 29: 2189–2198
2. Brodde OE, Anlauf M, Graben N, Bock KD (1982a) In vitro and in vivo down-regulation of human platelet α_2-adrenoceptors by clonidine. Eur J Clin Pharmacol 23: 403–409
3. Brodde OE, Anlauf M, Graben N, Bock KD (1982b) Age-dependent decrease of α_2-adrenergic receptor number in human platelets. Eur J Pharmacol 81: 345–347
4. Bylund DB, U'Prichard DC (1983) Characterization of alpha-1 and alpha-2 adrenergic receptors. Int Rev Neurobiol 24: 343–431
5. Cambridge D (1981) UK-14,304, a potent and selective α_2-agonist for the characterisation of α-adrenoceptor subtypes. Eur J Pharmacol 72: 413–415
6. Daiguji M, Meltzer HY, Tong C, U'Prichard DC, Young M, Kravitz H (1981) α_2-Adrenergic receptors in platelet membranes of depressed patients: no change in number or ^{3}H-yohimbine affinity. Life Sci 29: 2059–2064
7. Feldman HA (1972) Mathematical theory of complex ligand-binding systems at equilibrium. Some methods for parameter fitting. Anal Biochem 48: 317–338
8. Galant SP, Underwood S, Duriseti L, Insel PA (1978) Characterization of high-affinity β_2-adrenergic receptor binding of (−)-dihydroalprenolol to human polymorphonuclear cell particulates. J Lab Clin Med 92: 613–618
9. Grant JA, Scrutton MC (1980) Interaction of selective α-adrenoceptor agonists and antagonists with human and rabbit blood platelets. Br J Pharmacol 71: 121–134
10. Heidenreich KA, Weiland GA, Molinoff PB (1982) Effects of magnesium and N-ethylmaleimide on the binding of ^{3}H-hydroxybenzylisoproterenol to β-adrenergic receptors. J Biol Chem 257: 804–810
11. Hoffman BB, Michel T, Kilpatrick DM, Lefkowitz RJ, Tolbert MEM, Gilman H, Fain JN (1980) Agonist versus antagonist binding to α-adrenergic receptors. Proc Natl Acad Sci USA 77: 4569–4573
12. Hollister AS, Fitzgerald GA, Nadeau JH, Robertson D (1983) Acute reduction in human platelet α_2-adrenoceptor affinity for agonist by endogenous and exogenous catecholamines. J Clin Invest 72: 1498–1505
13. Jakobs KH, Aktories H, Schultz G (1981) Inhibition of adenylate cyclase by hormones and neurotransmitters. Adv Cyclic Nucleotide Res 14: 173–187
14. Lamble JW, Abbott AC (eds) (1984) Receptors, again. Elsevier, Amsterdam
15. Loftus DJ, Stolk JM, U'Prichard DC (1984) Binding of the imidazoline UK-14,304, a putative full α_2-adrenoceptor agonist, to rat cerebral cortex membranes. Life Sci 35: 61–69
16. Lynch CJ, Steer ML (1981) Evidence for high and low affinity α_2-receptors – Comparison of (^{3}H)norepinephrine and (^{3}H)phentolamine binding to human platelet membranes. J Biol Chem 256: 3298–3303
17. Motulsky HJ, Insel PA (1982) Adrenergic receptors in man – Direct identification, physiologic regulation, and clinical alterations. N Engl J Med 307: 18–29
18. Motulsky HJ, Shattil SD, Insel PA (1980) Characterisation of α_2-adrenergic receptors on human platelets using (^{3}H)yohimbine. Biochem Biophys Res Commun 97: 1562–1570
19. Motulsky HJ, O'Connor DT, Insel PA (1983) Platelet α_2-adrenergic receptors in treated and untreated essential hypertension. Clin Sci 64: 265–272

20. Newman KD, Williams LT, Bishopric NH, Lefkowitz RJ (1978) Identification of α-adrenergic receptors in human platelets by (^{3}H)dihydroergocryptine binding. J Clin Invest 61: 395-402
21. Perry BD, U'Prichard DC (1981) (^{3}H)Rauwolscine (α-yohimbine): a specific antagonist radioligand for brain α_2-adrenergic receptors. Eur J Pharmacol 76: 461-464
22. Pfeifer MA, Ward K, Malpass T, Stratton J, Halter J, Evans M, Beiter H, Harker LA, Porte D Jr (1984) Variations in circulating catecholamines fail to alter human platelet alpha-2-adrenergic receptor number or affinity for (^{3}H)yohimbine or (^{3}H)dihydroergocryptine. J Clin Invest 74: 1063-1072
23. Reinhardt D, Becker B, Nagel-Hiemke M, Schiffer R, Zehmisch T (1983) Influence of beta-receptor-agonists and glucocorticoids on alpha- and beta-adrenoceptors of isolated blood cells from asthmatic children. Pediatr Pharmacol (New York) 3: 293-302
24. Schloos J, Vogt C, Palm D (1985) Agonist-induced high-affinity state of α_2-adrenoceptors of human platelets characterized by ^{3}H-antagonist and ^{3}H-agonist binding. Naunyn Schmiedebergs Arch Pharmacol 330 [Suppl]: R61
25. Smith SK, Limbird LE (1981) Solubilization of human platelet α-adrenergic receptors: Evidence that agonist occupancy of the receptor stabilizes receptor-effector interactions. Proc Natl Acad Sci USA 7: 4026-4030
26. Starke K (1981) α-Adrenoceptor subclassification. Rev Physiol Biochem Pharmacol 88: 199-236
27. Sundaresan PR, Madan MK, Kelvie SL, Weintraub M (1985) Platelet alpha-2 adrenoceptors and the menstrual cycle. Clin Pharmacol Ther 37: 337-342
28. Tsai BS, Lefkowitz RJ (1979) Agonist-specific effects of guanine nucleotides on alpha-adrenergic receptors in human platelets. Mol Pharmacol 16: 61-68
29. U'Prichard DC, Snyder SH (1978a) Guanyl nucleotide influences on ^{3}H-ligand binding at α-noradrenergic receptors in calf brain membranes. J Biol Chem 253: 3444-3452
30. U'Prichard DC, Snyder SH (1978b) ^{3}H-Catecholamine binding to α-receptors in rat brain: Enhancement by reserpine. Eur J Pharmacol 51: 145-155
31. van Meel JCA, de Jonge A, Timmermans PBMWM, van Zwieten PA (1981) Selectivity of some alpha adrenoceptor agonists for peripheral alpha-1 and alpha-2 adrenoceptors in the normotensive rat. J Pharmacol Exp Ther 219: 760-767
32. Wellstein A, Palm D (1984) Theory of ligand-receptor interactions - Evidence for more than one site. In: Erdmann E (ed) Cardiac glycoside receptors and positive inotropy. Steinkopff, Darmstadt, pp 9-15
33. Wiemer G, Wellstein A, Palm D, von Hattingberg HM, Brockmeier D (1982) Properties of agonist binding at the β-adrenoceptor of the rat reticulocyte. Naunyn-Schmiedebergs Arch Pharmacol 321: 11-19
34. Wikberg JES (1979) The pharmacological classification of adrenergic α_1 and α_2 receptors and their mechanism of action. Acta Physiol Scand [Suppl] 468: 5-99
35. Yamamura HI, Enna SJ, Kuhar MJ (1978) Neurotransmitter receptor binding. Raven, New York
36. Yokoyama M, Kusui A, Sakamoto S, Fukuzaki H (1984) Age-associated increments in human platelet α-adrenoceptor capacity - Possible mechanism for platelet hyperactivity to epinephrine in aging man. Thromb Res 34: 287-295

Discussion

Brodde: You said that the K_I value or 50% of the inhibition of sodium in the high-affinity state is at 90 mol. Does that mean that at 135 mmol/liter in plasma the alpha$_2$ receptors on the platelets are present only in the low-affinity state?

Schloos: The problem with sodium is certainly that this high-affinity binding state is physiologically very short-lived. The system must be imagined as a sort of flip-flop circuit which the agonist induces. But then - and this we conclude from the binding experiments - when GTP binds to the regulatory subunit the receptor changes immediately to the low-affinity state. The agonist can again detach, which makes good sense physiologically when you consider that the signal transmission is frequency-coded and very rapid couplings are again required for this reason. This means that we have in principle an arbitrary system, in which by removing GTP we maintain a high-affinity binding state which does not exist physiologically in this situation. For this reason it is extremely difficult to say what the ultimate effect of sodium is. Is it analogous to the GTP effect? After all, GTP also switches the high-affinity to the low-affinity binding state. The GTP-dependent stimulation of adenylate cyclase is certainly controversial. We need it for the effector system, but for binding it is relatively unfavorable.

Regulation of the β-Adrenergic Receptor-Adenylate Cyclase System in Cardiac Membranes*

W. KRAWIETZ

Medizinische Klinik I, Zentralklinikum Augsburg, Lehrkrankenhaus der Ludwig-Maximilians-Universität München, 8900 Augsburg, FRG

Definition of Hormone or Drug Receptors

The idea that drugs react with receptors was initiated by Langley [47] and Paul Ehrlich [27]. In small concentrations, some drugs induce a biological effect, whereas other drugs with different structures cause a comparable effect only in much higher concentrations. Paul Ehrlich [28] introduced the hypothesis that drugs that are effective in small concentrations are bound to a specific membrane protein (receptor). He pronounced the well-known sentence: corpora non agent nisi fixata.

For the effectiveness of such drugs, a molecular structure complementary to its primary binding site (receptor) was postulated. Therefore, these drugs were called specific, referring to their structure [1, 2, 41]. Identical structure characteristics of different drugs thus explain their identical biological effects. Small changes in their chemical structure may influence their pharmacological effect, even leading to an antagonistic effect. The introduction of radiolabelled drugs enabled direct biochemical proof of specific membrane proteins [5, 6, 13, 14, 21, 34, 35, 50, 74].

Therefore, a drug or hormone receptor is defined today as a macromolecule which binds certain drugs and hormones with high affinity and high selectivity. The hormone-receptor or drug-receptor complex formed induces further steps of the drug or hormone effect after a possible change of the receptor conformation [8]. Receptors have accordingly been found in the cytoplasm of cells, e.g., for steroid hormones [8] and in cell membranes [23] e.g., for insulin [20, 31], histamin [68, 72], TSH [62], STH [51], acetylcholin [38], ACTH [30, 50], glucagon [7, 53], catecholamines [43, 48, 60], cardiac glycosides [4, 29], and opiates [69, 85].

A biological receptor is defined not only by a characteristic complementary structure, but also by a biological effect induced by the hormone or drug binding [37]. The following biochemical reactions after the drug or hormone were bound to their receptors were examined for only some hormones or drugs. Parallel measurements of receptor binding and enzyme activity revealed that binding of cardiac glycosides to their specific binding sites in cardiac tissue resulted in a concentration-dependent inhibition of the cardiac glycoside receptor-bound enzyme $(Na^+ + K^+)$ATPase. The concentration-dependent inhibition of the $(Na^+ + K^+)$ ATPase succeeded in an increase of the maximal force of contraction to the papillary muscle [15].

* This work was supported by grant Kra 679/3-1 of the *Deutsche Forschungsgemeinschaft*.

New Aspects in Hypertension: Adrenoceptors
M. Middeke and H. Holzgreve (Eds.)
Springer-Verlag Berlin Heidelberg New York 1986

A similar mechanism of signal transfer might exist for other receptor-enzyme systems [3]. A variety of biochemical approaches have been adopted to increase our understanding of how the β-adrenergic receptor interacts with the other components of the hormone-responsive adenylate cyclase system. In addition to the receptor (R), these other components include the catalytic moiety of the enzyme (C) and the regulatory protein (N). Considerable progress has been made in the characterization of the components and their regulation in different β-adrenergic receptor-adenylate cyclase systems: turkey erythrocytes [12, 80], frog erythrocytes [58], and lymphoma cells S49 [83]. Nevertheless, the sequence of molecular events has been only partially elucidated in myocardial membranes. The approach used for the elaboration of this β-receptor-adenylate cyclase system has been performed by showing the existence of different biochemical entities and their mutual interactions.

Experimental Characterization of the Three Components of the β-Adrenergic Coupled Adenylate Cyclase in Cardiac Membranes

Materials and Methods

Materials. Radiolabelled nucleotides were obtained from ICN Chemicals and Radioisotope Division (Irvine, Calif). Cholera toxin was from Schwarz/Mann (Orangeburg, NY). Other chemicals were the best grade commercially available.

Crude Cardiac Membrane Preparation. Rats were decapitated, and their hearts quickly removed and freed from connective tissue, atria, and valves. The ventricles were dissected and washed free from blood. The washed ventricular tissue was minced, and a crude membrane fraction was prepared [26]. For the adenylate cyclase assay the membranes were quickly frozen at −70 °C.

Preparation of Red Cell Membranes. Membranes were prepared by hypotonic lysis of red cells in 5 m*M* sodium phosphate buffer, pH 8.0 [40]. The membrane preparation was washed extensively in the same buffer and stored in aliquots equivalent to 2.0 mg protein in liquid nitrogen.

Cholera Toxin Treatment of Crude Cardiac and Erythrocyte Membranes. This was performed according to Kaslow et al. [39]. Membranes (1.5–4.0 mg per ml) were incubated with 12 m*M* potassium phosphate buffer, pH 7.5, 20 m*M* thymidine, 5 m*M* ADP-ribose, 20 m*M* arginine-HCl, 100 units/ml Trasylol, 0.1 m*M* GTP, 100 µg/ml cholera toxin (activated with 20 m*M* DTT at 30 °C for 10 min) and NAD (for labelling experiments (^{32}P)NAD$^+$ was 10 µ*M* (5–30 Ci/nmol), for other experiments NAD$^+$ was 1 m*M*).

After the addition of membranes, the mixture was incubated for 20 min at 30 °C. The reaction was terminated by addition of 10 vol ice-cold potassium phosphate buffer 15 m*M*, pH 7.5, and the cells were washed three times by centrifugation. The final pellet was resuspended in 10 m*M* Tris-HCl, pH 7.5, containing 1.0 m*M* $MgCl_2$ and assayed as indicated at 30 °C for 20 min.

Enzyme Assay. Adenylate cyclase activity was determined as previously described [43] using 0.125 m*M* ATP as substrate. Results are expressed as cAMP generated (pmol/mg protein per min) or as indicated and are the mean of triplicate determinations.

Binding Assay. Freshly prepared membrane suspensions (0.4–0.8 mg protein) were incubated at 37 °C in 7.5 m*M* Tris-HCl, pH 7.4, 2.5 m*M* $MgCl_2$ with (^{3}H)(−)dihydroalprenolol, and unlabelled (−)alprenolol (final volume 1 ml). At the given time (usually 15 min) membrane-bound and free ligands were separated by rapid filtration followed by two washes (10 ml each) on Whatman fiberglass filters (GF/C). Radioactivity on filters was determined by liquid scintillation counting (Insta Fluor, Fa. Zinsser, Frankfurt, FRG).

Unspecific binding was determined in the presence of unlabelled (−) and (+)alprenolol, 10^{-5} *M*. It amounted to about 50% of maximal binding, as described by Krawietz and Erdmann [42].

SDS-Polyacrylamide Gel Electrophoresis. With membranes (2–4 mg/ml) discontinuous SDS-polyacrylamide gel electrophoresis was performed by the method of Laemmli [46] as described by O'Farrell et al. [67], using 10% acrylamide gels, and electrophoresed at 400 V for 7 h. After staining, destaining, and drying, X-ray film was exposed to the gels. To identify the 42 K band, the cholera toxin specific target for ADP ribosylation, a short exposure was performed [39] with the disadvantage of a faint autoradiogram.

Protein. Protein was measured according to the method of Lowry et al. [59].

Characterization of a Specific Cardiac β-Adrenergic Receptor

^{3}H-DHA and increasing concentrations of unlabelled (−) and (+)alprenolol were incubated together with cardiac membranes of guinea pigs, and the inhibition of labelled alprenolol binding to its binding sites was measured (Fig. 1a). The effect of β-adrenergic antagonists on adenylate cyclase activity was measured by the concentrations of cAMP generated in the same membrane preparation (not shown). Concentration-response curves demonstrated a 100-fold greater potency of the (−) isomers as compared with the (+) isomers in inhibiting the binding of ^{3}H-DHA or in inhibiting the activated adenylate cyclase [43]. These experiments demonstrated further that the plots of the action of the (−) and (+) isomers of the β-adrenergic antagonists intersect at a concentration of 10^{-5} *M;* greater concentrations of (−) and (+) isomers no longer lead to stereospecific inhibition of binding.

Cardiac membranes were heated at 37 °C over 23 h (Fig. 1b) in order to distinguish and acquire further information on two apparent types of binding sites (one type of binding site where there is stereospecific inhibition of binding - obvious in the presence of concentrations $< 10^{-5}$ *M* - and one type of binding site where there is inhibition of binding of ^{3}H-DHA by alprenolol, but no stereospecificity - obvious with concentrations $> 10^{-5}$ *M*). At defined intervals these pretreated membranes were incubated with ^{3}H-DHA and in additional, parallel series with 10^{-5} *M*

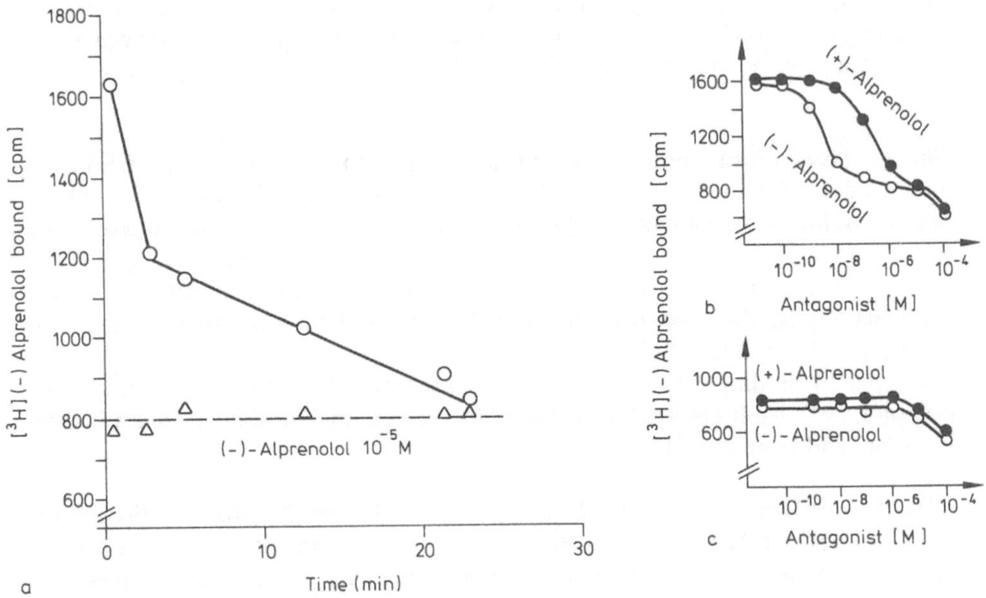

Fig. 1. **a** ^{3}H-DHA binding to cardiac membranes during prolonged incubation at 37 °C. The cardiac membranes were incubated at distinct intervals (O——O) with ^{3}H-DHA (1.6×10^{-12} mol/ml) and in parallel series with additional 10^{-5} *M* (−)alprenolol (Δ——Δ). The ^{3}H-DHA binding capacity decreased steadily, reaching that of "unspecific binding" after 23 h of incubation. **b** Concentration-dependent incubation of ^{3}H-DHA binding to crude cardiac cell membranes by (−) and (+)alprenolol. The incubation medium contained freshly prepared membranes, ^{3}H-DHA, and increasing concentrations of unlabelled (−) and (+)alprenolol. Concentration-response curves demonstrate a 100-fold greater potency of the (−) isomer as compared with the (+) isomer. **c** Inhibition of ^{3}H-DHA binding to cardiac cell membranes by (−) and (+)alprenolol. The cardiac cell membranes were heated for 23 h at 37 °C before incubation with ^{3}H-DHA and increasing concentrations of (−) and (+)alprenolol. At concentrations of 10^{-9}–10^{-5} *M* (−) or (+)alprenolol, there was no stereospecific inhibition of binding at all, at concentrations greater than 10^{-5} *M*, a nonstereospecific effect resulted

(−)alprenolol. Under these conditions, the maximal binding of ^{3}H-DHA diminished distinctly, but the binding capacity after addition of 10^{-5} *M* (−)alprenolol remained the same throughout the 23 h. Binding experiments with the (+) and (−) isomers of alprenolol with freshly prepared cardiac membranes are demonstrated in Fig. 1b. The same experiments performed with membranes heated at 37 °C for 23 h (Fig. 1c) did not show any alteration of binding in the presence of increasing concentrations up to 10^{-5} *M*. Concentrations of unlabelled β-blocking drugs greater than 10^{-5} *M* are able to inhibit binding of ^{3}H-DHA but without any stereospecific effect. About 50% of the total bound ^{3}H-DHA is inhibited from binding in such a manner. This amount is therefore termed "unspecific binding."

Heating of cardiac cell membranes might destroy the membrane proteins (= receptors) or change the affinity of specific binding sites, or both. Figure 2 demonstrates the result of equilibrium binding of ^{3}H-DHA and increasing concentrations of unlabelled alprenolol on freshly prepared cardiac membranes. The values plotted according to Scatchard [76] show a linear plot after subtraction of the amount of

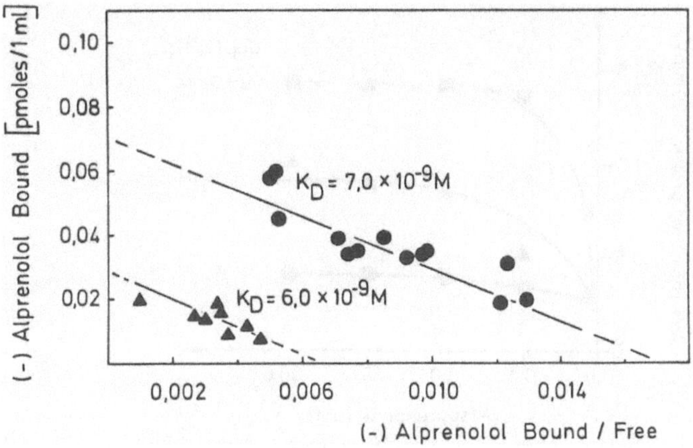

Fig. 2. Loss of specific ^{3}H-DHA binding sites after 8-h incubation of membranes at 37 °C for 8 h. Freshly prepared membranes were incubated for 15 min at 37 °C with ^{3}H-DHA (1.6×10^{-12} mol/ml) and increasing concentrations of (−)alprenolol. The result is plotted according to Scatchard. The same experiments were performed with cardiac cell membranes heated at 37 °C for 8 h and the data plotted in the same way. There was no change of receptor affinity for alprenolol, but a loss of binding sites

labelled alprenolol bound in the presence of 10^{-5} *M* (−)alprenolol. The dissociation constant (K_D) calculated from the slope of the plot is about 7×10^{-9} *M*. The intercept with the ordinate gives the maximal number of receptor sites (0.07 pmol/ml ≙ 0.15 pmol DHA/mg protein). The same experiment was performed after heating the membranes for 8 h. After plotting the results in the same way, a parallel slope indicates an identical dissociation constant ($K_D = 7 \times 10^{-9}$ *M*). The intercept of this slope, however, indicates a distinctly smaller number of receptor sites (0.06 pmol DHA/mg protein).

Essential for the evaluation of experimental binding data is a definition of "specific" and "unspecific" binding. Some criteria have been established to identify specific β-receptors in cell membrane preparations: binding has to be rapid, reversible, saturable, and stereospecific, and it has to exhibit high affinity for β-adrenergic agents [22, 36, 43]. In this respect, ^{3}H-DHA binding to cardiac cell membranes might be termed specific, as it is very rapid (completed within less than 4 min), reversible, and stereospecific. However, unspecific binding to these membranes may also be reversible, as shown in Fig. 1, where ^{3}H-DHA binding to heat-denatured membranes could be displaced easily by unlabelled alprenolol in concentrations above 10^{-5} *M*.

Thus, the results indicate that the loss of the stereospecificity in heat-denatured membranes and in native membranes correlates with specific binding of ^{3}H-DHA to cardiac membranes. It is quantitatively identical, with an unchanged amount of binding in heat-treated membranes. It is concluded that with the criteria for specific binding mentioned, stereospecificity is confirmed to be valid for specific ^{3}H-DHA binding to the β-adrenergic receptor.

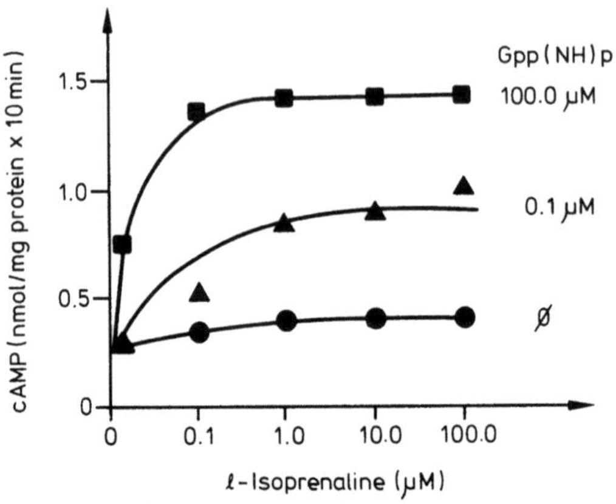

Fig. 3. Interaction of GppNHp and l-isoprenaline on the adenylate cyclase activity in cardiac membranes of guinea pigs. Cardiac membranes (80–160 μg/60 μl protein) were incubated with GppNHp and l-isoprenaline for 10 min at 0 °C, followed by incubation with a mixture mentioned in *Methods* for 10 min at 37 °C. The reaction was stopped with ATP and sodium dodecylsulfate. GppNHp stimulated the adenylate cyclase activity maximally in the presence of l-isoprenaline (1 μ*M*)

Characterization of Adenylate Cyclase Activity in Cardiac Membranes

A biological receptor is one that induces a biological effect after a drug or hormone has been bound. The enzyme linked to the β-adrenergic receptor is adenylate cyclase which transfers ATP into cAMP.

Incubation of native crude cardiac membranes with increasing concentration of l-isoprenaline (up to 50 μ*M*) shows a small stimulatory effect on adenylate cyclase activity (basal 250 pmol cAMP/mg protein × 10 min) up to 450 pmol cAMP/mg protein × 10 min (Fig. 3). Guanine nucleotides (GppNHp 10^{-4} *M*) added to the incubation medium stimulate the basal adenylate cyclase activity sevenfold, which indicates an amplification of the catecholamine effect by guanine nucleotides.

Solubilization of cardiac membranes reveals a stimulatory effect of guanine nucleotides bypassing the β-adrenergic receptor. Additional incubation with catecholamines shows no specific effect on the enzyme activity, indicating the absence of the β-adrenergic receptor. Nevertheless, the basal activity is increased tremendously by GppNHp (10^{-4} *M*) and fluoride (10^{-2} *M*) (Fig. 4). Even though fluoride also activates the enzyme in the absence of catecholamines, it remains to be seen whether fluoride stimulates the enzyme activity by the same binding site as guanine nucleotides.

Cardiac membranes were therefore incubated with and without GMP (10^{-4} *M*) and l-isoprenaline (10^{-4} *M*) (Table 1). Basal activity remained equal. The addition of GppNHp (10^{-4} *M*) showed a near fourfold stimulation compared with a twofold effect in control membranes. No significant difference was measurable by GppNHp (10^{-4} *M*) stimulation together with l-isoprenaline (10^{-4} *M*). In the presence of GMP (10^{-4} *M*) fluoride (10^{-2} *M*) stimulated the adenylate cyclase activity, but its effect was decreased in the presence of GTP (10^{-4} *M*).

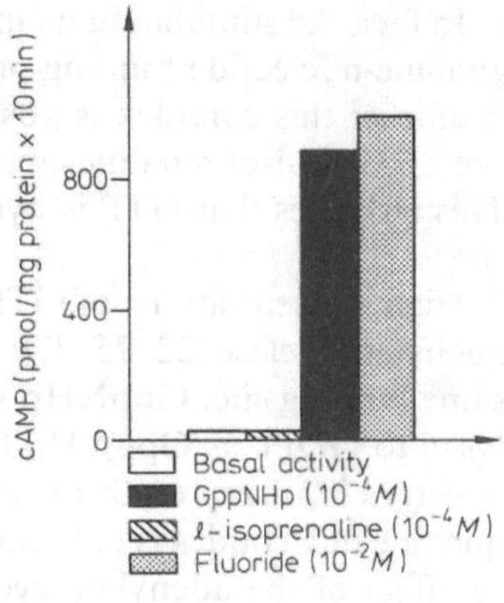

Fig. 4. Effect of l-isoprenaline, GppNHp, and fluoride on the adenylate cyclase activity in solubilized cardiac membranes. Cardiac membranes were solubilized in 1% Lubrol PX according to Levey [52]. Adenylate cyclase assay was performed as mentioned in *Methods*. GppNHp and fluoride demonstrated a significant stimulation of the basal adenylate cyclase activity (26- versus 28-fold) in solubilized cardiac membranes, whereas l-isoprenaline induced no stimulatory effect

Our results show that catecholamines stimulate the basal cardiac adenylate cyclase activity (1.8-fold). In the presence of guanine nucleotides, basal activity is increased 5-6-fold, indicating an exponential rather than an additional effect of guanine nucleotides to the stimulatory effect of catecholamines.

In another β-adrenergic receptor-adenylate cyclase system, viz. turkey erythrocytes, no activating by GppNHp alone could be shown [25, 73, 77, 79]. Only in the presence of catecholamines was enzyme activity increased 21-fold over basal. Catecholamines alone showed no effect on adenylate cyclase activity in turkey erythrocytes. On the basis of these experimental findings, it was suggested that catecholamines induce the binding of guanine nucleotides to their specific binding sites, the so-called guanine-nucleotide-binding protein (regulatory unit of the adenylate cyclase) [80].

Table 1. Effect of preincubation with GMP 10^{-4} *M* and l-isoprenaline 10^{-4} *M* on subsequent stimulation of adenylate cyclase activity in cardiac membranes[a]

Cardiac membranes	Basal activity	GppNHp 10^{-4} *M*	GppNHp 10^{-4} *M* l-isoprenaline 10^{4} *M*	F^- 10^{-2} *M*	F^- 10^{-2} *M* GTP 10^{-4} *M*
Control	256	473	1280	814	706
Preincubation with GMP 10^{-4} *M* and l-isoprenaline 10^{-4} *M*	240	1088	1440	940	620

[a] Preincubation resulted in a higher stimulatory effect for GppNHp alone than was observed in control membranes. Results are given in picomoles per milligram of protein per 10 min

In fact, the stimulating guanine nucleotide (^{3}H-GTP) is bound specifically to the guanine-nucleotide-binding protein only in the presence of catecholamines. Dissociation of this complex is possible only in the presence of catecholamines. In the presence of l-isoprenaline, about 80% of the released guanine nucleotides are GDP. This indicates that GTP is hydrolysed to GDP after binding to a specific binding site.

High concentrations of GTP decrease the stimulatory effect of GppNHp on the adenylate cyclase [22, 75, 77]. Both guanine nucleotides are therefore bound to the same binding site. GppNHp shows a greater stimulatory effect than GTP (hydrolysed to GDP), as GppNHp forms a persistent, activated complex of the enzyme. Whereas in turkey erythrocyte membranes stimulation of the adenylate cyclase by guanine nucleotides is only possible in the presence of catecholamines, a stimulatory effect of the adenylate cyclase in cardiac membranes is possible by catecholamines alone. This difference is due to a different membrane structure and therefore different access for the guanine nucleotides to their binding sites.

Table 1 clearly demonstrates that if incubated together, guanine nucleotides and fluoride interact, by stimulating adenylate cyclase. Experiments in turkey erythrocytes show an inhibition of the fluoride stimulatory effect in the presence of GMP, whereas in the presence of GTP stimulation was the same as without GTP. This indicates that in turkey erythrocytes, the stimulatory effect of fluoride depends on the guanine nucleotide bound to the guanine-nucleotide-binding protein.

From the interaction of guanine nucleotides and fluoride, it can be concluded that both guanine nucleotides and fluoride influence the adenylate cyclase activity through the same regulatory unit. The different effect of GMP or GTP on the fluoride stimulation of the adenylate cyclase in turkey erythrocytes and cardiac membranes suggests a different composition of the regulatory protein [84].

Cardiac Adenylate Cyclase Consists of a Regulatory Unit

So far, catecholamines bound to specific binding sites in cardiac membranes stimulate the activity of the adenylate cyclase. It has also been shown that guanine nucleotides and fluoride stimulate the enzyme without binding to the β-receptor, but binding to a specific protein, the guanine-nucleotide-binding protein (= regulatory unit, [71]). This binding protein contains an enzyme (GTPase) that dephosphorylates GTP to GDP. GDP is no longer able to stimulate the adenylate cyclase activity. The enzyme activity of the specific GTPase can be measured by the increased phosphate concentration:

$$\mathrm{GTP} \xrightarrow[\mathrm{GTPase}]{} \mathrm{GDP} + \mathrm{P_i}$$

This effect of GTPase is inhibited by cholera toxin [18].

Adenylate Cyclase Activity Measured in the Presence of Cholera Toxin and NAD

The GTPase activity is inhibited by cholera toxin in the presence of nicotinamide adenine dinucleotide (NAD) in different membranes [61, 65, 71, 78].

ADP ribose is formed by cholera-toxin-induced hydrolyses of NAD. After binding of ADP ribose to the GTPase, GTP is no longer dephosphorylated to GDP:

$$\text{NAD} + \text{Ⓝ} \xrightarrow[\text{Cholera toxin}]{} \text{ADP ribose} - \text{Ⓝ} + \text{Nicotinamide} + \text{H}^+$$

where Ⓝ is the regulatory unit with GTPase (guanin-nucleotide-binding protein). In cardiac membranes (Fig. 5) basal activity was nearly equal (14 pmol cAMP/mg protein × min) in cholera-toxin-treated membranes and control membranes (18.5 pmol cAMP/mg protein × min). GTP 10^{-4} *M* showed no stimulatory effect on basal activity, whereas in cholera-toxin-treated membranes an activity of 21.5 pmol cAMP/mg protein × min was measured.

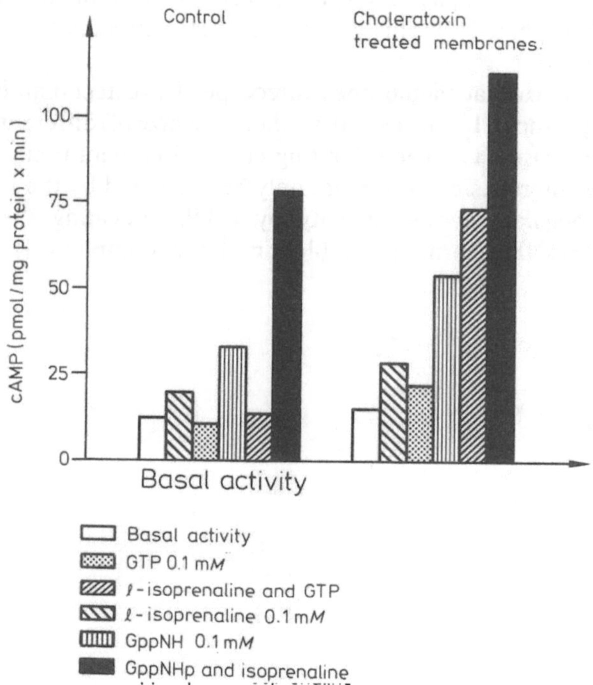

Fig. 5. Effect of l-isoprenaline, GTP, and GppNHp on the adenylate cyclase activity in cholera-toxin-treated cardiac membranes. Cardiac membranes (1.5–4.0 mg protein/ml) were incubated with 12 m*M* potassium phosphate buffer, pH 7.5, 20 m*M* thymidine, 5 m*M* ADP ribose, 20 m*M* arginine-HCl, 100 units/ml aprotinin, 0.1 m*M* GTP, 100 µg/ml cholera toxin (activated with 20 m*M* DTT at 30 °C for 10 min) and NAD^+ was 1 m*M*. Control membranes were treated identically without cholera toxin. The reaction was stopped by an excess of potassium phosphate buffer; adenylate cyclase assay followed. l-isoprenaline and GTP showed no stimulatory effect on the adenylate cyclase activity in control membranes, whereas in cholera-toxin-treated membranes the effect was comparable to the stimulation by l-isoprenaline and GppNHp in control membranes

GppNHp stimulated the adenylate cyclase activity up to 34 pmol cAMP/mg protein × min in control membranes and up to 53 pmol cAMP/mg protein × min in cholera-toxin-treated membranes. Whereas l-isoprenaline 10^{-4} *M* and GTP 10^{-4} *M* together had no stimulatory effect in control membranes, in cholera-toxin-treated membranes adenylate cyclase activity rose to 72 pmol cAMP/mg protein × min, indicating the same activity as shown in control membranes by l-isoprenaline 10^{-4} *M* and GppNHp 10^{-4} *M* (Fig. 5). In cholera-toxin-treated membranes, adenylate cyclase activity was increased up to 112 pmol cAMP/mg protein × min by l-isoprenaline and GppNHp together. The effect of fluoride on adenylate cyclase activity in cardiac membranes is shown in Fig. 6. In the presence of l-isoprenaline 10^{-4} *M* and GTP 10^{-4} *M*, adenylate cyclase activity in cholera-toxin-treated membranes was 75 pmol cAMP/mg protein × min, showing no effect in control membranes, whereas fluoride significantly stimulated adenylate cyclase activity in control membranes (87 pmol cAMP/mg protein × min) and was inhibited in cholera-toxin-pretreated cardiac membranes (53 pmol cAMP/mg protein × min).

Cholera toxin catalyses the hydrolysis of NAD and transfers the ADP ribose to the guanine nucleotide-binding protein [63, 64]. The inhibiting effect of cholera toxin to the GTPase activity is directly measurable by the reduction in the amount of phosphate [18]. This directly measured effect is correlated to adenylate cyclase activity.

In cardiac membranes, direct specific (catecholamine-stimulated) GTPase activity cannot be measured in the presence of different high amounts of unspecific NTPases [17]. The inhibiting effect of cholera toxin to GTPase activity in cardiac membranes can therefore only be measured by the increased stimulatory effect on adenylate cyclase activity by GTP, indicating the same stimulatory effect as GppNHp (forming a stable stimulatory complex). The reduced fluoride stimulatory

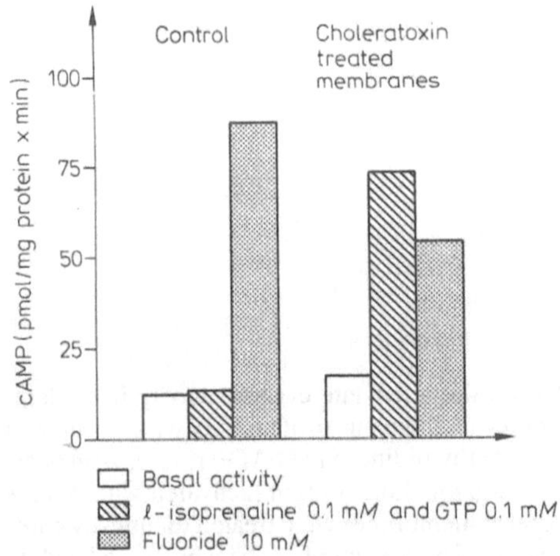

Fig. 6. Effect of fluoride on adenylate cyclase activity in cholera-toxin-treated cardiac membranes (Methods see Fig. 5). Fluoride stimulation in cholera-toxin-treated cardiac membranes was decreased

effect of cardiac adenylate cyclase activity (Fig. 6) in the presence of cholera toxin is a characteristic phenomenon for the cholera toxin effect in response to GTPase activity in different membranes, even though the basic mechanism therefore is unexplained [17, 80]. The inhibition of the fluoride effect remains unexplained by the cholera-toxin-induced inhibition of the GTPase. Even though the fluoride-induced effect on the adenylate cyclase activity is comparable in cardiac and turkey erythrocyte membranes, the effect of l-isoprenaline and GppNHp together is different. In turkey erythrocyte membranes, the same activity is reached in control and in cholera-toxin-treated membranes [80], whereas in cardiac membranes a different activity is obtained (72 pmol cAMP/mg protein × min in control membranes; 112 pmol cAMP/mg protein × min in cholera toxin-treated membranes; Fig. 5).

A possible explanation for this result might be a different access to the guanine-nucleotide-binding protein for GppNHp in cardiac and in turkey erythrocyte membranes. This hypothesis is supported by the fact that a change of guanine nucleotides at the guanine-nucleotide-binding protein in turkey erythrocyte membranes is only possible in the presence of catecholamines or after incubation with GMP, whereas in cardiac membranes the catecholamines only accelerate, instead of initiating, the exchange.

Cholera toxin therefore influences only the guanine-nucleotide-binding proteins that are in connection with a β-adrenergic receptor. Preincubation of cardiac membranes is performed in the presence of l-isoprenaline and GTP, and it might be that in the final incubation the high concentration of GppNHp causes an additional stimulatory effect on adenylate cyclase activity, even though these guanine-nucleotide-binding proteins are not linked to a β-receptor. Nevertheless, we can conclude that the guanine-nucleotide-binding protein in cardiac membranes is comparable to the functional unit in turkey erythrocytes.

Labelling of Cardiac Membranes by ^{32}P-NAD in the Presence of Cholera Toxin

In pigeon erythrocyte membranes, labelling of a protein in the presence of ^{32}P-NAD and cholera toxin was possible using SDS gelelectrophoresis in an autoradiogram [32, 33]. The same experimental procedure enabled the characterization of a guanine-nucleotide-binding protein in human erythrocytes [39, 40] and in turkey erythrocyte membranes [78].

We were able to show a similar labelled protein with a molecular weight of 42 000 in cardiac membranes [44]. Cardiac membranes were incubated as described with cholera toxin and labelled NAD, to succeed in ADP ribosylation of the regulatory unit (= guanine-nucleotide-binding protein).

The SDS gelelectrophoresis showed no difference of the protein bands with and without cholera-toxin-catalysed ADP ribosylation in erythrocyte membranes of man and rats or in cardiac membranes. The autoradiogram showed (Fig. 7) very distinct protein bands in different membranes. In human and rat erythrocyte membranes, a band with a molecular weight of 42 000 was shown (Fig. 7), whereas in cardiac tissue of rats and guinea-pigs, two specific ADP-ribosylated bands with a molecular weight of 42 000 and 46 000 were seen (Fig. 7).

In pigeon and human erythrocyte membranes, a specific cholera-toxin-catalysed ADP ribosylation of a protein with a molecular weight of 42 000 was shown. The

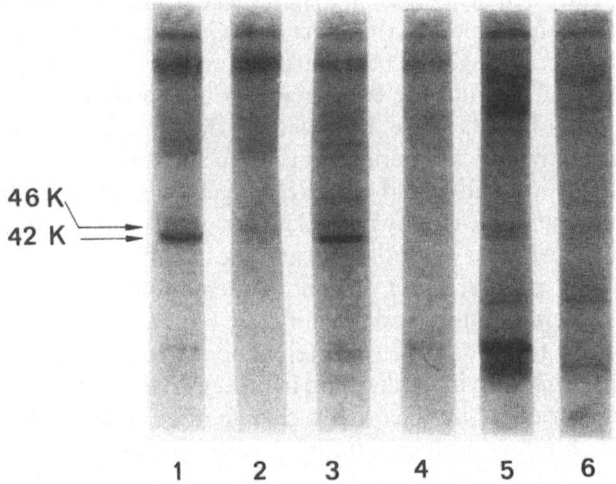

Fig. 7. Polyacrylamide gel analysis (autoradiogram) of radioactive products resulting from cholera-toxin-catalysed reaction of human erythrocyte membrane *(1, 2)*, rat erythrocyte membranes *(3, 4)*, and rat crude cardiac membranes *(5, 6)* with [^{32}P]NAD$^+$. Freshly prepared membranes were pelleted, incubated, washed, and electrophoresed as described under *Materials and Methods*

fact that it is identical with the guanine-nucleotide-binding protein can be explained as follows:

Cholera toxin inhibits the GTPase activity, and GTP stimulates the adenylate cyclase, comparable to GppNHp stimulation [17]. After pigeon erythrocyte membranes were incubated with ^{32}P-NAD and cholera toxin, the specific labelled membrane protein (mol.wt. 42000) could be eluted [16, 71]. If this eluate (containing the specific labelled ADP-ribosylated guanine-nucleotide-binding protein) is transferred in untreated pigeon erythrocyte membranes, GTP is able to stimulate the adenylate cyclase activity as if GTPase activity were inhibited [16]. Therefore, it can be concluded that the guanine nucleotide-binding protein and the specific ADP-ribosylated membrane protein (mol.wt. 42000) are identical in the presence of cholera toxin.

In cardiac membranes of rats and guinea-pigs two different bands are shown, referring to proteins with the molecular weights 42000 and 46000. Membranes of S49 lymphoma cells and hepatoma cells of rats (HTC-4) also show an additional cholera-toxin-specific labelled band (mol.wt. 52000–53000) [39], as do human fibroblasts (mol.wt. 47000) [86]. In the purified regulatory unit of liver cell membranes, obtaining three proteins with molecular weights 52000, 45000 and 35000, only the 52K and 45K bands referred to cholera toxin substrate.

In recent years, it has become clear that the stimulatory regulatory unit consists of three distinct subunits, designated alpha, beta, and gamma [81]. GTP binds to the alpha subunit, and when binding occurs, the alpha subunit dissociates from the beta and gamma subunits and activates the catalytic unit.

Interactions of the Three Units of the β-Receptor-Coupled Adenylate Cyclase System

The guanine-nucleotide-binding protein assumes a key function for the hormonal effect on the intracellular cAMP concentrations by influencing the binding affinity of the β-adrenergic receptor and the catalytic activity.

Incubation of cardiac membranes with l-isoprenaline together with and without the guanine nucleotide GppNHp 10^{-4} *M* is shown (Fig. 8). The competition curve for β-adrenergic agonists (in contrast to antagonist competition curve) is shallow, complex, and best fitted by a model for two classes of binding sites that have respectively high- and low-affinity sites for the agonist [24]. In the presence of the guanine nucleotide GppNHp, the curve is shifted to the right and steepened. Guanine nucleotide appear to convert all of the high-affinity-state receptors into low-affinity-state receptors.

In order to explain the small stimulatory effect of the guanine nucleotides on adenylate cyclase activity, the time-dependent stimulation by guanine nucleotides alone and in the presence of catecholamines was determined (Fig. 9). A stimulatory effect on basal adenylate cyclase activity was measurable after 4 min, whereas in the presence of catecholamines the adenylate cyclase activity was doubled after 2 min. This delay caused by guanine nucleotides alone to adenylate cyclase activity is explained by the fact that GDP (a nonstimulating guanine nucleotide) is bound to the guanine-nucleotide-binding protein. GppNHp has to replace GDP from its binding site in a time-dependent process [17, 18, 66, 70]. Catecholamines accelerate this process in cardiac and turkey erythrocyte membranes [19].

β-Blocking agents inhibit the effect of catecholamines, and only the effect of GppNHp should be measurable. Therefore, we looked for the inhibitory effect of β-blocking agents when the adenylate cyclase activity had already been stimulated

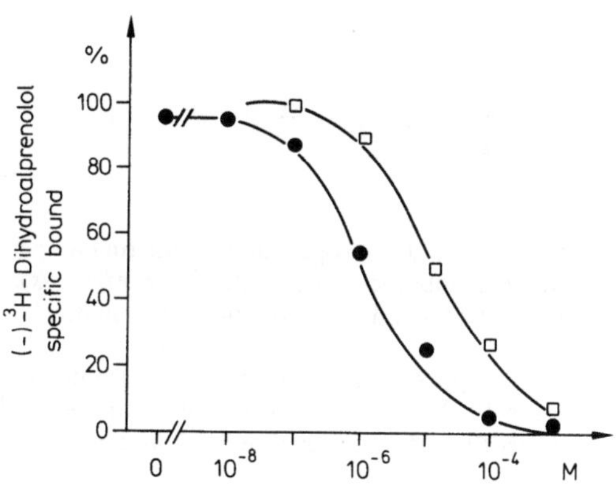

Fig. 8. Concentration-dependent inhibition of ^{3}H-DHA binding to cardiac membranes by increasing concentrations of l-isoprenaline. Cardiac membranes were incubated (see *Methods* for further details) with increasing concentrations of l-isoprenaline as indicated, ^{3}H-DHA, with and without GTP 1 m*M*. Incubation with GTP resulted in a shift of the concentration-inhibition curve to higher concentrations

●——● control; □——□ GTP 1 m*M*

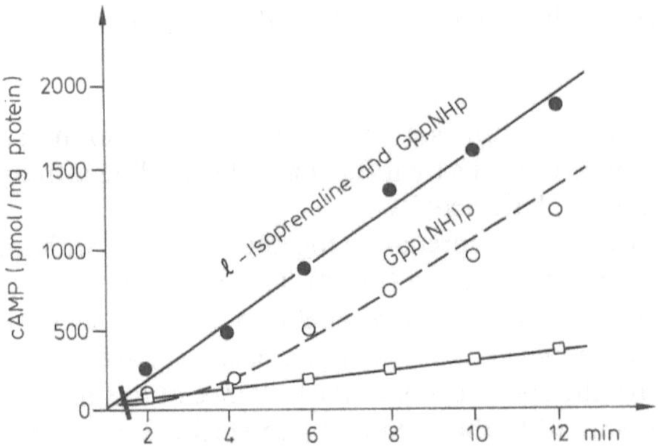

Fig. 9. Time-dependent effect of catecholamines on the guanine nucleotide stimulation of adenylate cyclase activity (for further details see *Methods*). In the presence of l-isoprenaline and GppNHp, a steady increase of adenylate cyclase activity was shown, whereas in the presence of GppNHp alone, adenylate cyclase activity increased after a lagphase

●——●, l-isoprenaline 10^{-4} *M* and GppNHp 10^{-4} *M*; ○——○, GppNHp 10^{-4} *M*; □——□, basal activity

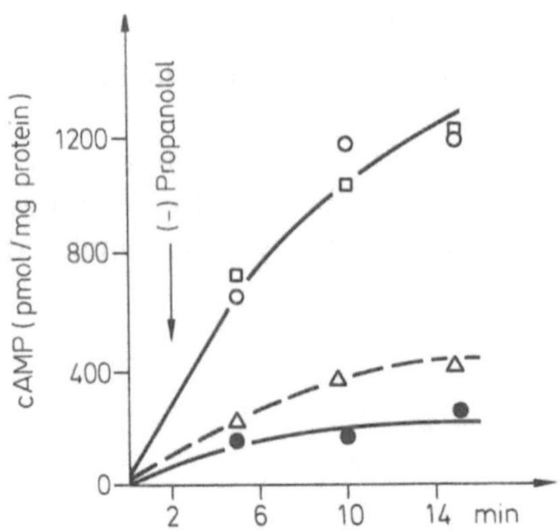

Fig. 10. Effect of (−)propranolol on the time-dependent stimulation on adenylate cyclase activity in cardiac membranes (further details in *Methods*). Addition of (−)propranolol after starting the incubation had no influence on the l-isoprenaline/GppNHp-stimulated adenylate cyclase activity

□——□, GppNHp 10^{-4} *M* and l-isoprenaline 10^{-4} *M*; ○——○, GppNHp 10^{-4} *M* and l-isoprenaline 10^{-4} *M*; addition of (−)propranolol 10^{-4} *M* 2 min after incubation started; △——△, GppNHp 10^{-4} *M*, l-isoprenaline 10^{-4} *M*, and propranolol 10^{-4} *M*; ●——●, basal activity

by l-isoprenaline and GppNHp. Incubation of cardiac membranes with and without β-blocking agents together with GppNHp and l-isoprenaline were measured at different time points (Fig. 10). In the presence of a β-blocking agent, GppNHp shows only a small effect on adenylate cyclase activity, since the catecholamine effect is blocked. GppNHp and l-isoprenaline together stimulate the adenylate cyc-

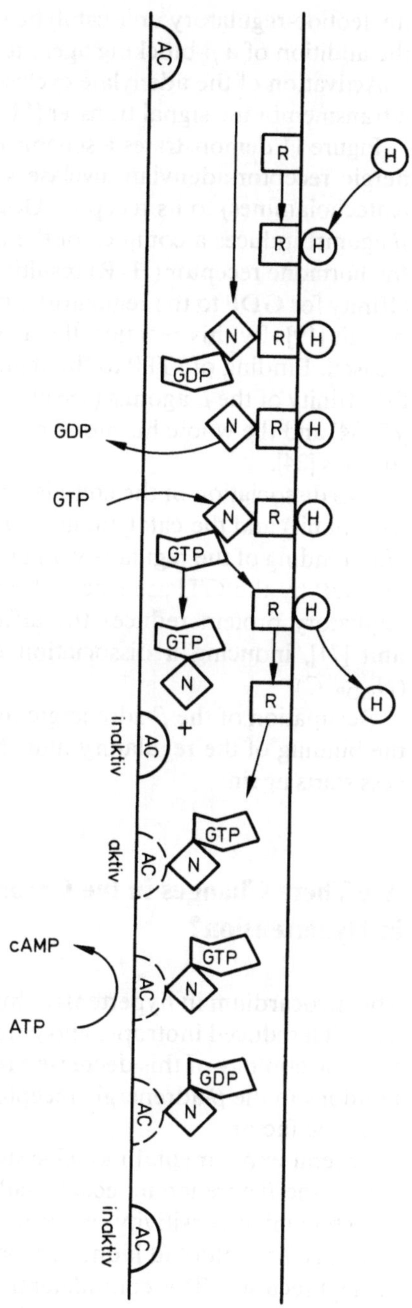

Fig. 11. Transmembranous signal transfer by the β-adrenergic-receptor-adenylate-cyclase system

lase activity 5- to 6-fold over the basal value. The addition of the β-blocking agent 2 min after start of incubation has no influence on the GppNHp/l-isoprenaline stimulated adenylate cyclase activity. This indicates that after a β-receptor-guanine-nucleotide-regulatory-unit complex has formed in the presence of catecholamines, the stimulation of the catalytic unit takes place immediately by forming a guanine nucleotide-regulatory unit-catalytic unit complex. This process is not influenced by the addition of a β-blocking agent to the incubation medium.

Activation of the adenylate cyclase system by a hormone can be characterized as a transmembrane signal transfer [11, 45, 49, 54, 56, 71, 80, 84].

Figure 11 demonstrates a scheme of the interaction of the subunits of the β-adrenergic receptor-adenylate cyclase system induced by the binding of a hormone (catecholamines) to its receptor. Occupation of the β-receptor (R) (see Fig. 11) by a β-agonist induces a complex of the regulatory unit (GDP bound to it – N_{GDP}) with the hormone receptor (H · R) resulting in H · R · N_{GDP} [57]. This complex reduces the affinity for GDP to the regulatory unit (N), and GDP dissociates from the regulatory unit [19]. By this reaction the affinity for GTP to the regulatory unit (N) is increased. Binding of GTP to the regulatory protein (N), on the other hand, reduces the affinity of the β-agonist (see also Fig. 8) and the regulatory unit to the β-receptor [82, 84] and the whole hormone-receptor-regulatory unit complex (H · R · N_{GTP}) dissociates [24].

This dissociation of the complex enables the association of the regulatory protein (α-subunit) and the catalytic unit ($\alpha N_{GTP} \cdot C$) [81]. The increased amount of cAMP after binding of the regulatory unit to the catalytic unit persists until GTP is reduced to GDP by the GTPase (located on the regulatory unit) [18]. GDP bound to the regulatory protein reduces the affinity between regulatory protein and catalytic unit [71], inducing a dissociation of the regulatory unit-catalytic unit complex ($N_{GDP} \cdot C$).

Occupation of the β-adrenergic receptor by a β-adrenergic agonist again induces the binding of the regulatory unit (N_{GDP}) to the β-receptor (H · R · N_{GDP}). The process starts again.

Are There Changes in the Cardiac β-Receptor-Adenylate Cyclase System in Hypertension?

The myocardium in hypertensive humans and in experimental animals is known to exhibit a reduced inotropic and chronotropic response to adrenergic stimulation [9, 87]. The etiology of this decreased responsiveness is probably multifactorial, but alterations in the β-adrenergic receptor-adenylate cyclase system appear to be a contributing factor.

Several experimental model systems have been employed to assess the possible role of the β-adrenergic receptor-adenylate cyclase system in mediating the altered catecholamine sensitivity in various tissues from hypertensive animals. One such model is the Goldblatt kidney preparation, in which rats are subjected to a unilateral nephrectomy. The contralateral renal artery is then stenosed by placing a clip around the artery. Woodcock et al. [88] found that when rats had become hypertensive there was a significant (~50%) fall in the number of myocardial β-adrenergic receptors compared with the number in sham-operated animals. Moreover, the isoprenaline-stimulated adenylate cyclase activity was also decreased, whereas the basal and fluoride-stimulated enzyme activities were unchanged. The alteration in cAMP production may therefore be specific for the β-adrenergic receptor-mediated pathway and does not represent a generalized alteration in the adenylate cyclase itself.

Woodcock's group [89] also demonstrated that when the β-adrenergic receptor concentration was decreased in the heart, there were no changes in β-adrenergic receptor number in either the lung or the kidney of these hypertensive animals. These bindings were interpreted as evidence that there was no generalized β-adrenergic receptor decrease associated with elevated circulating catecholamines in the hypertensive animals, but rather the downregulation of cardiac β-adrenergic receptors might be due to a specific increase in cardiac sympathetic tone with consequent increase in local norepinephrine levels. Using a different model of hypertension in which rats undergo unilateral nephrectomy and then are given high-salt diets and injections of the mineral corticoid deoxycorticosterone, Woodcock et al. [88, 89] found similar decreases in myocardial β-adrenergic receptor number and isoprenaline-stimulated adenylate cyclase activity.

A third model system frequently used to assess the relationship of β-adrenergic receptor and hypertension is that of the spontaneously hypertensive rat (SHR) and its control animal, the Wistar-Kyoto (WKY) rat. However, the results of β-adrenergic receptor-binding studies reported in this model have been contradictory. For example, Bhalla et al. [10] found that from 2 through 36 weeks of age, the number of myocardial β-adrenergic receptors was the same in the two strains of rats, but the number did decrease in parallel fashion with age in both strains. Although there were no interstrain differences in the number of β-adrenergic receptors in this study, there was a significant decrease in both basal and isoprenaline-stimulated myocardial adenylate cyclase activity in the hypertensive animals compared with the activity in controls at all time points assessed. In addition, the ability of l-isoprenaline to compete for specific ^{3}H-DHA-binding sites in heart membranes was decreased by three- to fourfold in SHR compared with WKY rats. This finding suggested to the authors that, at least in this model of hypertension, there may be impaired coupling of the receptors with the N protein. This decreased coupling might be responsible for the decreased sensitivity to catecholamines in these hypertensive animals rather than a simple decrease in receptor number (which was not observed in these studies).

Limas and Limas [55] have also used the SHRs and WKY rats to assess the relationship of hypertension and myocardial β-adrenergic receptors. They found the SHRs had significantly fewer myocardial β-adrenergic receptors than the WKY rats, whereas there was no alteration in the ability of l-isoprenaline to compete for ^{3}H-DHA sites. They also found that the differences in the number of β-adrenergic receptors between the two strains develops before the development of hypertension. The authors concluded that the fall in β-adrenergic receptor number is not a direct result of the hypertension process itself, but rather a part of the underlying process that produces the elevated blood pressure.

The reasons for these disparate results from various investigators are unknown. There does, however, seem to be general agreement that once hypertension develops, the catecholamine sensitivity of the heart is decreased. This decreased sensitivity is associated with a decreased ability of l-isoprenaline to activate adenylate cyclase. The decreased sensitivity may be a consequence of either decreased β-adrenergic receptor number, uncoupling, or both. In addition, it seems reasonable to assume that different model systems may produce different effects on the myocardial β-adrenergic receptor-adenylate cyclase system, so that the results with SHRs may not be the same as with the Goldblatt model.

Of overriding importance is the fact that no one has yet determined whether the downregulation or uncoupling phenomenon observed in these hypertensive animals is simply a consequence of excessive local or circulating catecholamines or whether the receptor alterations are independently mediated by distinct processes linked to the etiology of the hypertension.

Abbreviations:
regulatory unit = regulatory protein = guanine nucleotide - binding protein = G unit; NAD = β-Nicotinamid-adenin-dinucleotid; ^{3}H-DHA = [^{3}H](−)dihydroalprenolol; GppNHp = Guanylyl-5'-imidodiphosphat; GTP = Guanosin-5'-triphosphat; GDP = Guanosin-5'-diphosphat; GMP = Guanosin-5'-monophosphat; ATP = Adenosintriphosphate

References

1. Ahlquist RP (1948) A study of the adrenotropic receptors. Am J Physiol 153: 586-600
2. Ahlquist RP (1976) Adrenergic beta-blocking agents. Proc Drug Res 20: 27-42
3. Ahrén K, Albertsson-Wikland K, Isaksson O, Kostyo JL (1976) Cellular mechanism of the acute stimulatory effect of growth hormone. In: Pecile A, Müller EE (eds) Growth hormone and related peptides. Excerpta Medica, Amsterdam, pp 94-103
4. Akera T (1977) Membrane adenosinetriphosphatase: a digitalis receptor? Science 198: 596-574
5. Alexander RW, Davis JN, Lefkowitz RJ (1975) Direct identification and characterization of β-adrenergic receptors in the rat brain. Nature 258: 437-440
6. Aurbach GD, Fedak SA, Woodard CJ, Palmer JS, Hauser D, Troxler F (1974) β-Adrenergic receptor: stereospecific interaction of iodinated β-blocking agent with high affinity site. Science 186: 1223-1224
7. Bataille D, Freychet P, Rosselin G (1974) Interaction of glucagon, vasoactive intestinal polypeptide and secretin with liver and fat cell membranes: binding to specific sites and stimulation of adenylate cyclase. Endocrinology 95: 713-721
8. Baulieu EE (1975) Commentary. Steroid receptors and hormone receptivity: new approaches in pharmacology and therapeutics. Biochem Pharmacol 24: 1743-1748
9. Bertel O, Bühler FR, Kiowski W, Lütold BE (1980) Decreased β-adrenoceptor responsiveness as related to age, blood pressure, and plasma catecholamines in patients with essential hypertension. Hypertension 2: 130-138
10. Bhalla RC, Sharma RV, Ramanathan S (1980) Ontogenetic development of isoproterenol subsensitivity of myocardial adenylate cyclase and β-adrenergic receptors in spontaneously hypertensive rats. Biochim Biophys Acta 632: 497-506
11. Bilezikian JP, Aurbach GD (1973) β-Adrenergic receptor of the turkey erythrocyte: I. Binding of catecholamine and relationship to adenylate cyclase activity. J Biol Chem 248: 5577-5583
12. Bilezikian JP, Aurbach DD (1974) The effects of nucleotide on the expression of β-adrenergic adenylate cyclase in membranes from turkey erythrocytes. J Biol Chem 249: 157-161
13. Bristow M, Sherrod TP, Green RD (1970) Analysis of beta-receptor drug interactions in isolated rabbit atrium, aorta, stomach and trachea. J Pharmacol Exp Ther 171: 52-61
14. Brown EM, Aurbach GD, Hauser D, Troxler F (1976) β-Adrenergic receptor interactions: characterization of iodohydrooxybenzylpindolol as a specific ligand. J Biol Chem 251: 1232-1238
15. Brown L, Werdan K, Erdmann E (1983) Consequences of specific ^{3}H-ouabain binding to guinea pig left atria and cardiac cell membranes. Biochem Pharmacol 32: 423-435
16. Cassel D, Pfeuffer T (1978) Mechanism of cholera toxin action: covalent modification of the guanyl-nucleotide-binding protein of the adenylate cyclase system. Proc Natl Acad Sci USA 75: 2669

17. Cassel D, Selinger Z (1976) Catecholamine stimulated GTPase activity in turkey erythrocyte membranes. Biochim Biophys Acta 452: 538–551
18. Cassel D, Selinger Z (1977) Mechanism of adenylate cyclase activation by cholera toxin: inhibition of GTP hydrolysis at the regulatory site. Proc Natl Acad Sci USA 74: 3307–3311
19. Cassel D, Selinger Z (1978) Mechanism of adenylate activation through the β-adrenergic receptor: catecholamine-induced displacement of bound GDP by GTP. Proc Natl Acad Sci USA 75: 4155–4159
20. Cuatrecasas P (1973) Insulin receptor of liver and fat cell membranes. Fed Proc 32: 1838–1846
21. Cuatrecasas P (1974) Membrane receptors. Ann Rev Biochem 43: 169–214
22. Cuatrecasas P, Hollenberg MD (1975) Binding of insulin and other hormones to non-receptor materials: saturability, specificity and apparent "negative cooperativity". Biochem Biophys Res Commun 62: 31–41
23. Cuatrecasas P, Hollenberg MD (1976) Membrane receptors and hormone action. Adv Protein Chem 30: 251–451
24. De Lean A, Stadel JM, Lefkowitz RJ (1980) A ternary complex model explains the agonist-specific binding properties of the adenylate cyclase-coupled β-adrenergic receptor. J Biol Chem 255: 7108–7117
25. Downs RW, Spiegel AM, Singer M, Reen S, Aurbach GD (1980) Fluoride stimulation of adenylate cyclase is dependent on the guanine nucleotide regulatory protein. J Biol Chem 255: 949–954
26. Drummond GI, Severson DL (1974) Preparation and characterization of adenylate cyclase from heart and skeletal muscle. In: Hardman JG, O'Malley BW (eds) Methods in enzymology, vol 38. Academic, New York, pp 143–149
27. Ehrlich P (1909) Über den jetzigen Stand der Chemotherapie. Dtsch Chem Ges 42: 17
28. Ehrlich P (1913) Address in pathology on chemotherapeutics: scientific principles, methods, and results. Lancet 16: 445–451
29. Erdmann E (1977) Cell membrane receptors for cardiac glycosides in the heart. Basic Res Cardiol 72: 315–325
30. Finn FM, Widnell CC, Hofmann K (1972) Localisation of an adrenocorticotropic hormone receptor on bovine adrenal cortical membranes. J Biol Chem 247: 5695–5702
31. Forgue ME, Freychet P (1975) Insulin receptors in the heart muscle. Diabetes 24: 715–723
32. Gill DM (1975) Involvement of nicotinamide adenine dinucleotide in the action of cholera toxin in vitro. Proc Natl Acad Sci USA 72: 2064–2068
33. Gill DM, Meren R (1978) ADP-ribosylation of membrane proteins catalyzed by cholera toxin: basis of the activation of adenylate cyclase. Proc Natl Acad Sci USA 75: 3050–3054
34. Goodfriend T, Lin SY (1969) Angiotensin receptors. Clin Res 17: 243–248
35. Hall ZW (1972) Release of neurotransmitters and their interactions with receptors. Ann Rev Biochem 41: 925–952
36. Harden TK, Wolfe BB, Molinoff PB (1976) Binding of iodinated beta adrenergic antagonists to proteins derived from rat heart. Mol Pharmacol 12: 1–15
37. Hollenberg DM, Cuatrecasas P (1978) Membrane receptors and hormone action: recent developments. Prog Neuropsychopharmacol Biol Psychiatry 2: 287–302
38. Karlin A (1973) Molecular interactions of the acetylcholine receptor. Fed Proc 32: 1847–1853
39. Kaslow HR, Farfel Z, Johnson GL, Bourne HR (1979) Adenylate cyclase assembled in vitro: cholera toxin substrates determine different patterns of regulation by isoproterenol and guanosine 5'-triphosphate. Mol Pharmacol 15: 472–483
40. Kaslow HR, Johnson GL, Brothers VM, Bourne HR (1980) A regulatory component of adenylate cyclase from human erythrocyte membranes. J Biol Chem 255: 3736–3741
41. Korolkovas A (1974) Grundlagen der molekularen Pharmakologie. Thieme, Stuttgart, pp 7–9
42. Krawietz W, Erdmann E (1979) Specific and unspecific binding of ^{3}H-(−)-dihydroalprenolol to cardiac tissue. Biochem Pharmacol 28: 1283–1288
43. Krawietz W, Poppert D, Erdmann E, Glossmann H, Struck CJ, Konrad C (1976) β-Adrenergic receptors in guinea-pig myocardial tissue. Naunyn-Schmiedebergs Arch Pharmacol 295: 215–224
44. Krawietz W, Werdan K, Erdmann E (1982) Effect of thyroid status on β-adrenergic receptor, adenylate cyclase activity and guanine nucleotide regulatory unit in rat cardiac and erythrocyte membranes. Biochem Pharmacol 31: 2463–2469

45. Lad PM, Nielsen TB, Preston MS, Rodbell M (1980) The role of the guanine nucleotide exchange reaction in the regulation of the β-adrenergic receptor and in the actions of catecholamines and cholera toxin on adenylate cyclase in turkey erythrocyte membranes. J Biol Chem 255: 988–995
46. Laemmli VK (1975) Cleavage of structural proteins during the assembly of the head of bacteriophage T_4. Nature 227: 680–685
47. Langley JW (1906) On nerve endlings and on special exitable substances. Proc Roy Soc 78: 170–194
48. Lefkowitz RJ (1976) β-Adrenergic receptors: recognition and regulation. N Engl J Med 295: 323–328
49. Lefkowitz RJ, Williams LT (1978) Molecular mechanism of activation and desensitization of adenylate cyclase coupled beta-adrenergic receptors. Adv Cyclic Nucleotide Res 9: 1–17
50. Lefkowitz RJ, Pastan D, Roth J, Pricer W (1970) ACTH receptors in the adrenal: specific binding of ACTH-^{125}J and its relation to adenylate cyclase. Proc Natl Acad Sci USA 65: 745–752
51. Lesniak MA, Gorden P, Roth J, Gavin JR (1974) Binding of ^{125}J-human growth hormone to specific receptors in human cultured lymphocytes. Characterization of the interaction and a sensitive radioceptor assay. J Biol Chem 249: 1661–1667
52. Levey GS (1970) Solubilization of myocardial adenyl cyclase. Biochem Biophys Res Commun 38: 86–92
53. Levey GS, Fletcher MA, Klein I, Ruiz E, Schenk A (1974) Characterization of ^{125}I-Glucagon binding in a solubilized preparation of cat myocardial adenylate cyclase. J Biol Chem 249: 2665–2673
54. Levitzki A, Atlas D, Steer ML (1974) The binding characteristics and number of β-adrenergic receptors on the turkey erythrocyte. Proc Natl Acad Sci USA 71: 2773–2776
55. Limas C, Limas CJ (1978) Reduced number of β-adrenergic receptors in the myocardium of spontaneously hypertensive rats. Biochem Biophys Res Commun 83: 710–714
56. Limbird LE (1981) Activation and attenuation of adenylate cyclase. The role of GTP-binding proteins as macromolecular messengers in receptor-cyclase coupling. Biochem J 195: 1–13
57. Limbird LE, Lefkowitz RJ (1978) Agonist-induced increase in apparent β-adrenergic receptor size. Proc Natl Acad Sci USA 75: 228–232
58. Limbird LE, Gill DM, Lefkowitz RJ (1980) Agonist-promoted coupling of the β-adrenergic receptor with the guanine nucleotide regulatory protein of the adenylate cyclase system. Proc Natl Acad Sci USA 77: 775–779
59. Lowry OH, Rosenbrough NJ, Farr AL, Randall RJ (1951) Protein measurement with the folin phenol reagent. J Biol Chem 193: 265–275
60. Maguire ME, Ross EM, Gilman AG (1977) β-Adrenergic receptor: ligand binding properties and the interaction with adenylate cyclase. Adv Cyclic Nucleotide Res 8: 1–83
61. Malbon CC, Gill DM (1979) ADP-ribosylation of membrane proteins and activation of adenylate cyclase by cholera toxin in fat cell ghosts from euthyroid and hypothyroid rats. Biochim Biophys Acta 586: 518–527
62. Moore WV, Wolff J (1974) Thyroid-stimulating hormone binding to beef thyroid membranes. Relation to adenylate cyclase activity. J Biol Chem 249: 6255–6263
63. Moss J, Vaughan M (1979) Activation of adenylate cyclase by choleragen. Annu Rev Biochem 48: 581
64. Moss J, Stanley SJ, Lin MC (1979) NAD glycohydrolase and ADP-ribosyltransferase activities are intrinsic to the A_1-peptide of choleragen. J Biol Chem 254: 11993–11996
65. Nakaya S, Moss J, Vaughan M (1980) Effects of nucleotide triphosphate on choleragen-activated brain adenylate cyclase. Biochemistry 19: 4871
66. Nielson TB, Lad PM, Preston MS, Rodbell M (1980) Characteristics of the guanine nucleotide regulatory component of adenylate cyclase in human erythrocyte membranes. Biochim Biophys Acta 629: 143–155
67. O'Farrell PZ, Gold LM, Huang WM (1973) The identification of prereplicative bacteriophage T_4 protein. J Biol Chem 248: 5499–5501
68. Owen DAA (1977) Histamin receptors in the cardiovascular system. Gen Pharmacol 8: 141–156
69. Pasternak GW, Snyder SH (1975) Opiate receptor binding: enzymatic treatments that discriminate between agonist and antagonist interactions. Mol Pharmacol 11: 478–484

70. Pfeuffer T (1977) GTP-binding proteins in membranes and the control of adenylate cyclase activity. J Biol Chem 252: 7224-7243
71. Pfeuffer T (1979) Guanine nucleotide-controlled interactions between components of adenylate cyclase. FEBS Lett 101: 85-89
72. Powel JR, Brody MJ (1976) Identification and specific blockade of two receptors for histamine in the cardiovascular system. J Pharmacol Exp Ther 196: 1-14
73. Rodbell M (1980) The role of hormone receptors and GTP-regulatory proteins in membrane transduction. Nature 284: 17-22
74. Roth J (1973) Peptide hormone binding to receptors: a review of direct studies in vitro. Metabolism 22: 1059-1073
75. Salomon Y, Lin MC, Londons C, Rendell M, Rodbell M (1975) The hepatic adenylate cyclase system. I. Evidence for transition states and structural requirements for guanin nucleotide activation. J Biol Chem 250: 4239-4225
76. Scatchard G (1949) The attractions of proteins for small molecules and ions. Ann NY Acad Sci 51: 660-672
77. Spiegel AM, Aurbach GD (1974) Binding of 5′-guanylylimidodiphosphate to turkey erythrocyte membranes and effects on β-adrenergic-activated adenylate cyclase. J Biol Chem 249: 7630-7636
78. Spiegel AM, Downs RW (1981) Guanine nucleotides: key regulators of hormone receptor-adenylate cyclase interaction. Endocrine Rev 2: 275-305
79. Spiegel AM, Downs RW, Aurbach GD (1977) Guanosine 5′-α-β-methylene, triphosphate, a novel GTP analog, causes persistent activation of adenylate cyclase: evidence against pyrophosphorylation mechanism. Biochem Biophys Res Commun 76: 758-764
80. Spiegel AM, Downs RW, Levine MA, Singer MJ, Krawietz W, Marx SJ, Woodard CJ, Reen SA, Aurbach GD (1981) The role of guanine nucleotides in regulation of adenylate cyclase activity. Rec Prog Horm Res 37: 635-665
81. Spiegel AM, Gierschik P, Levine MA, Downs RW (1985) Clinical implications of guanine nucleotide-binding protein as receptor-effector couplers. N Engl J Med 312: 26-33
82. Stadel JM, Shorr RGL, Lefkowitz RJ (1981) Receptor associated guanine nucleotide regulatory protein reconstitutes GTP-γ-S stimulated adenylate cyclase activity. Adv Cyclic Nucleotide Res 14: 659
83. Sternweis PC, Gilman AG (1979) Reconstitution of catecholamine-sensitive adenylate cyclase. Reconstitution of the uncoupled variant of the S49 lymphoma cell. J Biol Chem 254: 3333-3340
84. Sternweis PC, Northup JK, Hanski E, Schleifer LS, Smigel MD, Gilman AG (1981) Purification and properties of the regulatory component (G/F) of adenylate cyclase. Adv Cyclic Nucleotide Res 14: 23-36
85. Teschemacher H (1978) Endogeneous ligands of opiate receptors (endorphins). In: Herz A (ed) Developments in opiate research. Dekker, New York, pp 68-125
86. Watkins PA, Moss J, Vaughan M (1980) Effects of GTP on choleragen-catalyzed ADP-ribosylation of membrane and soluble proteins. J Biol Chem 255: 3959-3963
87. Woodcock EA, Johnston CI (1980) Changes in tissue alpha- and beta-adrenergic receptors in renal hypertension in the rat. Hypertension 2: 156-161
88. Woodcock EA, Funder JW, Johnston CI (1979) Decreased cardiac β-adrenergic receptors in deoxycorticosterone-salt and renal hypertensive rats. Circ Res 45: 560-565
89. Woodcock EA, Ollson CA, Johnston CI (1980) Reduced vascular beta-adrenergic receptors in deoxycorticosterone-salt hypertensive rats. Biochem Pharmacol 29: 1465-1468

Discussion

Brodde: What species were used in your studies?

Krawietz: Guinea pigs and rats. No difference was noted.

Brodde: Today's view is that in most species not only $beta_1$, but also $beta_2$ receptors are present in the atria and - as many recent studies have shown and Dr. Göthert has correctly pointed out - in the ventricles as well. This applies particularly to humans. That, of course, is what interests us most. But this also holds true in guinea pigs, for example, so that actually a pure $beta_1$ system in the heart is no longer known in any animal species.

Krawietz: That is correct. There is the study by Molinoff, but there the percentage, which I do not recall at the moment, is considerably lower.

Brodde: I was just about to point that out myself. What Minneman published in 1980 cannot be taken as time value today, if only because they did not have such selective substances at the time. It is for this reason that Molinoff and Minneman wrote that only $beta_1$ receptors occur in the ventricles and only $beta_2$ receptors in the atria.

Krawietz: I used an unselective beta blocker for these measurements, and the displacement experiments were also performed with unselective blockers. I believe that it does not play a decisive role for the characterization of β-receptor adenylate-cyclase-system.

Göthert: There are often differences in the percentages given or the ratio of $beta_2$ to $beta_1$ receptors. The most recent issue of *American Journal of Pharmacology* includes a paper by the Molinoff group, in which it was even claimed that 45% of the cardiac receptors in the human atrium are $beta_2$ receptors. In this work Molinoff used pindolol. I believe you used IodoCYP?

Brodde: I think the decisive factor is not the ligand, although today one would no longer use dihydroalprenolol. But whether cyanopindolol, hydroxybenzylpindolol, or pindolol itself is used is of no matter. The majority of authors forget this and also fail to describe what pathologic condition the heart was in. We performed a study on end-stage cardiomyopathy, in which elevated catecholamine levels were found, primarily norepinephrine, and in fact we found 60% $beta_1$ and 40% $beta_2$ receptors. Two things must always be considered: First, the pathologic state plays an important role; secondly and just as importantly, so does the amount of time that has elapsed between the removal of the specimen from the heart and the time of binding. Steven Nahorski and Gerry Stiles have shown very nicely that if a specimen is left to stand the number of $beta_2$ receptors continues to undergo a relatively small increase, because the $beta_1$ receptors are so labile and $beta_2$ receptors stable. This accounts for the differences in numbers.

Göthert: May I interject a short comment? I am familiar with your work as well as with that of Stiles, and I found what you wrote must convincing. But in the study by Molinoff, which I just quoted from and which is really new, he also explicitly stated that healthy hearts were involved. He practically eliminated the failing heart, and I am therefore astonished that these high figures are introduced into the discussion. Possibly differences due to various ligands are at issue. Iodopindolol, which he uses, is certainly the optimal ligand.

Brodde: Iodopindolol is certainly the optimal ligand.

Göthert: Is it better than IodoCYP?

Brodde: Iodopindolol has the advantage that it does not have the crazy kinetics of IodoCYP.

Frequency Regulation in the Sinoatrial Node: Function of β_1- and β_2-Receptors

U. BORCHARD, D. HAFNER and D. SCHÜTZ
Institut für Pharmakologie der Universität Düsseldorf, Moorenstr. 5, 4000 Düsseldorf 1, FRG

Introduction

Since the subclassification of β-adrenoceptors by Lands et al. [13], the coexistence of β_1- and β_2-adrenoceptors has been shown in different organs [1, 8]. β_1- and β_2-adrenoceptors have been identified in the ventricular myocardium by means of binding experiments as well as concentration-response curves for the positive inotropic action of β-agonists in the absence and presence of partially selective antagonists [4, 7, 10, 11, 14].

The coexistence of β_1- and β_2-receptors has also been demonstrated in the right atria [2-4, 6, 9, 11, 12, 15]. However, it is still an open question whether β_1- and/or β_2-receptors of the sinus node are involved in the positive chronotropic action of β-agonists, especially with respect to variations among different species. Therefore, experiments were carried out on isolated, spontaneously beating rat and guinea pig right atria in order to investigate the role of β-adrenoceptor subtypes in the frequency regulation of the heart using substances with a high degree of selectivity for β_1- or β_2-receptors. Concentration-response curves for the β_1- and β_2-selective agonists norepinephrine and procaterol were registered in the absence and presence of the β_1- and β_2-selective antagonists bisoprolol and ICI 118551, respectively.

Methods

Rats (90-110 g body weight) and guinea pigs (250-350 g body weight) were pretreated with 10 mg/kg reserpine 24 h prior to the experiment. The preparations were incubated in organ baths containing 25 ml of a modified Krebs-Henseleit solution oxygenated with a gas mixture of 95% O_2 and 5% CO_2 at a temperature of 31 °C.

The spontaneous contractions of isolated right atria were registered by means of a force tranducer. Phenoxybenzamine 5 µmol/liter was added 1 h before the start of the experiment. Then, concentration-response curves for procaterol or L-norepinephrine (in the presence of 50 µmol/liter ascorbic acid) were plotted. After washing the preparations, the β-adrenoceptor-blocking drugs bisoprolol or ICI 118551 were added and allowed to equilibrate for 1 h. Thereafter, a second concentration-response curve for the β-agonist was performed. In one preparation, one or two consecutive concentrations of the β-antagonist were tested.

New Aspects in Hypertension: Adrenoceptors
M. Middeke and H. Holzgreve (Eds.)
Springer-Verlag Berlin Heidelberg New York 1986

The degree of the β_1- or β_2-adrenoceptor blockade at the 50% maximum response level of the agonists was calculated for the different concentrations of the antagonists in terms of the ratio CR = EC_{50} in the presence of the antagonist/EC_{50} in the absence of the antagonist. From these results pA_2 values were calculated (Schild plot).

Results

Bisoprolol antagonized the effects of norepinephrine in guinea pig right atria in a competitive manner, as shown by Fig. 1. From the Schild plot a pA_2 value of 8.8 was calculated, the regression and correlation coefficients being 0.94 and 0.93, respectively ($n = 9$).

ICI 118551 up to 10^{-8} mol/liter did not effect a shift to the right of the concentration-response curves for norepinephrine. At higher concentrations only a minimal shift occurred, which was indicated by an increase of CR (see *Methods*) to 1.3 at 3×10^{-8} mol/liter ($n = 4$) and to 2.5 at 10^{-7} mol/liter ($n = 2$). These results demonstrate that ICI 118551 is a selective β_2-antagonist and/or that the positive chronotropic effect of norepinephrine in the guinea pig sinus node is mainly due to stimulation of β_1-receptors.

Bisoprolol inhibited competitively the action of norepinephrine on the spontaneous rate of rat right atria (Fig. 2). From the shift to the right of the concentration-response curves, a pA_2 value of 8.3 was calculated by means of the Schild plot, the regression and correlation coefficients being 1.2 and 0.99, respectively ($n = 4$).

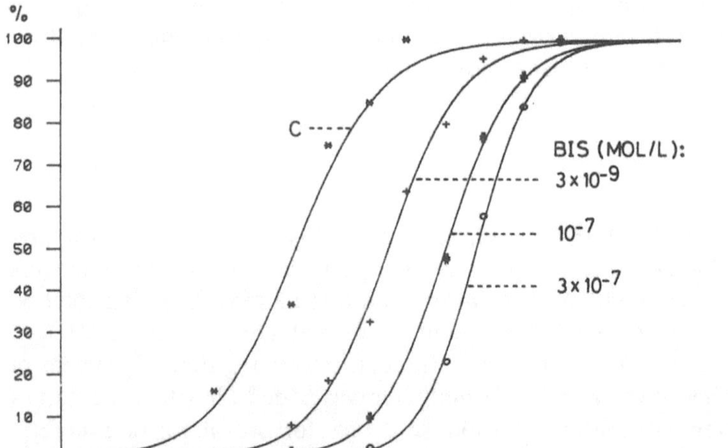

Fig. 1. Bisoprolol effects a shift to the right of the concentration-response curve for the positive chronotropic effect of norepinephrine in spontaneously beating guinea pig right atria. *Ordinate,* increase in beat frequency as percent of maximum response ($n = 1$-3). *, control (C); +, 3×10^{-9} mol/liter bisoprolol #, 10^{-7} mol/liter bisoprolol; O, 3×10^{-7} mol/liter bisoprolol

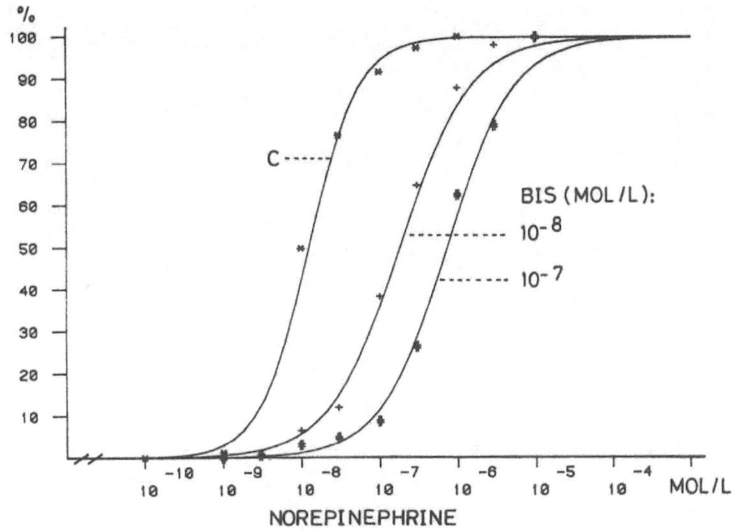

Fig. 2. Bisoprolol effects a shift to the right of the concentration-response curve for the positive chronotropic effect of norepinephrine in spontaneously beating rat right atria. *Ordinate*, increase in beat frequency as percentage of maximum response ($n=2$-4); *, control (C); +, 10^{-8} mol/liter bisoprolol; #, 10^{-7} mol/liter bisoprolol

However, ICI 118551 did not influence the effects of norepinephrine up to 10^{-8} mol/liter. At 3×10^{-8} mol/liter CR was increased to 2.9 ($n=2$) and at 10^{-7} to 2.0 ($n=1$). This indicates the high degree of β_2-selectivity of ICI 118551 in rat right atria; this has already been shown for the guinea pig.

Procaterol in a concentration range from 10^{-10} to 10^{-7} mol/liter increased spontaneous rate of guinea pig right atria, the EC_{50} being $(3.2 \pm 0.63) \times 10^{-9}$ mol/liter ($n=4$; Fig. 3). The preparations were preincubated with 3×10^{-7} mol/liter bisoprolol prior to the administration of ICI 118551 in order to prevent stimulation of β_1-adrenoceptors by procaterol. Bisoprolol 3×10^7 mol/liter induced a minor shift to the right of the concentration-response curves, which led to an increase in CR to 5.3 (Table 1), indicating the partial β_1-selectivity of bisoprolol. However, application of increasing concentrations of ICI 118551 shifted the concentration-response curve to the right and increased CR (Fig. 3, Table 1). At procaterol concentrations above 10^{-6} mol/liter, i.e., in the presence of ICI 118551 concentrations $\geq 3 \times 10^{-9}$ mol/liter, the concentration-response curves became biphasic. This may be explained by a replacement of bisoprolol from β_1-receptors by procaterol. The results clearly indicate that stimulation of β_2-receptors may contribute to the positive chronotropic effect in the guinea pig sinus node.

Procaterol led to an increase in spontaneous frequency in rat right atria (Fig. 4) which, in contrast to the guinea pig, occurred in a concentration range from 3×10^{-8} to 3×10^{-6} mol/liter, the EC_{50} being $(4.1 \pm 1.7) \times 10^{-7}$ mol/liter ($n=4$). Application of ICI 118551 from 10^{-9} to 10^{-8} mol/liter did not influence the effects of procaterol. Preincubation with 3×10^{-7} mol/liter bisoprolol in order to prevent stimulation of β_1-receptors prior to the application of ICI 118551 induced a large

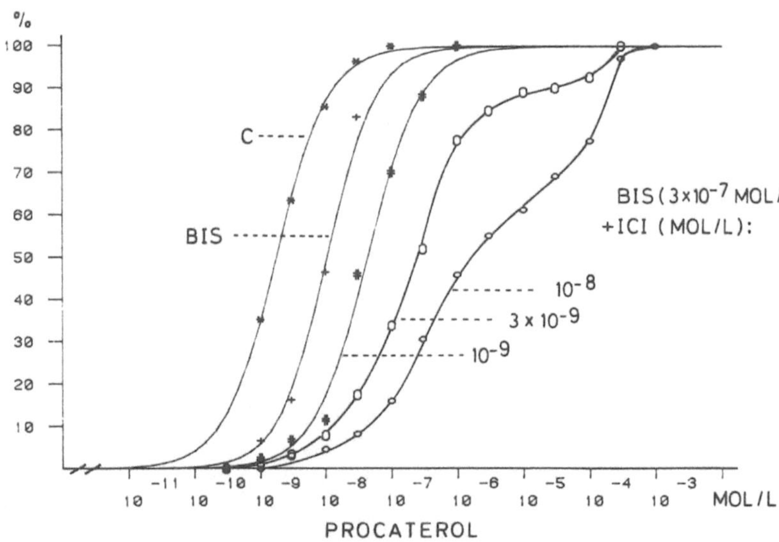

Fig. 3. Procaterol ($C=*$) at concentrations $>10^{-10}$ mol/liter increases spontaneous rate in guinea pig right atria. Bisoprolol ($BIS=^{+}$) 3×10^{-7} mol/liter effects a shift to the right of the concentration-response curve for procaterol. A further shift to the right of the concentration response curve in the presence of 3×10^{-7} mol/liter bisoprolol is brought about by ICI 118551. #, 10^{-9} mol/liter; ◯, 3×10^{-9} mol/liter; O, 10^{-8} mol/liter; *ordinate*, increase in beat frequency as percent of maximum response ($n=1$-4). Note the biphasic shape of the curves at concentrations of ICI 118551 > 10^{-9} mol/liter

Table 1. Inhibition of the positive chronotropic action of procaterol in the presence of bisoprolol alone or with additional ICI 118551 in guinea pig (GP) or rat right atria, as indicated by the corresponding concentration ratios of EC_{50} values

n	Biso[a] (mol/l)	EC_{50} (Proc[b]/Biso) / EC_{50} (Proc)	+ICI[c] (mol/l)	EC_{50} (Proc/Biso/ICI) / EC_{50} (Proc/Biso)
GP				
1	3×10^{-7}	7.2	10^{-9}	3.8
2	3×10^{-7}	7.0	3×10^{-9}	31.0
3	3×10^{-7}	3.0	10^{-8}	386.0
4	3×10^{-7}	4.0	3×10^{-8}	622.7
$\bar{X}\pm s_{\bar{X}}$		5.3 ± 2.1		
Rat				
1	3×10^{-7}	106.4	10^{-9}	1.2
2	3×10^{-7}	102.7	3×10^{-9}	1.1
3	3×10^{-7}	227.6	3×10^{-8}	0.8
4	3×10^{-7}	186.0	10^{-7}	1.5
$\bar{X}\pm s_{\bar{X}}$		155.7 ± 26.6		

[a] Bisoprolol 3×10^{-7} mol/liter
[b] Procaterol
[c] Bisoprolol 3×10^{-7} mol/liter plus ICI 118551

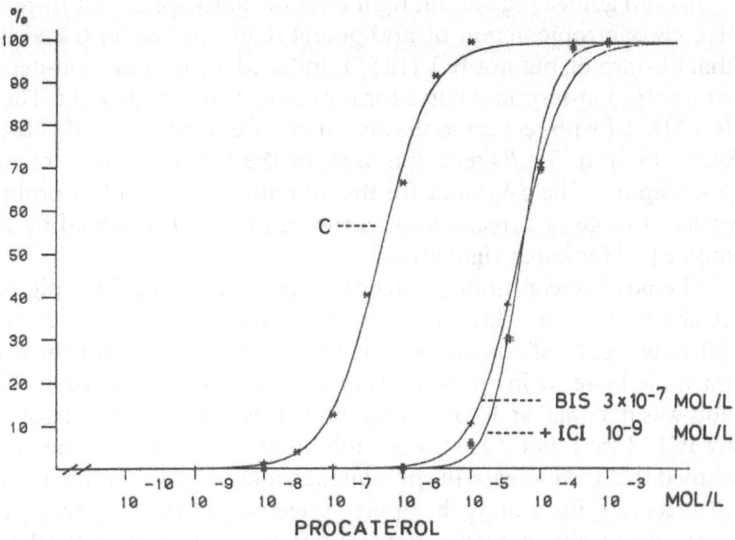

Fig. 4. Procaterol ($C = *$) at concentrations $> 10^{-8}$ mol/liter increases spontaneous rate in rat right atria. Bisoprolol 3×10^{-7} mol/liter (+) induces a shift to the right of the concentration-response curve of procaterol. ICI 118551 10^{-9} mol/liter (#) in the presence of bisoprolol has no additional effect. *Ordinate,* increase in beat frequency as percentage of maximum response ($n = 4$)

shift of the concentration-response curves to the right, as indicated by an increase in CR to 155.7 (Table 1). Consecutive application of increasing concentrations of ICI 118551 did not bring about a further shift to the right of the concentration-response curves as shown by the corresponding CR values (Fig. 4, Table 1). Similar results were obtained after preincubation with 3×10^{-8} mol/liter bisoprolol. These results indicate that there is no functional evidence for the existence of β_2-adrenoceptors in the sinoatrial node of the rat.

Discussion

Binding studies in the right atria of guinea pig [6] and of rat hearts [14] have shown the coexistence of β_1- and β_2-receptors, the β_1: β_2 ratio being 76.7%:23.3% in the guinea pig and 83%:17% in the rat. However, values for right atria may not be representative for the sinoatrial node. As the distinct region of the sinoatrial node is not yet accessible to binding studies, indirect evidence for the participation of β_1- and/or β_2-receptors in the regulation of heart rate may be obtained from the positive chronotropic action of β_1- and β_2-selective agonists in the absence and presence of β_1- and β_2-selective antagonists.

In the present investigations, norepinephrine and procaterol were used - two substances that are known to preferentially stimulate β_1- and β_2-adrenoceptors, respectively [16, 18, 19]. Furthermore, bisoprolol and ICI 118551 were applied, which have been reported to be antagonists highly selective for β_1- and β_2-receptors, respectively [5, 11, 17].

In both guinea pig and rat right atria the participation of β_1-receptors in the positive chronotropic action of norepinephrine was demonstrated by the observation that bisoprolol, but not ICI 118551, induced a concentration-dependent shift of the concentration-response curve for norepinephrine to the right. The ineffectiveness of ICI 118551 with respect to the action of norepinephrine indicates the high selectivity of the drug for β_2-receptors and/or the high selectivity of norepinephrine for β_1-receptors. The pA_2 value for the inhibitory action of bisoprolol in the guinea pig of 8.8 is in good agreement with the value of 8.7 observed by Kaumann and Lemoine [11] for kitten right atria.

The positive chronotropic action of procaterol in guinea pig right atria occurred at about 10^{-10} mol/liter and was maximal at 10^{-7} mol/liter, which is consistent with the results of Johansson and Persson [9] reported for the same tissue. In contrast, the increase in spontaneous rate in rat right atria began at 3×10^{-8} mol/liter and was maximal at 3×10^{-6} mol/liter. This effect of procaterol was not influenced by ICI 118551, but was strongly inhibited by bisoprolol. Therefore, it may be concluded that the increase in spontaneous rate by procaterol in the rat is mediated via β_1-receptors, illustrating the limited selectivity of the drug for β_2-receptors. Furthermore, the results show that there is no functional evidence for the existence of β_2-receptors in the rat sinoatrial node.

In guinea pig right atria, however, the positive chronotropic action of procaterol was inhibited by ICI 118551 even if the β_1-receptors were blocked by bisoprolol. These results demonstrate that β_2-receptors were involved in the increase in heart rate in the guinea pig, in contrast to the rat. The shift of the concentration-response curve for procaterol to the right by 3×10^{-7} mol/liter bisoprolol is probably due to an inhibition of β_2-receptors, showing the partial β_1-selectivity of the antagonist. In the presence of bisoprolol and ICI 118551, the concentration-response curves of procaterol became biphasic at concentrations $> 10^{-6}$ mol/liter. This effect may be explained by the partial β_2-selectivity of procaterol, which then replaced bisoprolol from β_1-receptors. The limited selectivity of procaterol has also been shown by Johannsson and Persson [9] for the positive chronotropic response in guinea pig right atria. These authors observed biphasic concentration-response curves, which were attributed to the consecutive stimulation of β_2- and β_1-receptors by procaterol. The second slope of the concentration-response curves of procaterol insensitive to ICI 118551 was attributed by the authors to the stimulation of β_1-receptors and occurred at procaterol concentrations $> 10^{-7}$ mol/liter. This is consistent with our findings in rat right atria that an increase in spontaneous rate by procaterol was observed at concentrations $\geq 10^{-7}$ mol/liter, the EC_{50} being 4.1×10^{-7} mol/liter.

Our results in guinea pig right atria are contradictory to those of O'Donnell and Wanstall [15], who report the lack of functionally active β_2-receptors in the guinea pig sinoatrial node. But these authors used fenoterol as β_2-selective agonist, and α-methylpropranolol as β_2-selective antagonist - substances with a rather limited degree of selectivity for the β-receptor subtypes as compared with the substances used in this study. Furthermore, the authors conclude from their results that both β_1- and β_2-receptors coexist in the cat sinoatrial node. On the other hand, Kaumann [10] found 94% β_1- and 6% β_2-receptors in this tissue, so that one should expect a negligible effect mediated via β_2-receptors. This has been confirmed by the observation that in kitten sinoatrial pacemaker β_1-adrenoceptors contribute 97% to the stimulus induced by (-)-noradrenaline [11].

The coexistence of β_1- and β_2-receptors has also been shown for the rabbit sinoatrial node by Dukes and Vaughan Williams [4]. However, these authors used only one high concentration of the subtype-selective antagonist, so that selective blockade of the corresponding receptor subtype is questionable.

The development of still more selective agonists and antagonists for β_1- or β_2-receptors could provide the tools to study the functional role of these receptor subtypes in more detail, although the substances used in this study already possess a high degree of selectivity.

Summary

Investigations were carried out in isolated spontaneously beating rat and guinea pig right atria to test the role of β-adrenoceptor subtypes in the regulation of heart rate.

The highly β_1- and β_2-selective antagonists bisoprolol and ICI 118551, respectively, were used. Concentration-response curves for the increase in frequency by the agonists in the absence and presence of the antagonists were recorded. In rat and guinea pig right atria, β_1-receptor stimulation with norepinephrine was antagonized by bisoprolol but not by ICI 118551, the pA_2 values of bisoprolol being 8.3 and 9.0, respectively. The increase in spontaneous frequency by procaterol in guinea pig atria was inhibited by ICI 118551, but not by bisoprolol. However, the procaterol-induced positive chronotropic action in the rat, which occurred at concentrations two orders of magnitude higher than in the guinea pig, was antagonized by bisoprolol but not by ICI 118551. The results indicate that the increase in heart rate is mediated via β_1- and β_2-receptors in the guinea pig, but only by β_1-receptors in the rat. In conclusion, there is no functional evidence for the existence of β_2-receptors in the rat sinoatrial node.

References

1. Ariens EJ, Simonis AM (1983) Physiological and pharmacological aspects of adrenergic receptor classification. Biochem Pharmacol 32 (10): 1539-1545
2. Brodde OE, Leifert FJ, Krehl HJ (1982) Coexistence of β_1- and β_2-adrenoceptors in the rabbit heart: quantitative analysis of the regional distribution by (-)- ^{3}H dihydroalprenolol binding. J Cardiovasc Pharmacol 4: 34-43
3. Bryan LJ, Cole JJ, O'Donnell SR, Wanstall JC (1981) A study designed to explore the hypothesis that beta-1 adrenoceptors are "innervated" receptors and beta-2 adrenoceptors are "hormonal" receptors. J Pharmacol Exp Ther 216: 395-400
4. Dukes ID, Vaughan Williams EM (1984) Effects of selective α_1, α_2, β_1 and β_2-adrenoceptor stimulation on potentials and contractions in the rabbit heart. J Physiol (Lond) 355: 523-546
5. Goldie RG, Paterson JW, Spina D, Wale JL (1984) Classification of β-adrenoceptors in human isolated bronchus. Br J Pharmacol 81: 611-615
6. Hedberg A, Minnemann KP, Molinoff PB (1980) Differential distribution of beta-1 and beta-2 adrenergic receptors in cat and guinea-pig heart. J Pharmacol Exp Ther 212: 503-508
7. Heitz A, Schwartz J, Velly J (1983) β-adrenoceptors of the human myocardium: determination of β_1 and β_2 subtypes by radioligand binding. Br J Pharmacol 80: 711-717

8. Hoffman BB, Lefkowitz RJ (1980) Radioligand binding studies of adrenergic receptors: new insights into molecular and physiological regulation. Ann Rev Pharmacol Toxicol 20: 581–608
9. Johansson LH, Persson H (1983) β_2-adrenoceptors in guinea-pig atria. J Pharm Pharmacol 35: 804–807
10. Kaumann AJ (1983) Herz-β-Rezeptoren – experimentelle Standpunkte. Z Kardiol 72: 63–82
11. Kaumann AJ, Lemoine H (1985) Direct labelling of myocardial β_1-adrenoceptors. Naunyn-Schmiedebergs Arch Pharmacol 331: 27–29
12. Kaumann AJ, Marano M (1982) On equilibrium dissociation constants for complexes of drug-receptor subtypes. Naunyn-Schmiedebergs Arch Pharmacol 318: 192–201
13. Lands AM, Arnold A, McAucliff JP, Luduena FP, Brown TG (1967) Differentiation of receptor systems activated by sympathomimetic amines. Nature 214: 597–598
14. Minnemann KP, Hegstrand LR, Molinoff PB (1979) Simultaneous determination of beta-1 and beta-2 adrenergic receptors in tissues containing both receptor subtypes. Mol Pharmacol 16: 34–46
15. O'Donnell SR, Wanstall JC (1979) pA_2-values of selective β-adrenoceptor antagonists on isolated atria demonstrate a species difference in the β-adrenoceptor populations mediating chronotropic responses in cat and guinea-pig. J Pharm Pharmacol 31: 686–690
16. O'Donnell SR, Wanstall JC (1979) The importance of choice of agonist in studies designed to predict β_2:β_1 adrenoceptor selectivity of antagonists from pA_2-values on guinea-pig trachea and atria. Naunyn-Schmiedebergs Arch Pharmacol 308: 183–190
17. O'Donnell SR, Wanstall JC (1980) Evidence that ICI 118551 is a potent, highly beta$_2$-selective adrenoceptor antagonist and can be used to characterize beta-adrenoceptor populations in tissues. Life Sci 27: 671–677
18. Takayangi I, Kondo N, Yamashita H, Hongo T, Takagi K (1977) New selective β_2-adrenoceptor stimulants 5-(1-hydroxy-2-ethylaminobutyl)-8-hydroxycarbostyril hydrochlorides (OPC-2009 and OPC-2030) and cyclic AMP concentration. J Pharm Pharmacol 29: 187–189
19. Yamashita S, Takai M, Yabundi Y (1978) Actions of procaterol (OPC-2009), a new β_2-adrenoceptor stimulant, on pulmonary resistance, contractions of the soleus muscle, and cardiovascular system of the anaesthetized cat. J Pharm Pharmacol 30: 273–279

Discussion

Göthert: You work only with selective beta$_2$ agonists. Have you ever tried to work with selective beta$_1$ agonists, for example by blocking beta$_2$ receptors or using norepinephrine or the less sufficient substances like the ones I mentioned earlier, such as prenalterol or dobutamine?

Borchard: No, we haven't tried them. We started right off with highly selective substances. I have discussed norepinephrine here; and earlier we blocked the beta$_2$ receptors.

Brodde: Dr. Borchard, a short comment on norepinephrine and bisoprolol. The curves are not parallel. The bisoprolol curves diverge. Doesn't this indicate that norepinephrine possesses a beta$_2$ activity that is not inhibited by bisoprolol?

Borchard: I think we have to consider the following: I could only show one control curve for different experiments. We performed them in such a way that we never had three four or five concentrations in one preparation. In other words, we selected a control curve that matched the other experiments as well as possible. Of course, to calculate the Schild plot we always used the pairs. These pairs are absolutely parallel.

Brodde: Excuse me; I think the findings are wonderful, but your last comment does not convince me: That is not the case in rats. In rats they are all parallel.

Borchard: I'd like to repeat what Dr. Göthert has already pointed out. We also performed the converse experiment: we took ICI and then in the presence of ICI repeated the concentration-effect curve of norepinephrine. There is no right shift.

Göthert: You found different PA_2 values for bisoprolol in rats and guinea pigs: 8.8 in one case and 8.3 in the other. How do you account for that?

Borchard: That is not difficult to explain. If you look through the literature, you'll find that the PA_2 value differs for various tissues by a half or almost a full log unit. I would say that the overall system is not the same for all animals or animal species, as has been repeatedly claimed.

Göthert: My question was meant only in the context of Dr. Brodde's question. I too noticed that your curves really are much steeper when you perform just these experiments. They diverge. Perhaps that has an effect on the PA_2 calculation.

Borchard: I would rule that out as in each experiment the control and test concentration response curves were absolutely parallel.

Mechanisms of Stimulatory and Inhibitory Coupling to Adenylate Cyclase*

M. Minuth, S. Bauer, R. Grandt, C. Greiner, P. Zubin, and K. H. Jakobs

Pharmakologisches Institut der Universität Heidelberg, Im Neuenheimer Feld 366, 6900 Heidelberg, FRG

Introduction

Neurotransmitters, peptide and protein hormones, and a variety of regulatory and growth-promoting hormones, the receptors for which are localized at the plasma membrane, transmit their regulatory functions into target cells by specific signal transduction systems, also localized within the lipid bilayer of the plasma membrane. These signal transduction systems can be classified into four subtypes: (a) receptors that are ion channels and induce flux of specific ions, such as the nicotinic acetylcholine receptor and the GABA receptor; (b) receptors that possess tyrosine kinase activity and are assumed to act on the basis of this property, such as receptors for insulin and epidermal growth factor; (c) receptors that induce the formation of inositolphosphates and diacylglycerol by activating the phospholipase C, such as α_1-adrenoceptors and receptors for vasopressin (V_1) and many other hormones; and (d) receptors that regulate the formation of cyclic AMP by the adenylate cyclase. This signal transduction system is composed of several interacting subunits integrated within the plasma membrane: the hormone receptors, two guanine-nucleotide-binding coupling proteins called N_s and N_i or G_s and G_i proteins, and the adenylate cyclase catalytic subunit. The purpose of this review is to give a short overview of the transduction mechanisms involved in the coupling of stimulatory and inhibitory hormone receptors with the adenylate cyclase. (For recent reviews see [1-3]).

Stimulatory and Inhibitory Hormone Receptors

Receptors that on occupancy by their specific agonist ligands regulate cyclic AMP formation can be subclassified into two subtypes: receptors (R_s) which increase cyclic AMP levels by stimulating the enzyme adenylate cyclase and receptors (R_i) which decrease cyclic AMP accumulation by inhibition of the cyclic AMP-forming enzyme. There is a wide variety of R_s and R_i type of receptors (examples are shown in Table 1). Receptor subtypes have been identified for some of the hormone ago-

* This work was supported by the *Deutsche Forschungsgemeinschaft* and an Alexander von Humboldt Foundation fellowship to Palmira Zubin.

New Aspects in Hypertension: Adrenoceptors
M. Middeke and H. Holzgreve (Eds.)
Springer-Verlag Berlin Heidelberg New York 1986

Table 1. Stimulatory *(R_s)* and inhibitory *(R_i)* hormone receptors

Agonists	R_s	R_i
Adrenaline/Noradrenaline	β_1, β_2	α_2
Dopamine	D_1	D_2
Acetylcholine		M_2
Histamine	H_2	
Adenosine	A_2	A_1
Vasopressin	V_2	V_1
Glucagon	+	
ACTH	+	
LH, FSH	+	
Somatostatin		+
Opioids		+
Bradykinin		+

nists that regulate adenylate cyclase activity. No receptor subtype can both stimulate and inhibit adenylate cyclase. There seems to be some overlap between receptors mediating adenylate cyclase inhibition and those stimulating phosphoinositide breakdown (see below). Usually, both stimulatory and inhibitory hormone receptors (one or more of each subtype) are found at a given cell. Even stimulatory and inhibitory hormone receptor subtypes for one given agonist can be found at a single cell, e.g., β- and α_2-adrenoceptors in adipocytes, platelets, and some other cells.

The receptors involved in the regulation of adenylate cyclase activity display some characteristic common features. Towards agonist ligands, the receptors exhibit two distinct affinity states (high- and low-affinity states). As best shown with the β- and α_2-adrenoceptors, there is a good correlation between the high-affinity binding and the intrinsic activity of agonists to regulate adenylate cyclase activity (stimulation or inhibition) [4, 5]. Furthermore, the receptor affinity for agonists is regulated on addition of guanine nucleotides (GTP, GDP, or their analogues), provided the receptor binds the hormone in a reversible fashion. This regulation is apparently caused by the N_s and N_i proteins interacting with the receptors. However, there are apparently some differences between stimulatory and inhibitory hormone receptors with regard to regulation by guanine nucleotides. First, guanine nucleotides generally reduce agonist affinity of stimulatory hormone receptors, while examples have shown that guanine nucleotides can even cause an increase of agonist binding affinity at inhibitory hormone receptors [6]. Secondly, at stimulatory hormone receptors, GDP is usually as potent as or, as recently shown with the rat liver glucagon receptor [7], even much more potent than GTP in reducing agonist binding. These data suggest that the stimulatory receptor loses affinity for the agonist upon formation of $N_s \cdot GDP$, the inactive form of N_s, and that after release of GDP, the receptor may reassociate with N_s and increase affinity for the agonist [3, 7]. At inhibitory hormone receptors, GTP or its analogues are more potent than GDP in regulating agonist binding, suggesting that the guanine-nucleotide-free form of N_i or the N_i.GDP form is associated with the inhibitory receptors and induces high-affinity agonist binding, whereas upon formation of the active $N_i \cdot GTP$ form the receptor loses affinity for the agonist. Finally, at stimulatory hormone receptors, guanine nucleotides affect only agonist binding, as best shown with β-adrenoceptors [4], whereas guanine nucleotides can also regulate antagonist binding at inhibitory hormone receptors, as shown with dopamine D_2 and muscarinic acetylcholine receptors [8]. All these data indicate that in spite of many similarities there are some fundamental differences in the mechanisms by which stimulatory and inhibitory hormone receptors couple to their respective N proteins.

Stimulatory and Inhibitory Coupling Proteins

The coupling proteins N_s (G_s) and N_i (G_i), which act as transducers between the sensors (i.e., the receptors) and the effector (i.e., the adenylate cyclase), have recently been isolated and purified [1, 3]. These proteins are heterotrimeric in structure, consisting of a larger α-subunit and two smaller subunits (β- and γ-subunit) (Table 2). Whereas the β- and γ-subunits of N_s and N_i are very similar, if not identical, the α-subunits are clearly distinct polypeptides. The α-subunits bind guanine nucleotides and are the targets for ADP ribosylation by cholera toxin (α_s) and pertussis toxin (α_i). ADP ribosylation of α_s by cholera toxin requires the presence of a membrane-bound ADP-ribosylation factor (ARF) [9], which may have an additional, as yet unknown, function in the adenylate cyclase system. In many systems, an additional α_s-subunit (52000 daltons) is found with yet unknown function. While the β-subunit appears to act as an inhibitor of the α-subunit (α_s), the role of the γ-subunit is not yet defined. It may act as an anchor for the N proteins in the lipid bilayer of the membrane [1, 3].

Both N proteins possess an allosteric binding site for Mg^{2+} required for activation. Furthermore, both N_s and N_i not only bind GTP but also exhibit the capacity to hydrolyze it, as shown in membrane preparations and with purified components [1–3, 10, 11]. Increased GTP hydrolysis observed in the presence of the appropriate hormones seems to come about simply as a result of increased cycling of the N proteins between the inactive GDP-bound and the active GTP-bound state. For expression of the GTP-hydrolyzing activity, the adenylate cyclase catalytic subunit is not required, while the role of the individual subunits is not yet defined. ADP ribosylation of the α-subunits by cholera and pertussis toxin blocks the GTPase activity of N_s and N_i, respectively. However, cholera toxin apparently blocks the GTP-hydro-

Table 2. Some properties of the N proteins

1) Consist of 3 subunits:
   α: 45000 (α_s, ADP-ribosylated by CT)
   41000 (α_1, ADP-ribosylated by PT)
   β: 35000 (inhibitory subunit?)
   γ: 8000 (unknown function)
2) Bind guanine nucleotides (α); hydrolyze GTP
3) Interact with receptors; regulate receptor affinity for agonists
4) Interact with adenylate cyclase

CT, cholera toxin; *PT*, pertussis toxin

lyzing capacity of N_s directly, whereas the blockade of the GTPase activity of N_i by pertussis toxin is apparently due to a blockade of the formation of the active $N_i \cdot GTP$ species [2].

Stimulatory and Inhibitory Coupling Mechanisms

Stimulatory and inhibitory hormones, respectively, increase and decrease adenylate cyclase activity by a receptor-dependent activation of N_s and N_i (Fig. 1). From studies in membrane preparations and with purified components, it is evident that the GTP-bound form of the N proteins is the active species, although binding of GTP or its analogs such as GTPγS and Gpp(NH)p, which are resistent to hydrolysis by the N-associated GTPase activities, is not sufficient for activation. This process apparently requires some further changes, which may represent a dissociation of the subunits of N_s and N_i into the respective α- and $\beta\gamma$-subunits. This has been shown to occur with the purified components in detergent solutions upon addition of stable GTP analogs [1, 3]. However, it is not yet clear whether the subunit disso-

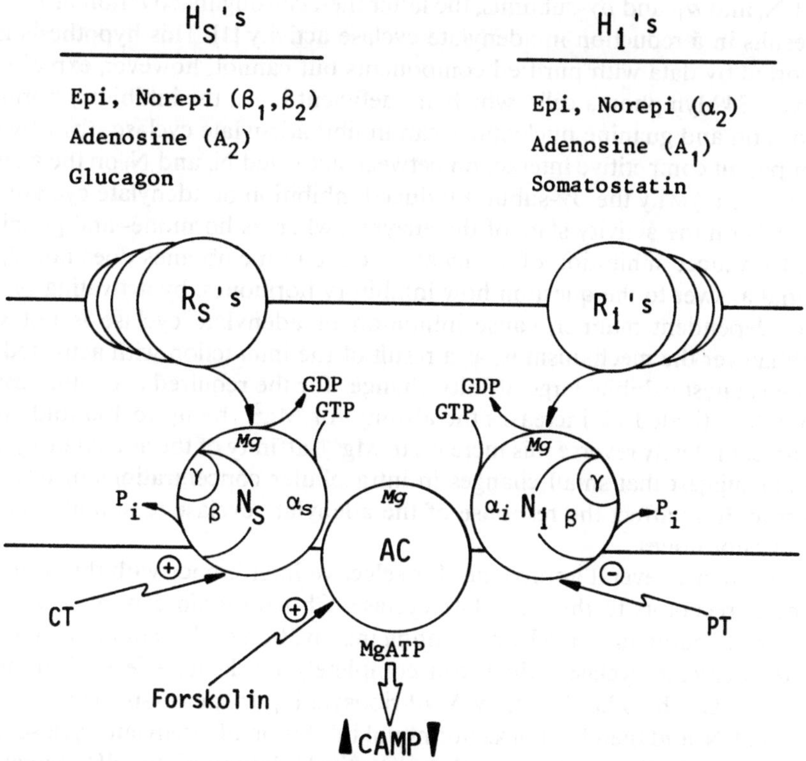

Fig. 1. Constituents of the hormone-sensitive adenylate cyclase system. H_s, H_i, R_s, R_i, N_s, N_i, stimulatory and inhibitory hormones *(H)*, receptors *(R)* and guanine-nucleotide-binding coupling proteins *(N)*; *AC*, adenylate cyclase catalytic moiety; *CT*, cholera toxin; *PT*, pertussis toxin. For further explanations see text

ciation reaction occurs with GTP, is obligatory for stimulation and inhibition of adenylate cyclase, and occurs at all with stimulatory and inhibitory hormones within the intact membrane [3]. Pfeuffer et al. [12] recently reported purification of the Gpp(NH)p-activated adenylate cyclase from rabbit myocardium. They found that the final purification product consisted of two major peptides of M_r 150000 and M_r 42000, apparently representing the catalytic moiety (AC) and the α_s component, respectively. Furthermore, since the $\beta\gamma$-subunits have been shown by Gilman's group to inactivate activated N_s [1], the presently available evidence indicates that activation of adenylate cyclase by N_s is brought about by dissociation of N_s into α_s and $\beta\gamma$, followed by association of activated α_s with AC, which then exhibits increased cyclic AMP-forming activity. The process is apparently terminated by reassociation of α- and $\beta\gamma$-subunits and hydrolysis of α_s-bound GTP to GDP [1, 3].

In the case of N_i, similar dissociation reactions have been described with purified components in detergent solutions as with N_s upon addition of stable GTP analogues [1, 3]. However, it is presently unclear which of the subunits of N_i is inhibitory to the adenylate cyclase and how this inhibition is brought about. Since the activated α_i is a poor inhibitor of the catalyst and since the $\beta\gamma$-subunit of N_i can inhibit adenylate cyclase - but only in the presence of (activated) N_s - it has been proposed that the mechanism of adenylate cyclase inhibition involves a dissociation of N_i into α_i- and $\beta\gamma$-subunits, the latter then causing inactivation of N_s (α_s), which results in a reduction in adenylate cyclase activity [1]. This hypothesis is also supported by data with purified components but cannot, however, explain (a) why in cyc^- S49 lymphoma cells, which are deficient in α_s, the inhibitory hormone somatostatin and guanine nucleotides can inhibit adenylate cyclase; (b) why there is no apparent competitive interaction between activated N_s and N_i on the adenylate cyclase; or (c) why the $\beta\gamma$-subunit-induced inhibition of adenylate cyclase largely depends on the activity state of the enzyme, whereas hormone- and guanine nucleotide-induced inhibition of adenylate cyclase in membranes does not [2]. Thus, the final answer to the question how inhibitory hormones, by activating N_i in a receptor-dependent manner, cause inhibition of adenylate cyclase is not yet known. Whatever the mechanism is, as a result of the interaction with activated N_s and N_i the catalyst exhibits large affinity changes for the required activating cation Mg^{2+}. While activated N_s increases the affinity for Mg^{2+} by up to 100-fold, activated N_i can completely reverse this increase in Mg^{2+} affinity of the adenylate cyclase. These data suggest that small changes in intracellular concentrations of free Mg^{2+} may profoundly affect the response of the adenylate cyclase to stimulatory and inhibitory hormones.

There are several approaches for selective interference with the coupling of hormone receptors to the adenylate cyclase. Cholera toxin can, by ADP-ribosylating the α_s-subunit and thereby preventing inactivation of this component, fully activate the adenylate cyclase, which can completely mask the effect of stimulatory hormones. On the other hand, by ADP-ribosylating α_i, pertussis toxin prevents activation of N_i and thereby blocks hormonal inhibition of adenylate cyclase. N_i or its action can, furthermore, be rather selectively impaired by SH reagents such as *N*-ethylmaleimide and diamide and by several proteolytic enzymes. The site of action of the SH reagents is apparently the α_i-subunit, whereas the target of the proteolytic enzymes in preventing adenylate cyclase inhibition is unknown [2].

Interaction of the Adenylate Cyclase System with Other Signal Transduction Systems

As mentioned above, there seems to be some overlap between the hormone receptors that mediate adenylate cyclase inhibition and those that induce phosphoinositide breakdown, as shown, e.g., with vasopressin, platelet-activating factor and thrombin in human platelets, with bradykinin in neuroblastoma × glioma hybrid cells, and with angiotensin II in adrenal cells [13]. These hormones inhibit adenylate cyclase in membrane preparations by an N_i-mediated process. However, they do not induce the expected fall in cyclic AMP levels in intact cells, where the same hormones increase the formation of inositolphosphates and diacylglycerol by activation of the phospholipase C. These data lead us to study the question as to whether one of the effector systems of the phosphoinositide system, namely the Ca^{2+}-activated, phospholipid-dependent protein kinase (protein kinase C), which is activated by diacylglycerol [14], may interfere with the adenylate cyclase system. As recently reported, activated protein kinase C can prevent inhibitory hormone-induced, N_i-mediated inhibition of adenylate cyclase apparently by phosphorylation of the α-subunit of N_i [15, 16].

These data indicate that the hormone-sensitive adenylate cyclase system can be regulated by phosphorylation-dephosphorylation reactions, a subject not studied so far in great detail, and that the two hormonal signal transduction systems, namely the adenylate cyclase and the phosphoinositide system, are closely linked to each other. There are also some indications that, on the other hand, cyclic AMP can interfere with the phosphoinositide system in human platelets via activation of the cyclic AMP-dependent protein kinase(s). Further studies may even reveal that there are also interactions between the hormone-sensitive adenylate cyclase system and the two other signal transduction systems of membrane-bound receptors, i.e., those receptors that possess tyrosine kinase activity and those acting as specific ion channels.

References

1. Gilman AG (1984) G Proteins and dual control of adenylate cyclase. Cell 36: 577–579
2. Jakobs KH, Aktories K, Minuth M, Schultz G (1985) Inhibition of adenylate cyclase. Adv Cyclic Nucleotide Protein Phosphor Res 19: 137–150
3. Birnbaumer L, Codina J, Mattera R, Cerione RA, Hildebrand JD, Sunyer T, Rojas FJ, Caron MG, Lefkowitz RJ, Iyengar R (1985) Regulation of hormone receptors and adenylyl cyclases by guanine nucleotide binding N proteins. Rec Prog Horm Res 41: 41–94
4. Stiles GL, Caron MG, Lefkowitz RJ (1984) β-Adrenergic receptors: Biochemical mechanisms of physiological regulation. Physiol Rev 64: 661–743
5. Hoffman BB, Michel T, Brenneman TB, Lefkowitz RJ (1982) Interactions of agonists with platelet α_2-adrenergic receptors. Endocrinology 110: 926–932
6. Grandt R, Aktories K, Jakobs KH (1982) Guanine nucleotides and monovalent cations increase agonist affinity of prostaglandin E_2 receptors in hamster adipocytes. Mol Pharmacol 22: 320–326
7. Rojas FJ, Birnbaumer L (1985) Regulation of glucagon receptor binding. Lack of effect of Mg and preferential role for GDP. J Biol Chem 260: 7829–7835

8. Martin MM, Smith MM, Harden TK (1984) Modulation of muscarinic cholinergic receptor affinity for antagonists in rat heart. J Pharmacol Exp Ther 230: 424-430
9. Kahn RA, Gilman AG (1984) Purification of a protein cofactor required for ADP-ribosylation of the stimulatory regulatory component of adenylate cyclase by cholera toxin. J Biol Chem 259: 6228-6234
10. Cassel D, Selinger Z (1976) Catecholamine-stimulated GTPase activity in turkey erythrocyte membranes. Biochem Biophys Acta 452: 538-551
11. Aktories K, Jakobs KH (1981) Epinephrine inhibits adenylate cyclase and stimulates a GTPase in human platelet membranes via α-adrenoceptors. FEBS Lett 130: 235-238
12. Pfeuffer E, Dreher RM, Metzger H, Pfeuffer T (1985) Catalytic subunit of adenylate cyclase: Purification and identification by affinity crosslinking. Proc Natl Acad Sci USA 82: 3086-3090
13. Jakobs KH, Watanabe Y, Bauer S (in press) Interactions between the adenylate cyclase system and the phosphoinositide-metabolizing pathway in human platelets. J Cardiovasc Pharmacol
14. Nishizuka Y (1984) The role of protein kinase C in cell surface signal transduction and tumour promotion. Nature 308: 693-698
15. Jakobs KH, Bauer S, Watanabe Y (1985) Modulation of adenylate cyclase of human platelets by phorbol ester. Impairment of the hormone-sensitive inhibitory pathway. Eur J Biochem 151: 425-430
16. Katada T, Gilman AG, Watanabe Y, Bauer S, Jakobs KH (1985) Protein kinase C phosphorylates the inhibitory guanine nucleotide-binding regulatory component and apparently suppresses its function in hormonal inhibition of adenylate cyclase. Eur J Biochem 151: 431-437

Discussion

Neyses: Clinical experience has shown that beta receptor blockers can have very many desirable but also very many undesirable side effects. Is there any possibility of interfering pharmacologically somewhere in the cAMP system? How would you judge this prospect in the future?

Jakobs: There is one substance, forskolin, which is already undergoing clinical tests. Forskolin, which stimulates adenylate cyclase (Fig. 1) and, if I'm not mistaken, is used in the treatment of glaucoma, appears to be a very useful substance. It has also been tried in heart failure, but I don't think it lived up to expectations. The toxins certainly couldn't work. Some SH-group reagents act selectively on N_i components - again not a possibility that can be used clinically. I am not aware of any such substances, although some may exist.

Göthert: Would it be therapeutically sensible at all to use those substances that interfere with N_s or N_i; a host of systems would be affected, when you consider all the neurotransmitters and hormones involved.

Jakobs: Yes, one might suppose that such substances not only affect parts of the organism. In pseudohypoparathyroidism the N_s components are reduced to activity levels of under 50%. Nevertheless, consider the sodium-potassium ATPase in the cell membrane, which is also a universal system and is needed everywhere. We can influence the activity of this enzyme therapeutically with the cardiac glycosides.

Brodde: Do you know of any other pathologic conditions besides hypoparathyroidism?

Jakobs: Not in humans. There was recently a report on so-called obese mice in whose adipocytes the function of N_i was reported to be disturbed. Otherwise I'm not aware of any.

Aspects of the Pathogenesis of Essential Hypertension

H. Holzgreve

Medizinische Poliklinik, Universität München, Pettenkoferstr. 8 a, 8000 München 2, FRG

Introduction

As early as 2300 B.C. the Yellow Emperor, a lengendary Chinese physician of the Ming Dynasty, made a statement on the cause of high blood pressure that still holds today. He had observed that the constant consumption of highly salted foods "makes the pulse hard" and - replacing his graphic description with succinct modern terms - may lead to stroke and aphasia.

Although this presumably first insight into the cause of elevated blood pressure is now 4000 years old, research of the pathogenesis of hypertension is still beset with problems. The rare, but highly interesting, secondary or symptomatic forms of hypertension have contributed to our knowledge of how blood pressure is regulated in normal and pathologic states. They have taught us that several different causes underlie a persistent increase in blood pressure. To this day, however, our knowledge of the exact cause of the far commoner form of hypertension, essential or primary

Table 1. Possible factors involved in the pathogenesis of essential hypertension

Adrenoceptor status
Alcohol consumption
Baroreceptor reflexes
Body weight
Catecholamines and their metabolism
Cellular transport of electrolytes
Diet (sodium, potassium, calcium)
Drugs (e.g., hormonal contraceptives)
Emotional, psychosocial factors and stress
Genetic factors
Hormonal inhibition of cellular transport
Intracellular cation concentrations
Kidney diseases
Neuroendocrine factors (e.g., vasopressin, endorphine, serotonin)
Renal functional abnormalities
Renin-angiotensin-aldosteron-system
Salt sensitivity
Vascular reactivity
Vasodepressorfunction (e.g., prostaglandins)

New Aspects in Hypertension: Adrenoceptors
M. Middeke and H. Holzgreve (Eds.)
Springer-Verlag, Berlin Heidelberg New York 1986

hypertension, is still inadequate (2; 13). The current state of incomplete knowledge is still best described by the "mosaic theory of hypertension" as formulated by Page in 1963 in which many facets of blood pressure control are pictured [21].

In recent years a number of findings on the cause of essential hypertension have been presented. The studies dealing with this problem have been considerably advanced from an experimental point of view by the recognition of so-called spontaneously hypertensive rats (SH rats) as a model for essential hypertension in humans. All of the factors and mechanisms cited in Table 1 are thought to be involved in the pathogenesis of hypertension, although the list is not meant to be exhaustive. In interpreting the experimental and clinical research results two persistent questions arise for which definitive answers have yet to be found.

- Is a specific finding the primary cause of essential hypertension or only a manifestation of the elevated blood pressure?
- Is a specific finding the cause of hypertension or only a permissive factor of another, perhaps still unknown, anomaly?

Despite these difficulties, an attempt will be made in the following to schematically order the manifold findings on the pathogenesis of essential hypertension (Fig. 1).

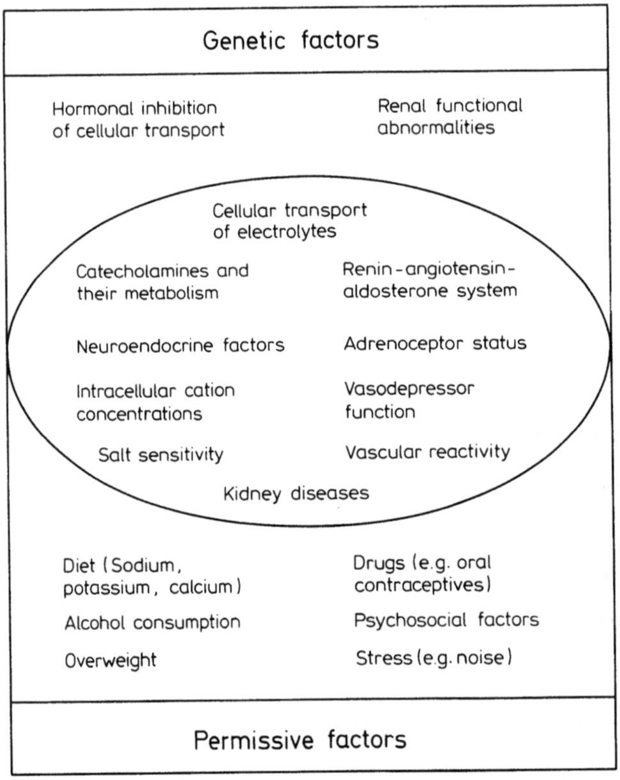

Fig. 1. Pathogenesis of essential hypertension

Genetic Factors

The history of persons with high blood pressure should always include the question as to whether hypertension is present in the family. Indeed, a number of findings have pointed to a hereditary component in the pathogenesis of essential hypertension - not only in laboratory animals but also in humans (17). For example, there is a marked correlation of blood pressure between parents, children and siblings. The relationship between parents and children has been shown in newborns just 5 days after birth [25]. Studies with twins have also shown an agreement in blood pressure with a correlation coefficient of 0.55-0,58 in monozygotic twins and 0.25-0.27 in dizygotic twins [9].

On the other hand, between spouses, between parents and adopted children, and between natural and adopted children of a family the correlation of blood pressure behavior is either extremely low or nonexistent [6, 10, 14, 15, 20].

Thus, the familial aggregation of essential hypertension is not due to common life styles, e.g., nutrition, but rather to genetically determined factors. Despite some differences of opinion, it is generally assumed today that essential hypertension is inherited polygenically and that hereditary factors determine the development of essential hypertension to an extent of 30%-80%. The decisive question is how can this genetic predisposition for essential hypertension be detected morphologically, biochemically, or functionally. At present two possibilities exist: (1) Hormonal inhibition of transmembrane electrolyte transport; and (2) renal functional disturbances.

1. Hormonal inhibition of transmembrane electrolyte transport. As early as 1960, Losse and coworkers reported on elevated concentrations of sodium in the erythrocytes of patients with essential hypertension [18]. Following a long latency period, these findings were taken up, largely confirmed, and expanded, first by French and American groups [7, 12] and then by a number of other researchers [16]. These studies indicated that sodium-lithium countertransport was enhanced and sodium-potassium cotransport depressed in patients with essential hypertension. Later, a substance was identified in the serum of patients with essential hypertension that inhibits the activity of sodium-potassium ATPase [19] and impairs the transport of sodium out of cells in both hypertensive and normotensive persons, leading to elevated intracellular sodium concentrations [22]. The calcium concentration in the erythrocytes and thrombocytes of hypertensives have also been reported to be elevated [8, 30].

It cannot be conclusively decided which of these changes are primary or secondary. Possibly the altered concentration of the hormone that inhibits sodium transport at the cell membrane is the primary, genetically determined defect. In that case, essential hypertension would constitute an "endocrinopathy," and the transmembrane electrolyte transport disturbance and elevated intracellular sodium and calcium concentrations would be a consequence of the endocrine disturbance. However, both phenomena, namely the presence of the hormone-like substance and the disturbed transmembrane electrolyte transport, are certainly the expression of a genetic predisposition and not a result of high blood pressure, because electrolyte transport disturbances and elevated intracellular sodium and calcium concentrations are found not only in patients with manifest essential hypertension, but also in persons with a family history of hypertension who are still normotensive. They are not found in patients with secondary forms of high blood pressure or in normotensive subjects without a genetic disposition [7, 12, 30].

2. Renal functional disturbances. Another body of evidence suggests a different possibility, namely that the genetic predisposition for essential hypertension manifests itself primarily in a renal functional disturbance. A rat strain bred in Milan develops high blood pressure that is very similar to essential hypertension in humans. When the kidneys of these animals are transplanted into normal rats, the blood pressure of the recipient rises. On the other hand, the elevated blood pressure drops when the kidneys of normal rats are implanted in animals with a genetic predisposition for hypertension [3]. In addition, these animals exhibit a renal functional disturbance that disappears as soon as the hypertension becomes manifest.

Similar findings have been observed in normotensive persons between 14 and 30 years of age with a familial predisposition for hypertension. The offspring of parents, both of whom had blood pressure values of 150/95 mmHg or above, were compared with the offspring of parents with blood pressure values below 140/90 mmHg. In subjects who were still normotensive themselves but whose parents had hypertension, the glomerular filtration rate, renal plasma flow, and 24-h urine volume were increased and the plasma renin activity depressed [4, 5]. There is no doubt that in the long term, hypertension leads to kidney damage. However, since such changes are apparently detectable only in the prehypertensive state and disappear after manifestation of the hypertension, they cannot be the consequence but must rather be the cause of the hypertension.

According to the current state of knowledge, the aforementioned hormonal inhibition of transmembrane sodium transport and the renal functional disturbances are very probably the direct expression of a genetic predisposition, especially since they are already present in the prehypertensive phase of essential hypertension. The most convincing evidence for this hypothesis would surely be if one could reliably predict the later manifestation of essential hypertension by demonstrating the presence of MacGregor's hormone, the transmembrane transport disturbance or the renal functional disturbance in the prehypertensive stage.

Permissive Factors

It has long been known that a genetic disposition alone is not sufficient for the development of hypertension and that other factors also play a role. The factors known as permissive factors, which are shown at the lower end of Fig. 1, are of special practical significance because only they - and not a genetic disposition and its direct consequences - are amenable to antihypertensive prophylaxis and therapy.

Epidemiologic studies on numerous population groups have shown that the incidence of hypertension is related to salt intake (Fig. 2). In certain populations, such as the Carajas in Brazil, the Eskimos, members of the Kung tribe in Botswana, and the Pukapukas in Polynesia, who consume less than 4 g salt per day, high blood

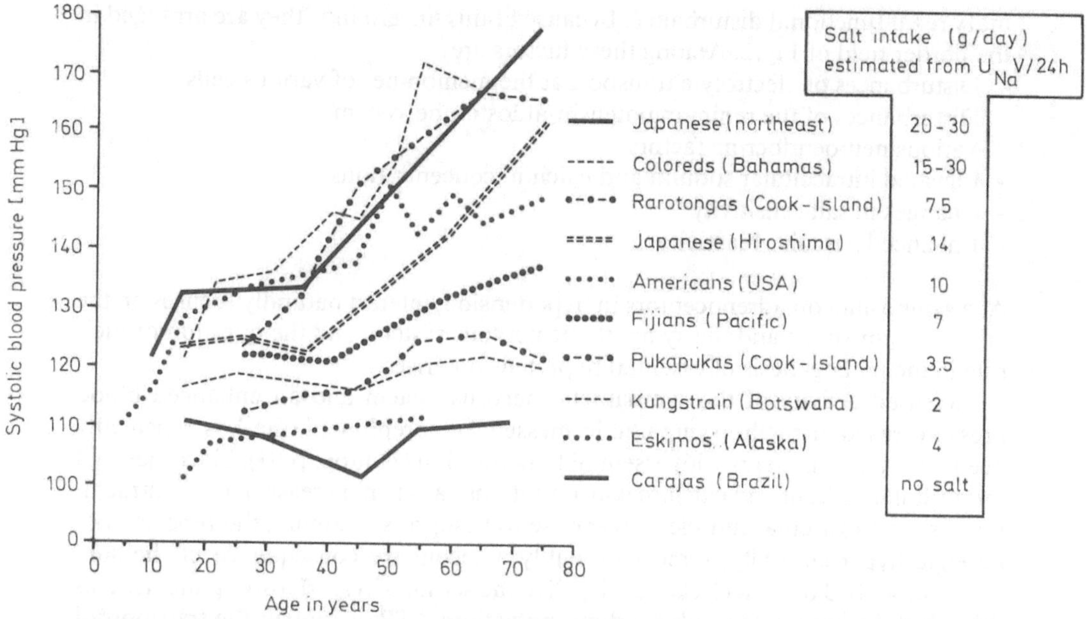

Fig. 2. Correlation between daily salt consumption (in g) and mean systolic blood pressure (mmHg) in different age groups and several populations

pressure is virtually unkown, even in advanced age. By contrast, populations that consume large quantities of salt, e.g., people in northeast Japan and the black population on the Bahamas, are among those with the highest incidence of hypertension.

In terms of conception and consequence, it appears expedient to define the above-described hormonal changes and electrolyte transport disturbance as the primary genetic defect and the high salt intake as a permissive factor.

A further permissive factor is overweight [23, 24, 28]. Adipose persons have a two- to eightfold higher risk of having hypertension or of developing it in the course of the next few years. According to this classification, numerous other factors, e.g., alcohol consumption, certain drugs (e.g., oral contraceptives), psychosocial factors, and stress [1; 27; 29], perhaps also dietary calcium, are regarded as permissive factors.

Secondary Consequences of a Genetic Predisposition

A number of other changes and disturbances have been described in patients with essential hypertension, and sometimes also in normotensive subjects with a familial predisposition for hypertension, which theoretically could also constitute the functional or biochemical substrate of the genetic predisposition but which are probably only the consequence of the hormonal inhibition of sodium transport or the pri-

mary renal functional disturbance. Because of this uncertainty, they are arranged in the border field of Fig. 2. Among these factors are:
- Disturbances of electrolyte transport at the membranes of various cells
- Disturbances of the renin-angiotensin-aldosterone system
- Various neuroendocrine factors
- Elevated intracellular sodium and calcium concentrations
- Changes in salt sensitivity
- Enhanced vascular reactivity

At a symposium on adrenoceptors in hypertension, interest naturally focuses on the adrenoceptor status and the sympathetic nervous system, and the question of their role in the pathogenesis of essential hypertension arises.

Increased activity of the sympathetic nervous system and an enhanced blood pressure reaction to the sympathetic messenger norephinephrine has repeatedly been reported in patients with essential hypertension (Philipp, p. 91). Since elevated intracellular sodium and calcium concentrations cause an increase in the contractility of smooth vascular muscle in response to vasopressor stimuli, the reported adrenergic hypersensitivity is most probably a secondary consequence of the substance described by MacGregor et al. [19] in the serum of hypertensive patients. This substance is reported to inhibit sodium-potassium ATPase, impair the transport of sodium out of the cell, and produce an increase in intracellular sodium and calcium concentrations.

The adrenoceptor status of hypertensive patients could be analogous. Altered receptor density and disturbed regulation could readily be incorporated in the pathogenetic chain "hormonal disturbance - impairment of transmembrane electrolyte transport - elevated sodium and calcium concentrations - enhanced vascular reactivity" in patients with essential hypertension (Middeke, p. 103). Fraser et al. found that an increase in salt intake from 10 to 400 mval/l resulted in an increase in lymphocytic beta$_2$-adrenoceptors [11]. Accordingly, the altered adrenoceptor status could be a secondary consequence of the elevated intracellular electrolyte concentrations and a tertiary consequence of the substance described by MacGregor et al. [19]. In this case, the disturbed transmembrane electrolyte transport, the increase in intracellular electrolyte concentrations, the increase in adrenoceptor density, and the enhanced vascular reactivity would all be consequences of a genetically determined endocrinopathy.

Summary

An attempt is made to arrange the numerous findings concerning the pathogenesis of essential hypertension in an ordered system. Accordingly, the various pathogenetic mechanisms can be assigned to three levels:

1. Disturbances that are direct morphologic, biochemical, or functional expressions of a genetic predisposition, e.g., a hormonal disturbance of transmembrane sodium transport or a genetically determined renal functional disturbance, as described by Bianchi et al. [3, 4].

2. Changes that are secondary consequences of the primary genetical predisposition, e.g., enhanced vascular reactivity or changes that are a consequence of the elevated blood pressure, e.g., nephropathy.
3. Permissive factors that promote the manifestation of the genetic predisposition, e.g., high salt intake.

References

1. Andren L, Piros S, Hansson L (1982) Different hemodynamic reaction patterns during noise exposure in normotensives with and without heredity for essential hypertension. 9th Scientific meeting of the international society of hypertension, Mexico, Abstract 20, February 21-24, 1982
2. Berglund G, Andersson O, Wilhelmsen L (1976) Prevalence of primary and secondary hypertension: Studies in a random population sample. Br Med J 554
3. Bianchi G, Fox U, di Francesco GF, Giovanetti AM, Pagetti D (1974) Blood pressure changes produced by kidney cross transplantation between spontaneously hypertensive rats and normotensive rats. Clin Sci Mol Med 47: 435
4. Bianchi G, Gatti M, Ferrari P, Picotti GB, Colombo G, Velis O, Cusi D, Lupi GP, Barlassina C, Bracchi G, Gori D, Mazzei D (1979) A renal abnormality as a possible cause of "essential" hypertension. Lancet 1: 173
5. Bianchi G, Cusi D, Barlassina C, Lupi P, Gatti M, Salvioli G, Ferrari P, Picotti GB, Elli A (1982) Renal function difference between young normotensive offspring of two hypertensive and two normotensive parents. 9th Scientific meeting of the international society of hypertension, Mexico, Abstract 43, February 21-24, 1982
6. Biron P, Mongeau J, Bertrans D (1976) Familial aggregation of blood pressure in 558 adopted children. Can Med Assoc J 115: 773
7. Canessa M, Adragna N, Solomon HS, Connolly TM, Tosteson DC (1980) Increased sodium-lithium countertransport in red cells of patients with essential hypertension. N Engl J Med 302: 772
8. Erne P, Bolli P, Bürgisser E, Bühler FR (1984) Correlation of platelet calcium with blood pressure. Effect of antihypertensive therapy. N Engl J Med 310: 1084
9. Feinleib M, Garrison R, Borhani N, Rosenman R, Christian J (1975) Studies of hypertension in twins. In: Paul O (ed) Epidemiology and control of hypertension. Thieme, Stuttgart, p 3
10. Feinleib M, Robert PH, Garrison RJ (1979) The contribution of family studies to the partitioning of population variations of blood pressure. In: Genetic analysis of common diseases. Liss, New York, p 653
11. Fraser J, Nadeau J, Robertson D, Wood AJJ (1981) Regulation of human leukocyte beta receptors by endogenous catecholamines. Relationship of leucocyte beta receptor density to the cardiac sensitivity to Isoproterenol. J Clin Invest 67: 1777
12. Garvy RP, Elghozi J-L, Dagher G, Meyer P (1980) Laboratory distinction between essential and secondary hypertension by measurement of erythrocyte cation fluxes. N Engl J Med 302: 769
13. Greminger P, Vetter W, Zimmermann K, Beckerhoff R, Siegenthaler W (1977) Primäre und sekundäre Hypertonie in einem poliklinischen Patientengut. Schweiz Med Wochenschr 107: 605
14. Hamilton M, Pickering CW, Roberts JAF, Sowry CSC (1954) The aetiology of essential hypertension. 4. The role of inheritance. Clin Sci 13: 273
15. Hayes CG, Tyroler HA, Cassel JC (1971) Family aggregation of blood pressure in Evans County, Georgia. Arch Intern Med 128: 965
16. Hilton PJ (1986) Cellular sodium transport in essential hypertension. N Engl J Med 314: 222
17. Klaus D (1981) Genetische Disposition - eine Ursache der essentiellen Hypertonie. Dtsch Med Wochenschr 106: 1523
18. Losse H, Wehmeyer H, Wessels F (1960) Der Wasser- und Elektrolytgehalt von Erythrozyten bei arterieller Hypertonie. Klin Wochenschr 38: 393
19. MacGregor GA, Fenton S, Alaghband-Zadeh J, Markandu N, Roulston JE, de Wardener HE (1981) Evidence for a raised concentration of a circulating sodium transport inhibitor in essential hypertension. Br Med J 283: 1355

20. Miall WE, Heneage P, Khosla T, Lovell HG, Moore F (1967) Factors influencing the degree of resemblance in arterial pressure of close relatives. Clin Sci 33: 271
21. Page IH (1963) The nature of arterial hypertension. Arch Intern Med 111: 103
22. Poston L, Sewell RB, Wilkinson SP, Richardson PJ, Williams R, Clarkson EM, MacGregor GA, de Wardener HE (1981) Evidence for a circulating sodium transport inhibitor in essential hypertension. Br Med J 282: 847
23. Ramsay LE, Ramsay MH, Hettiarachchi J, Davis DL, Winchester J (1978) Weight reduction in a blood pressure clinic. Br Med J 244
24. Reisin E, Abel R, Modan M, Silverberg DS, Eliahou HE, Modan B (1978) Effect of weight loss without salt restriction. N Engl J Med 298: 1
25. Scherer B, Friedmann B, Dumbs A, Holzmann K, Weber PC (1981) Urinary prostaglandins in human neonates: relationship to kidney function and blood pressure. Klin Wochenschr 58: 449
26. Skrabal F (1981) Prävention und nicht-medikamentöse Therapie des Hochdrucks. Münch Med Wochenschr 123: 1791
27. Schulte W, Neus H, von Eiff AW (1981) Blutdruckreaktivität unter emotionalem Streß bei unkomplizierten Formen des Hochdrucks. Klin Wochenschr 59: 1243
28. Tyroler HA, Heyden S, Hames CG (1975) Weight and hypertension: Evans county study of blacks and whites. In: Paul O (ed) Epidemiology and control of hypertension. Thieme, Stuttgart, p 177
29. von Eiff AW, Neus H (1980) Verkehrslärm und Hypertonie-Risiko. Münch Med Wochenschr 122: 894
30. Zidek W, Losse H, Dorst KG, Zumkley H, Vetter H (1982) Intracellular sodium and calcium in essential hypertension. Klin Wochenschr 60: 859

Discussion

von Eiff: In recent studies we saw that in children there is not only a relationship between blood pressure at rest and the heredity of blood pressure, but most notably that children with a genetic predisposition show hyperactivity though reacting differently to emotional and psychic stress factors. Boys and girls react differently even before puberty; but with regard to heredity, at the time of puberty boys' blood pressure rises while that of girls remains at the same level due to an estrogenic protective mechanism. On the basis of all the studies we have conducted so far I believe that the factor is ultimately hypothalamic. This would certainly fit in with your theory about the sodium inhibition factor, which might also be controlled hypothalamically. The experiments we carried out do in fact support the view that hypersensitivity – which can be found from childhood to adult age in normotonic persons with a genetic predisposition and in essential hypertensives – primarily involves not a hyperreactivity of the vascular system but rather a central hyperactivity. The permissive factors would then also interfere in this mechanism. I think that should be added as a third possibility.

Holzgreve: I'm not so sure it's really needed as a third possibility. If, for example, the primary genetically determined defect is an intracellular change of electrolyte concentrations, this is certainly a systemic defect. Then it would have to be present in the brain as well.

Unidentified: If the inhibition of active sodium-potassium transport is of decisive importance in the genesis of hypertension, then we should expect that patients receiving long-term digitalis medication, in whom 10%–30% of the sodium-potassium transport is inhibited for years, would develop hypertension. Are there any studies on whether these patients have elevated blood pressure?

Holzgreve: Digitalis therapy is no risk factor for hypertension.

Philipp: There are, after all, various ATPases; it need not necessarily be the oubain-inhibitable sodium-postassium ATPase. As far as I am aware, there are various studies that show that oubain-inhibitable ATPase does not differ between hypertensive patients and normotensives. It is certainly conceivable that other sodium-potassium ATPases are inhibited by this suspected natriuretic factor.

Lemmer: You keep referring to the substance described by McGregor. Have we meanwhile learned a bit more about it?

Holzgreve: That's the problem where we're just not getting any farther. Larry Early, I think, first spoke of an additional third factor in the mid-1960s. Then came all the studies by de Wardener, but I don't have the impression that these older studies or the more recent McGregor studies have identified a substance that you can really take and synthesize or that has been analyzed and is available. At least I'm not aware of any.

Koella: Let's assume that in hypertension due to some genetically determined factors we have a disturbance in the central and peripheral adrenosympathetic system. Now we know that the central adrenergic system performs a host of functions. My question: Are there studies in which an attempt has been made to determine whether certain additional typical clinical pictures (typical in the sense of a disturbances, say, of the central adrenergic system) lead to hypertension? A banal example: We have some justification for assuming that depression is probably due to an underfunctioning of central noradrenergic functions. Is there a possibility of finding such a disturbance at the same time or in a large percentage of hypertensives?

Holzgreve: Basically you are asking whether the patient with essential hypertension has an additional disease or an additional symptom that characterizes him as a hypertensive. The answer is no, unless one analyzes the long list of various changes which I tried to assign an order to. Which are the primary, which the secondary effects? But if I understood your question correctly, whether hypertensives have a special syndrome, a characteristic sign that would characterize them as hypertensives, I'm not aware of any. We'd certainly like to have something of that nature. Then we could recognize a person at birth as a potential hypertensive.

Koella: I didn't mean it in the sense of an obligatory accompanying symptom – more in the sense of an aggregation of certain diseases that might also be related to disturbances of central adrenergic systems.

Holzgreve: I'd answer this question with no, unless we confuse secondary diseases with hypertension, unless we designate something as a secondary disease of hypertension which in reality is a disease entity in its own right.

von Eiff: Dr. Koella, that was extremely interesting. I interpreted your question somewhat differently. You would presuppose if, for example, a central hyperactivity of the sympathetic system is present, that the blood pressure is low during a depression. That would be exactly the opposite of the actual situation. That's how I interpreted your question. And that is the ultimate question: What happens in the initial phase of hypertension? These central signs of hyperactivity are present only in the initial phase. Afterwards the peripheral mechanisms have gained so much dominance that the central mechanisms play a role at most again in the development of malignant hypertension. So, your question is whether a change in the clinical picture takes place in the initial phase of hypertension with concurrent endogenous depression. Have I understood your question correctly?

Koella: Absolutely. You could also turn it around. Since reduced central adrenergic activity is expected in depression, one could say that hypertensive patients typically have no depression. Or now in a positive light, we have evidence indicating that anxiety is associated with a central adrenergic underactivity. It is therefore conceivable that there is typically a high incidence of anxiety in hypertensives?

Göthert: I'd like to comment on one other point. In the whole of the discussion so far and also in your scheme only the sympathoadrenergic system is mentioned among the neurogenic factors. I believe one must also include serotonin in this consideration of the development of hypertension. It has been demonstrated in a whole series of experiments that in spontaneously hypertensive rats, for example, stimulation of the dorsal raphe nuclei can produce a much stronger hypertensive reaction than in Wistar Kyoto control rats. There is another body of evidence that indicates that the serotonin system may also be involved in the development of hypertension. For example, a new antihypertensive based on 5HT2 receptor blockade has been introduced into therapy.

Holzgreve: I can only thank you for this addition. I did not mention that and wanted to unite serotonin and everything else under the key word neuroendocrine factors, which also includes the endorphines. The question still remains, Dr. Göthert, as to whether that is to be classified as an expression of the primary defect. Or could these all be secondary effects of another principle we are looking for?

Sympathetic Nervous System in Essential Hypertension: Activity and Reactivity

T. PHILIPP

Universitätsklinikum Steglitz, Medizinische Klinik u. Poliklinik, Freie Universität Berlin
Hindenburgdamm 30, 1000 Berlin 45, FRG

Introduction

So far, only partial aspects of the pathogenesis of essential hypertension (EH) are known. Many findings indicate an increased activity of the sympathetic nervous system in patients with EH. Pathophysiological considerations of the role of the sympathetic nervous system in essential hypertension are based on two findings:

1. The sympathetic nervous system plays a decisive part in maintaining and regulating normal blood pressure.
2. Drugs which interfere with the sympathetic nervous system, such as ganglionic blockers, reserpine, clonidine, methyldopa, and α- and β-blockers are particularly effective in lowering high blood pressure.

Methods for the Registration of Sympathetic Activity

Direct registration of the sympathetic neural activity can be done by measuring the electric potentials of the sympathetic nerve fibers, a method which can now also be used in humans [1, 2]. Indirect measurements of the sympathetic nervous system activity are obtained on the basis of plasma and urinary levels of catecholamines and their derivatives. During the last few years, there has been an intensive scientific dispute over the value of direct nerve activity measurements [3], on the one hand, and the determination of plasma catecholamines [4] on the other. It is obvious that exact and direct registration of the sympathetic nervous system activity is achieved by measuring the nerve potentials. It is, however, not clear whether the sympathetic nerve fibers of the skin and muscles, whose potentials can be registered at present, are representative of the activity of the entire sympathetic nervous system [4]. In addition, this procedure is complicated and can only be performed by few centers.

There is also much criticism of plasma catecholamine determination for analyzing sympathetic neural activity [3]. The main objection is based on the fact that plasma noradrenaline concentration represents only a minor portion (less than 5%) of the noradrenaline released by the synaptic cleft. Depending on the metabolism, the noradrenaline level could lead to an over- or underestimation of sympathetic activi-

New Aspects in Hypertension: Adrenoceptors
M. Middeke and H. Holzgreve (Eds.)
Springer-Verlag Berlin Heidelberg New York 1986

ty [3]. Animal experiments, however, have shown that stimulation of the sympathetic fibers leading to the heart result in a directly proportional increase in plasma catecholamines [5]. Furthermore, simultaneous determination of sympathetic neural activity and plasma catecholamine levels shows a good positive correlation [6, 7].

Finally, modern procedures permit reproducible and exact determinations of urinary and plasma catecholamines. The determinations are often repeatable and can be done everywhere, so that on the basis of the present state of knowledge a sufficiently exact assessment of sympathetic neural activity by determining plasma and urinary levels of catecholamines is possible.

Urinary Catecholamines in Essential Hypertension

In an overview, de Champlain [8] compiled the results of 22 studies comparing catecholamine excretion of patients with EH with that of normotensive subjects. Seven of these studies described an increased excretion of noradrenaline and/or adrenaline. Eleven studies did not reveal any difference between the two groups, and in four studies reduced excretion was found in patients with EH (Table 1). However, the studies describing reduced excretion were done before 1964, so that their methodologic evaluation is limited.

We determined noradrealine excretion in 59 patients with essential hypertension during nightly rest and a defined 3-h period in an upright position, and compared the results with the levels measured in 20 normotensive and age-matched controls [9]. This study showed that noradrenaline excretion of patients with EH and normal plasma renin activity ($n=36$) was increased during rest and particularly during standing for a defined period of time (Fig. 1). Patients with EH and low plasma renin activity, on the other hand, did not differ from normotensive controls.

Sympathetic activity in the patient group with low plasma renin activity is generally assumed to be decreased [10], so that in this group of mostly older persons, consequences of hypertension are more often seen as the cause [10].

Table 1. Results of representative studies assessing pathophysiological importance of sympathetic nervous activity in EH

Catecholamine excretion	7 × ↑, 11 × n, 4 × ↓
Plasma catecholamines	9 × ↑, 3 × n
Plasma norepinephrine	25 × ↑, 39 × n
Plasma epinephrine	15 × ↑, 16 × n
Plasma dopamine	6 × n
Conjugated catecholamines	↑
Dopamine-β-hydroxylase	3 × ↑, 5 × n, 1 × ↓
Norepinephrine spillover rate	(↑), n

Most of the data are summarized in the literature [8, 12].
n, no difference between hypertensives and normotensives.

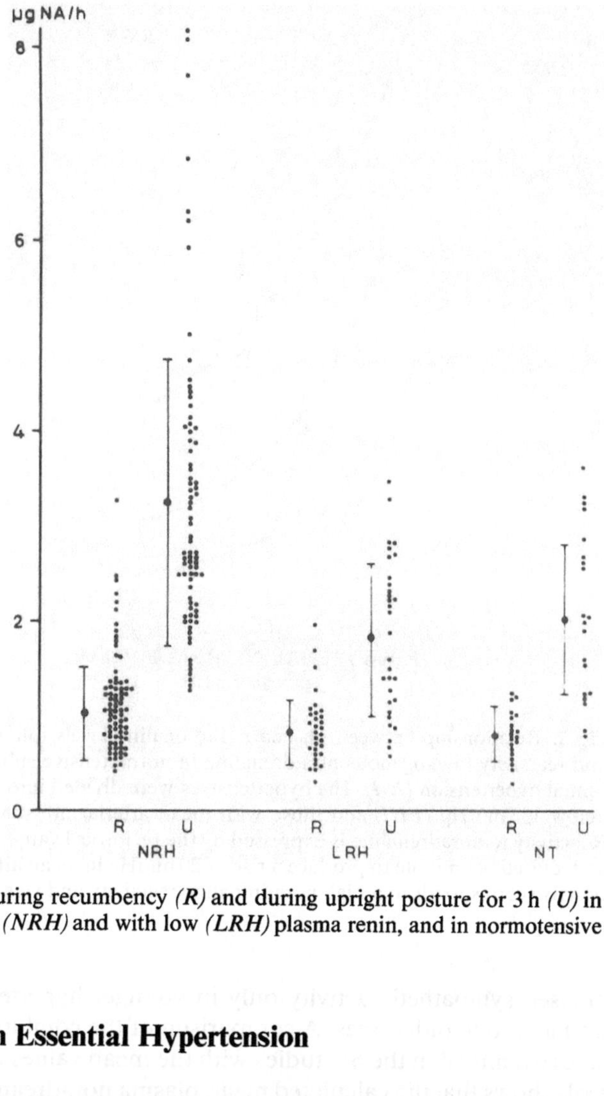

Fig. 1. Noradrenaline excretion during recumbency *(R)* and during upright posture for 3 h *(U)* in hypertensive patients with normal *(NRH)* and with low *(LRH)* plasma renin, and in normotensive control subjects *(NT)*

Plasma Catecholamines in Essential Hypertension

In the last few years, Goldstein has published various papers analyzing the numerous studies dealing with the question of whether plasma catecholamine concentration is increased in EH. The statements of various studies given in Fig. 2 are mainly based on the analyses by Goldstein [11, 12, 13]. Of the older studies, which mainly determined total plasma catecholamine concentrations, the majority described an increase in plasma catecholamines in aptients with EH. As more precise determination methods (radioenzymatic test, HPLC) were developed, the percentage of studies demonstrating an increased sympathetic neural activity in patients with EH decreased. Furthermore, many studies did not pay sufficient attention to the fact that plasma catecholamine levels increase in older normotensives and that consequently the age of the control group is of particular importance. Goldstein [13] was also able to show that all studies had demonstrated relevant characteristics of in-

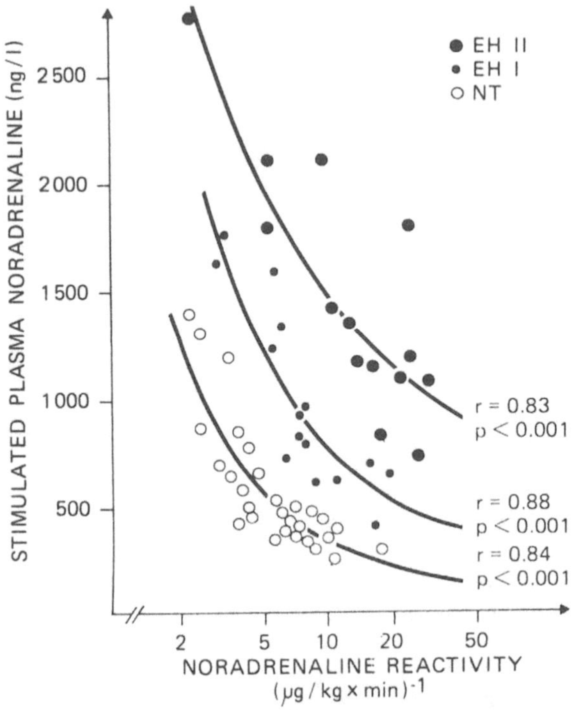

Fig. 2. Relationship between plasma noradrenaline levels following ergometry (100 W for 2 min) and reactivity to exogenous noradrenaline in normotensive subjects *(NT)* and in patients with essential hypertension *(EH)*. The hypertensives were divided into those with mean arterial pressures below 135 mmHg *(EHI)* and those with mean arterial pressures of 135 mmHg or more *(EHII)*. Reactivity to noradrenaline is expressed by the reciprocal values of the amounts of noradrenaline/kg required per minute to produce a rise of 20 mmHg in mean arterial pressure. A high value on the *abscissa* corresponds to a high noradrenaline reactivity and vice versa. [35]

creased sympathetic activity only in younger hypertensives (under the age of 40) and less so in older ones. A comparison of the combined data of all 2932 hypertensives examined in the 64 studies with the mean values of all 1825 normotensive controls shows that the calculated mean plasma noradreanline level of all hypertensives (280 ± 140 pg/ml) is almost 25% higher than the level of the normotensive controls (225 ± 10 pg/ml; $p < 0.001$).

Goldstein's analysis of the adrenaline levels shows that an increase was found in 50% of the studies. However, in most studies which did not find a statistically confirmed difference between hypertensives and normotensives ($n = 16$), the mean adrenal levels of hypertensive patients were higher ($n = 11$) than the control levels. It is possible that, in essential hypertension, adrenal levels are of particular pathophysiological importance [14].

Few studies have examined the common precursor of catecholamines, plasma dopamine. None of these studies, however, has revealed a difference between hypertensive patients and normotensive controls. This may mean that dopamine-β-hydroxylase, the enzyme which catalyzes the transformation of dopamine to noradrenaline, plays a decisive pathophysiological role. Some authors [15, 16, 17] found increased dopamine-β-hydroxylase in patients with EH, and Geffen et al. [18] described a direct positive correlation between diastolic blood pressure and serum dopamine-β-hydroxylase activity. We [9] and the vast majority of other authors [19-22] have not been able to demonstrate a difference in dopamine-β-hydroxylase activity between hypertensives and normotensives. Lawton et al. [23] even found lower dopamine-β-hydroxylase activity in hypertensives.

Individual reports indicate that conjugate plasma catecholamines are elevated in patients with EH [24] and that catecholamine clearance is increased [25] or the spillover rate of noradrenaline is higher [26] in borderline hypertension.

Increased Sympathetic Nervous System Activity and Essential Hypertension

Considering the data presented above, the sympathetic nervous activity in patients with essential hypertension seems to be slightly increased. The fact that elevated levels of plasma noradrenaline are especially found in younger patients [11] and in patients with normal renin activity [11] but not in older patients with low renin activity [14] supports the assumption that an increased sympathetic activity could be related to the development of hypertension and declines in importance with the progress of hypertensive disease.

Nevertheless, the minor increase in sympathetic nervous activity alone cannot be responsible for the blood pressure elevation, since in patients with pheochromocytoma where the dependency of the blood pressure on the elevated catecholamine level is obvious, plasma catecholamine levels have been described to be 10- to 1000-fold higher than in patients with essential hypertension [27]. On the other hand, increased plasma noradrenaline levels comparable to those in patients with essential hypertension have also been observed in patients with normal or even low blood pressure, e.g., in patients with hypothyroidism [28], adrenal insufficiency [29], or endogenous depression [30].

Therefore, if increased sympathetic tone is thought to be of importance in high blood pressure, it should be assumed that the pressor response to the sympathetic neurotransmitter noradrenaline is concomitantly increased.

Reactivity in Essential Hypertension

Goldenberg et al. [31] were the first to observe that patients with arterial hypertension responded to i.v. administration of noradrenaline with a more pronounced blood pressure increase than normotensive patients. The increased circulatory reactivity to noradrenaline in patients with EH could often be confirmed in the following years [32, 33, 34, 35]. Hypertensives also revealed an increased reactivity to noradrenaline in smaller vascular regions, such as the forearm [36], the capillary bed of the nail fold [37], and the digital circulation [38]. An observation common to all investigations, however, is that a distinctly increased reactivity to noradrenaline could only be confirmed in a certain number of patients, while 30%-60% of patients revealed unaltered responsiveness compared with normotensive controls. The reasons for the increased vascular reactivity are unclear. Basically, two diverging interpretations may be possible: on the one hand, the increased reactivity may have been due to structural organic changes [39]. These considerations are based upon the fact that a decrease in vascular lumen and particularly an increase in the ratio of vascular wall to vessel lumen in fourfold potency leads to increased flow resistance. Thus, even slight structural changes may result in a distinct reactivity increase in a vascular region. On the other hand, the increase in reactivity may be due to functional changes: an increased intracellular calcium content [40, 41], which is thought to be present in smooth vascular muscles of hypertensives, and an increase of intracellular calcium-transporting proteins [42], or a change of the adrenoceptor function [43] can contribute to a functional reactivity increase. Structural vascular changes, however, should lead to an unspecific increase of reactivity-like changes of intracellular calcium content or calcium-transporting proteins. Alterations in specific adrenoceptors would inevitably result in a selective reactivity increase for catecholamines.

Our own findings [35] point to a selective increase in noradrenaline reactivity in EH.

Sympathetic Nerve Activity and Noradrenaline Reactivity in Essential Hypertension

Neither the moderate and inconstant increase of sympathetic nerve activity nor the only slight increase of circulatory reactivity to noradrenaline alone can explain the blood pressure rise in EH. Taking both parameters into consideration, it can be demonstrated [35] that there is an inverse relationship between both parameters in normotensive patients. High sympathetic nerve activity (high plasma noradrenaline concentration) is accompanied by low reactivity to noradrenaline and vice versa. This relation seems to be based on automatic regulatory characteristics which are to maintain blood pressure at a normotensive level. In patients with EH there was a fundamental disorder in this automatic regulatory correlation of both parameters (Fig. 2).

In the presence of increased sympathetic nerve activity, no adequate decrease in noradrenaline reactivity can be observed and vice versa. With rising blood pressure values, the relationship between both parameters appears to be more and more impaired. By means of multiple regression, we were able to prove that blood pressure levels are largely determined by the reciprocal relationship of the two parameters (Fig. 3). Thus, the inadequate adjustment of noradrenaline reactivity to the normal or slightly increased sympathetic nerve activity seems to play an important role in blood pressure increase in EH.

An inverse relationship can also be found between increased plasma renin activity, which is known to be a reliable measure of the angiotensin II level, and reactivity to angiotensin II [44, 45, 46]. In patients with EH, however, this relation is maintained in a modified pattern [35], so that structural organic changes in the vascular system cannot be applied to describe this pathophysiological concept.

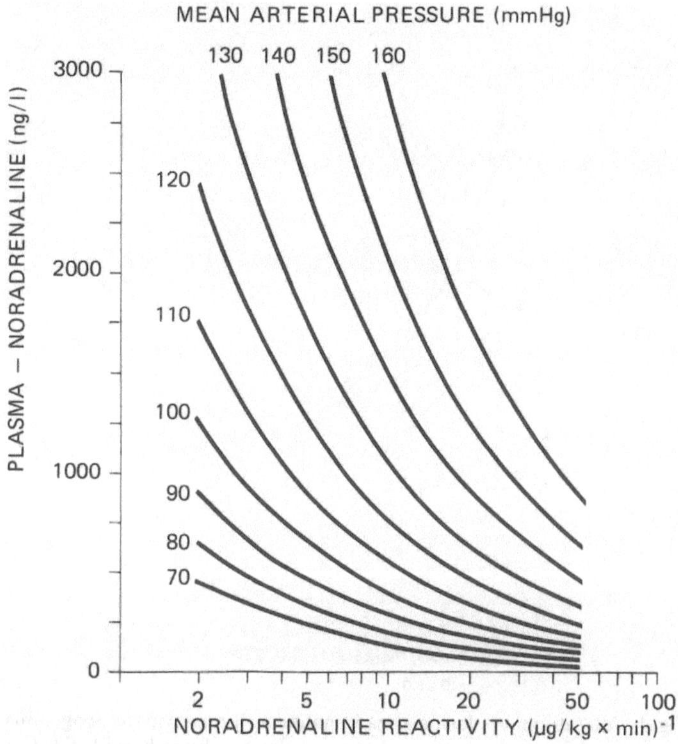

Fig. 3. Relationship between plasma noradrenaline and reactivity to exogenous noradrenaline. The two factors combined determine the level of blood pressure. Computer graph from the data given in Fig. 2. [35]

As mentioned above, the inverse relationship between sympathetic nerve activity and reactivity represents an automatic control system. This assumption is supported by studies in which we could demonstrate [47] that increased sympathetic nerve activity leads to a decrease of the reactivity to noradrenaline and vice versa. This dynamic change of both parameters could be observed in patients who had undergone total strumectomy for thyroid carcinoma. These patients are conventionally substituted with tyroxine in such a way as to suppress TSH, thus preventing possible TSH-induced metastatic spread. They are thus in a discretely hyperthyroid metabolic condition. In 6-month intervals, the possible occurrence of metastases is checked by whole-body iodine scanning. For this examination, the substitution therapy must be discontinued for a certain period, the patients being in a distinctly hypothyroid metabolic condition at this stage. There is evidence for the assumption that patients in a hyperthyroid metabolic condition reveal low [48] and patients in a hypothyroid metabolic condition high sympathetic nerve activity [28]. Therefore, combined sympathetic nerve activity was determined by measuring the plasma noradrenaline concentration and reactivity to noradrenaline in ten patients in the described hyper- and hypothyroid metabolic situation. With nearly unaltered blood pressure values, there was a distinct drop in the plasma noradrenaline concentra-

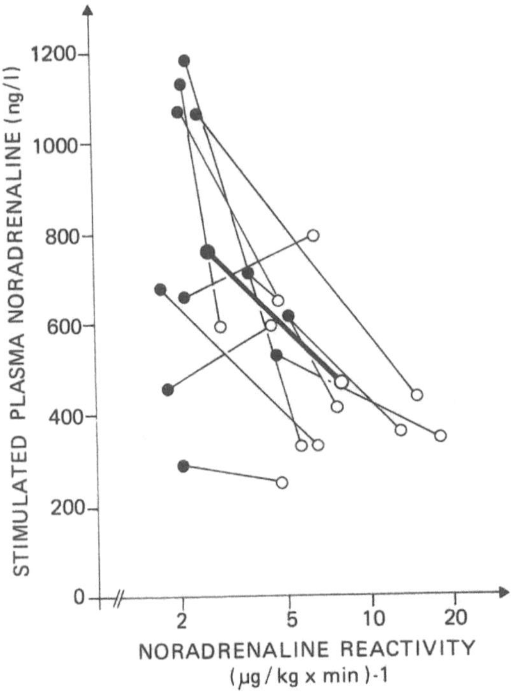

Fig. 4. Alterations in plasma noradrenaline and reactivity to exogenous noradrenaline in patients who passed from a hyperthyroid *(open circles)* to a hypothyroid *(filled circles)* stage

tion during the hyperthyroid metabolic period in all patients, accompanied by a significant increase in noradrenaline reactivity (Fig. 4).

Inverse changes in sympathetic nerve activity and reactivity can also be found under various antihypertensive substances. A decrease in noradrenaline reactivity was thus described during diuretic treatment [49, 50], while the values of plasma noradrenaline were distinctly increased. However, under substances which suppress sympathetic nerve activity, such as guanfacin, there was a significant increase in reactivity to noradrenaline, while plasma noradrenaline values decreased as expected [51]. During diuretic treatment, the decrease in noradrenaline reactivity is supposed to contribute to the antihypertensive effect of the substance and constitutes the primary change. Therefore, the increase in plasma noradrenaline values and hence of sympathetic nerve activity can be interpreted as a compensation phenomenon. Conversely, the decrease in plasma noradrenaline values and thus in sympathetic nerve activity is the primary pharmacological mechanism of guanfacin, while the increase in reactivity must be interpreted as a compensation phenomenon [51].

References

1. Delius W, Hagbarth KE, Hongell A, Wallin BG (1972) Manouevres affecting sympathetic outflow in human muscle nerves. Acta Physiol Scand 84: 82
2. Wallin BG, Delius W, Sundlöf G (1973) Comparison of sympathetic nerve activity in normotensive and hypertensive subjects. Circ Res 33: 9
3. Folkow B, Di Bona GF, Hjemdahl P, Torén PH, Wallin BG (1983) Measurements of plasma norepinephrine concentrations in human primary hypertension. A word of caution of their applicability for assessing neurogenic contributions. Hypertension 5: 399
4. Goldstein D (1983) Commentary to Folkow et al., ref. 3. Hypertension 5: 402
5. Yamaguchi N, De Champlain J, Nadeau R (1975) Correlation between the response of the heart to sympathetic stimulation and the release of endogenous catecholamines into the coronary sinus of the dog. Circ Res 36: 662
6. Wallin BG, Sundlöf G, Eriksson BM, Dominiak P, Grobecker H, Lindblad LE (1981) Plasma noradrenaline correlates to sympathetic muscle nerve activity in normotensive man. Acta Physiol Scand 111: 69
7. Goldstein DS, McCarty R, Polinsky RJ, Kopin IJ (1983) Relationship between plasma norepinephrine and sympathetic neural activity. Hypertension 5: 552
8. de Champlain J (1978) The contribution of the sympathetic nervous system to arterial hypertension. Can J Physiol Pharmacol 56: 341
9. Philipp T, Distler A, Hecking E, Lindmar R, Planz J, Schumann G, Wolff HP (1975) Reactivity to tyramine and norepinephrine, plasma dopamine-β-hydroxylase activity and norepinephrine excretion in hypertensive patients with normal and with low plasma renin concentration. Front Int Med 86, Karger-Verlag, Basel
10. Distler A, Philipp T (1980) Role of sympathetic nervous system in essential hypertension. Contrib Nephrol 23: 150
11. Goldstein DS (1981) Plasma norepinephrine in essential hypertension. Hypertension 3: 48
12. Goldstein DS (1983) Plasma catecholamines and essential hypertension. An analytical review. Hypertension 5: 86
13. Goldstein DS, Lake CR, Chernow B, Ziegler MG, Coleman MD, Taylor AA, Mitchell JR, Kopin IJ, Keiser HR (1983) Age-dependence of hypertensive-normotensive differences in plasma norepinephrine. Hypertension 5: 100
14. Bolli P, Amann FW, Hulthen L, Kiowski W, Bühler FR (1981) Elevated plasma adrenaline reflects sympathetic overactivity and enhanced α-adrenoceptor-mediated vasoconstriction in essential hypertension. Clin Sci 61: 161s
15. Louis WJ, Doyle AE, Anavekar SN, Johnston CI, Geffen LB, Rush R (1974) Plasma catecholamine, dopamine-beta-hydroxylase, and renin levels in essential hypertension. Circ Res 34/35 [Suppl 1]: 57
16. Stone RA, Gunnells JC, Robinson RR, Schanberg SM, Kirshner N (1974) Dopamine-beta-hydroxylase in primary and secondary hypertension. Circ Res 34 [Suppl 1]: 1-47
17. Aoki K, Tazumi K, Takikawa K (1975) Serum dopamine-β-hydroxylase activity in essential hypertension and in chronic renal failure with hypertension. Jpn Circ J 39: 1111
18. Geffen LB, Rush RA, Louis WJ, Doyle AE (1973) Plasma dopamine-β-hydroxylase and noradrenaline amounts in essential hypertension. Clin Sci 44: 617
19. Alexandre JM, London GM, Chevillard C, Lemaire P, Safar ME, Weiss Y (1975) The meaning of dopamine β-hydroxylase in essential hypertension. Clin Sci Mol Med 49: 573
20. Horwitz D, Alexander RW, Lovenberg W, Keiser HR (1973) Human serum dopamine-β-hydroxylase. Circ Res 32: 594
21. Aberg H, Wetterberg L, Ross SB, Froden O (1974) Dopamine-β-hydroxylase in hypertension. Acta Med Scand 196: 17
22. Noth RH, Mulrow PJ (1976) Serum dopamine β-hydroxylase as an index of sympathetic nervous system activity in man. Circ Res 38: 2
23. Lawton WJ, Fitz A, Grant C, Witte DL (1979) Dopamine beta-hydroxylase and plasma renin activity in patients with low-, normal-, and high-renin essential hypertension. Circulation 59: 1063
24. Kuchel O, Buu NT, Hamet P, Larochelle P, Bourque M, Genest J (1981) Essential hypertension with low conjugated catecholamines imitates pheochromocytoma. Hypertension 3: 347

25. Kuchel O, Cuche JL, Hamet P, Tolis G, Messerli FH, Barbeau A, Boucher R, Genest J (1975) Labile (borderline) hypertension - new aspects of a common disorder. Angiologie 26: 619
26. Esler M, Jackman G, Leonard P, Bobik A, Skews H, Jennings G, Kelleher D, Korner P (1970) Determination of noradrenaline uptake, spillover to plasma and plasma concentration in patients with essential hypertension. Clin Sci 59: 311s
27. Engelman K, Portnoy B, Sjoerdsma A (1970) Plasma catecholamine concentration in patients with hypertension. Circ Res 27 [Suppl 1]: 141
28. Christensen NJ (1972) Increased levels of plasma noradrenaline in hypothyroidism. J Clin Endocrinol 35: 359
29. Cordes U, Keller H, Beyer J (1975) Der diagnostische Wert der Plasmakatecholaminbestimmung bei primärer Nebenniereninsuffizienz. Verh Dtsch Ges Inn Med 81: 1540
30. Portnoy B, Engelman K, Wyatt R (1969) Plasma catecholamines in hypertensive and psychiatric disorders. Clin Res 17: 258
31. Goldenberg U, Pines KL, Baldwin EDF, Greene DG, Roh CE (1948) The hemodynamic response of man to norepinephrine and epinephrine and its relation to the problem of hypertension. Am J Med 5: 792
32. Safar ME, London GM, Weiss YA, Milliez PL (1975) Vascular reactivity to norepinephrine and hemodynamic parameters in borderline hypertension. Am Heart J 89: 480
33. London GM, Safar ME, Weiss YA (1976) The spectrum of pressor response to norepinephrine in normotensive and hypertensive patients. Biomedicine 24 (3): 178
34. Nestel PJ, Esler MD (1970) Patterns of catecholamine excretion in urine in hypertension. Circ Res 26/27 [Suppl 2]: 75
35. Philipp T, Distler A, Cordes U (1978) Sympathetic nervous system and blood-pressure control in essential hypertension. Lancet 2: 959
36. Doyle AE, Fraser JRE, Marshall RJ (1959) Reactivity of forearm vessels to vasoconstrictor substances in hypertensive and normotensive subjects. Clin Sci 18: 441
37. Greisman SE (1952) The reactivity of the capillary bed of the nailfold to circulating epinephrine and norepinephrine in patients with normal blood pressure and with essential hypertension. J Clin Invest 31: 782
38. Mendlowitz M, Naftchi NE, Wolf RL, Gitlow SE (1965) Vascular responsiveness in hypertensive and hypotensive stages. Geriatrics 20: 797
39. Folkow B, Grimby G, Thulesius O (1958) Adaptive structural changes of the vascular walls in hypertension and their relation to the control of the peripheral resistance. Acta Physiol Scand 44: 255
40. Erne P, Bolli P, Bürgisser E, Bühler FR (1984) Correlation of platelet calcium with blood pressure. Effect of antihypertensive therapy. N Engl J Med 310: 1084
41. Zidek W, Vetter H, Dorst KG, Zumkley H, Losse H (1982) Intracellular Na^+ and Ca^{2+} activities in essential hypertension. Clin Sci 63: 41s
42. Block LH, Jaksche H, Erne P, Bolli P, Bühler FR (1985) Adrenalin-induced, calcium-dependent phosphorilation of proteins in human platelets. J Clin Invest 75: 1600
43. Brodde OE, Stuka N, Demuth V, Fesel R, Bergerhausen J, Daul A, Bock KD (1985) Alpha- and beta-adrenoceptors in circulating blood cells of essential hypertensive patients: increased receptor density and responsiveness. Clin Exp Theory Pract A7: 1135
44. Weidmann P, Endres P, Siegenthaler W (1968) Plasma renin activity and angiotensin pressor dose in hypertension: correlation and diagnostic implications. Br Med J 3: 154
45. Distler A, Barth Ch, Liebau H, Vescei P, Wolff HP (1970) The effect of tyramine, noradrenaline and angiotensin on the blood pressure in hypertensive patients with aldosteronism and low plasma renin. Eur J Clin Invest 1: 196
46. Chinn RH, Düsterdieck G (1972) The response of blood pressure to infusions of angiotensin II: Relation to plasma concentrations of renin and angiotensin II. Clin Sci 42: 489
47. Philipp T, Brokamp B, Cordes U, Lüth B, Distler A (1979) Sympathikusaktivität und pressorische Wirkung von Noradrenalin bei Patienten mit hypo- und hyperthyreoter Stoffwechsellage. Verh Dtsch Ges Inn Med 85: 1047
48. Stoffer SS, Jiang NS, Gorman CA, Pikler GM (1973) Plasma catecholamines in hypothyroidism and hyperthyroidism. J Clin Endocrinol Metab 36: 587
49. Philipp T, Zschiedrich H, Renschin G, Distler A (1986) Pressorreaktionen unter Diuretika. Springer, Berlin Heidelberg New York Tokyo (in press)

50. Weidmann P, Grimm M, Meier A, Glück Z, Keusch G, Minder I, Beretta-Piccoli C (1980) Cardiovascular pressor reactivity as related to plasma catecholamines: role in the pathogenesis of essential hypertension and in the antihypertensive mechanism of diuretic treatment. In: Philipp T, Distler A (eds) Hypertension, mechanism and management. Springer, Berlin Heidelberg New York
51. Zschiedrich H, Renschin G, Lüth JB, Philipp T, Distler A (1982) Veränderungen von Sympathikusaktivität und Blutdruckwirksamkeit von exogenem Noradrenalin unter pharmakologischer Blutdrucksenkung. Verh Dtsch Ges Inn Med 88: 747

Discussion

Unidentified: When you give the synthesized choline ester of acetyl choline to a human there is the following possible reaction. First there is a blood pressure drop and, depending on the activity state, an overcompensating blood pressure rise until the normal level is reached again. If you do that with a large collection, then the subjects under 40 years of age show a behavior that corresponds to a normal distribution. There are hyporeactors, a larger portion of normoreactors corresponding to a normal distribution, and hyperreactors, who are characterized by the hypotension at the beginning being mild and the hyperreaction being very pronounced. Normally people under 45 years of age never have a hyperreaction, except for hypertensives. The central reactivity determined in this manner is normally reduced in elderly people unless a certain state, such as hypertension, is present.

Secondly, I wanted to say something with regard to the term stress. It depends very much on how the stress acts and with what intensity in the prehypertension state. In normotensives with a genetic predisposition a marked hyperreactivity is found only in response to emotional and physical stress with a very low watt age but not with stronger stress. In a later stage we then find such changes in genetically predisposed normotensives with stronger stress as well. It should probably always be stated in the prehypertensive stage how intense the physical stress is.

Philipp: Our applied stress was 200 W for 2 min at the time. The statement as to the inverse relationship in normotensives holds even when we regard the catecholamine levels at rest. As to the second point, please do not misunderstand me, I am concerned with the relatively specific phenomenon of nonadapted reactivity reduction, that is only with the norepinephrine effect, in order to close the circle to the adrenoreceptors, which is the subject of discussion here. If you consider what happens in the same patient groups with another vasopressor substance, for example with angiotensin, you'll again find an inverse relationship; a low angiotensin level is associated with a high renin activity - that's nothing new - and a low renin activity is associated with an elevated angiotensin effect. Since normotensives and hypertensives do not differ at all in this respect, the disturbance in this reaction remains limited to the sympathoadrenergic system.

Brodde: A short comment and a question. One should exercise caution when one says that thyroid hormones change the receptors. I don't think one can state that so globally. In hyperthyroidism the beta receptors are high and the alpha receptors low, and in hypothyroidism the beta receptors are low but there is disagreement about the alpha receptors. I don't think one can say, as you did, that they are high in hyperthyroidism and low in hypothyroidism.

Now the question: Is there really a disturbance between plasma norepinephrine and reactivity? What you showed is the same old curve - with increasing norepinephrine the reactivity drops. The higher the plasma norepinephrine level, the more norepinephrine must be given, and with increasing plasma norepinephrine the reactivity decreases, even in hypertensives. You showed that too. The difference is only that the one curve begins at 400 pg per ml and the other not until 1000. Does this mean there is a disturbance, or is there simply a shift of the normal level when regulation is resumed?

Philipp: No, we have to correct the numbers somewhat. In hypertensives smaller quantities of norepinephrine are required to increase the blood pressure. This is expressed in the increased reactivity shown. This applies to about 50%-60%, and I shall limit myself to this statement alone. But the regulatory system as a whole, which I have been able to show fairly clearly in normotensives with this inverse relationship, is fundamentally disturbed. We see this curve only when we take a group of hypertensives with comparable blood pressures. In these patients the regulatory cycle exists at a different level.

Schulte: In the last but one slide you showed that enhanced norepinephrine reactivity may lead to hypertension. According to my knowledge of the literature, norepinephrine activity is obviously enhanced only if manifest hypertension, that is, vascular damage, has already occurred according to the study by Safar, for example. This means that no pathogenetic mechanism is characterized, but rather a pathophysiologic state that has already set in.

Philipp: That's the old conundrum of the chicken and the egg. At the moment I am only considering the fact that the blood pressure was first measured and subsequently the reactivity, which was indeed investigated by Safar in various collectives. In this study, which is some ten years old, borderline hypertension and severe hypertension were compared with each other. And he never performed long-term studies. Safar's collectives differed in the blood pressure level. Thus the reactivity, which is to say the increase, became really striking only in the severe hypertensives and was not yet present in the subjects with mild hypertension. And what he derived from these observations about the reactivity of hypertension consequences, basing his conclusions on studies by the group headed by Folkow, was that structural changes are the basic cause of a reactivity change. In this context I should also like to point out that structural changes may of course lead to enhanced reactivity, but the disturbance in the relationship to each other should be just as apparent when we regard angiotensin and the plasma renin activity. That is a factor specific for the sympathoadrenergic system.

Adrenoceptors in Hypertension

M. MIDDEKE

Medizinische Poliklinik der Ludwig-Maximilians-Universität, Pettenkoferstraße 8 a, 8000 München 2, FRG

Introduction

Hypertension is characterized by several hemodynamic abnormalities, such as an increase in cardiac output and an enhanced peripheral resistance. In the sustained hypertensive state, the increase in total peripheral resistance is predominant (Fig. 1). Peripheral resistance is modulated mainly by α- and β-adrenoceptors located at the sympathetic nerve terminal (presynaptic) and at the arteriolar vascular smooth muscle (postsynaptic). While much information is available about peripheral adrenergic mechanisms, the role of central nervous adrenergic mechanisms in developing and maintaining hypertension is poorly understood. Much attention has been focused on the presynaptic β_2-adrenoceptor and its role in facilitating neurotransmitter release and vasoconstriction in recent years [3, 18, 21, 22]. By using radioligand binding studies to characterize and quantify adrenoceptors, we hope to increase our understanding of the role of sympathico-adrenergic system in the pathogenesis of hypertension and how it may be altered during antihypertensive therapy.

Experimental Studies on Animal Models

Many attempts have been made to determine the densities of α- and β-adrenoceptors in various tissues of different models of hypertension in the rat. Table 1 summarizes the alteration in receptor density, compared with normotensive control rats, observed in these studies. Whereas most studies documented a decrease [19, 36, 43] in α- or β-adrenoceptor number in myocardial tissue, one study reported an increase [29] and two reported no alteration [5, 6]. Similarly, all studies reported a decrease in β-adrenoceptor number in vascular tissues. However, the findings for β-adrenoceptors in the kidney are not clear, and α-adrenoceptors in the brain seem, in contrast, to be elevated. Thus, there is no clear evidence to indicate in what way adrenoceptors are altered by experimental or spontaneous hypertension in the rat.

New Aspects in Hypertension: Adrenoceptors
M. Middeke and H. Holzgreve (Eds.)
Springer-Verlag, Berlin Heidelberg New York 1986

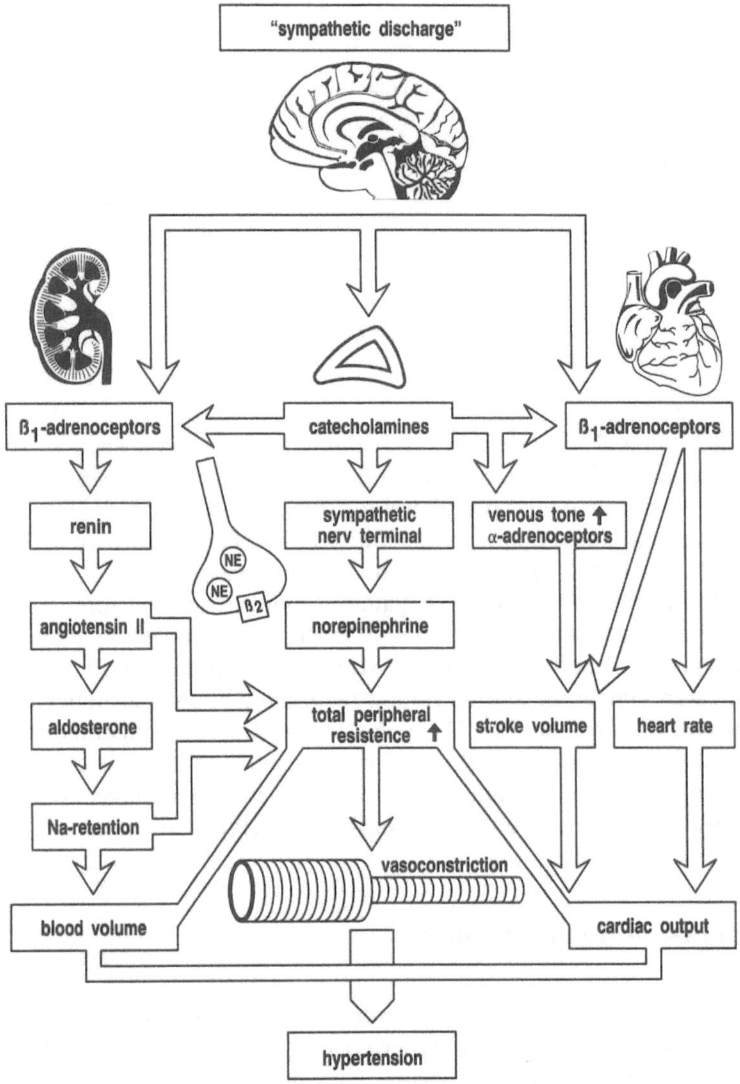

Fig. 1. Sympatho-adrenergic regulation of blood pressure: Distribution of peripheral adrenoceptors contributing to blood pressure regulation by influencing blood volume, cardiac output, and total peripheral resistance

Essential Hypertension in Man

There are no models to investigate adrenoceptors in innervated organs ex vivo at present, but both the lymphocytic β-adrenoceptor-adenylate cyclase-cAMP system and the platelet α_2-adrenoceptor system can be used to study adrenoceptor density and affinity in vivo. Table 2 summarizes the differences found in adrenoceptor density between hypertensives and normotensives. Using lymphocyte mem-

Table 1. α- and β-Receptor density in various tissues of different models of hypertension in the rat, compared with normotensive control animals

Experimental model	Tissue	Adrenoceptors alpha	beta	References
SHR	Myocardium		▼	Limas and Limas 1978 [19]
	Myocardium		---	Bhalla et al. 1980 [5]
	Myocardium		▼	Robberecht et al. 1981 [36]
	Myocardium	---	---	Blumenthal et al. 1982 [6]
	Myocardium	▼	▼ β_1	Yamada et al. 1984 [43]
	Myocardium		▲	Mochizuki and Ogawa 1984 [29]
	Aorta		▼	Limas and Limas 1979 [20]
	Aorta		▼	Bruschi et al. 1985 [10]
	Cava inf.		▼	Limas and Limas 1979 [20]
	Cerebral vessels	▲ α_1		Kobayashi et al. 1985 [15]
	Brain stem	▲ α_2	---	Palermo et al. 1981 [34]
	Hypothalamus	▲ α_1		Palermo et al. 1981 [34]
SHR	Myocardium		---	Murkherjee et al. 1980 [33]
stroke prone	Myocardium	▼	▼ β_1	Yamada et al. 1984 [43]
	Kidney		▲	Yamada et al. 1982 [42]
	Platelets	▲ α_2		Minuth and Jakobs 1983 [28]
DOCA	Myocardium		▼	Woodcock et al. 1979 [39]
	Mesenteric artery		▼	Woodcock et al. 1980 [40]
Goldblatt	Myocardium	▼	▼	Woodcock and Johnston 1980 [41]
	Lung		---	Woodcock and Johnston 1980 [41]
	Kidney	---	---	Woodcock and Johnston 1980 [41]

Receptor density increased (▲), decreased (▼), or unchanged (---) compared with normotensive control rats

Table 2. α- and β-Receptor density and affinity in peripheral blood cells of patients with essential hypertension compared with normotensive controls

Reference	Cells	Adrenoceptors alpha	beta	Affinity	Radioligand
Kafka et al. 1979 [14]	Platelets (M) ♀	▲		---	^{3}H-Dihydroergocryptine
	Platelets (M) ♂	---		---	^{3}H-Dihydroergocryptine
Motulsky et al. 1983 [31]	Platelets (M)	---		---	^{3}H-Yohimbine
Boon et al. 1983 [7]	Platelets (M)	---		---	^{3}H-Yohimbine
Brodde et al. 1985 [9]	Platelets (M)	▲		---	^{3}H-Yohimbine
Kafka et al. 1979 [14]	Lymphocytes (M)		---		^{3}H-Dihydroalprenolol
Doyle et al. 1982 [12]	Lymphocytes (M)		---	---	^{3}H-Dihydroalprenolol
Middeke et al. 1983 [23]	Lymphocytes (M)		---	---	125-Iodocyanopindolol
	Lymphocytes (C)		▲	---	125-Iodocyanopindolol
Brodde et al. 1983 [8]	Lymphocytes (C)		▲	---	125-Iodocyanopindolol
Landmann et al. 1983 [17]	Lymphocytes (?)		▲	---	^{3}H-Dihydroalprenolol
Bruschi et al. 1984 [10]	Lymphocytes (C)		▲	---	125-Iodocyanopindolol

(M), membrane fractions; *(C)*, intact cells; ▲, increase, ---, no difference compared with normotensives

brane fractions, no alterations in β_2-adrenoceptor density or affinity were found in essential hypertension [12, 14, 23] but in intact mononuclear leukocytes several investigators have shown a significantly higher β_2-adrenoceptor density [8, 10, 17, 23]. No difference in the number of α-adrenoceptors on platelets were found in two studies [7, 31]; in one study a 1.5-fold increase in α-adrenoceptors was observed in hypertensive women but not in hypertensive men [14], whereas another study describes a significant (twofold) increase in hypertensive subjects [9].

In order to examine these discrepancies further, adrenoceptors were measured on intact lymphocytes *and* on membrane fractions from normotensives and hypertensives. The results are summarized in Table 3. Patients with essential hypertension showed a twofold increase in β_2-adrenoceptor density when intact mononuclear cells were used, but no increase was found when membrane fractions were used [23]. The receptor affinity *(K_d)* was not different between the groups.

There was a significant positive correlation ($r = 0.73$) between mean arterial pressure and β_2-adrenoceptor density of intact mononuclear leukocytes (Fig. 2). In addition, there was a weak positive correlation between age and β_2-adrenoceptor density (Fig. 3). Testing mean arterial blood pressure, age, and sex together using factorial analysis revealed a significant correlation only between β_2-adrenoceptor density and blood pressure but not between sex or age and receptor number [25]. The positive correlation between age and β_2-adrenoceptor density was consistent with the findings of one earlier study [35], whereas other studies have shown no age-dependent alteration in β_2-adrenoceptor density [2, 12, 16] or even a decrease in receptor number with age [37]. These discrepancies may be explained by differences in the method or by the failure to take blood pressure into account, which strongly influences the β_2-adrenoceptor number.

As a consequence of the increased β_2-adrenoceptor density in patients with elevated blood pressure, the responsiveness of the β-adrenoceptor-adenylate cyclase-cAMP system was enhanced. The intracellular cAMP concentration after iso-

Table 3. β-Adrenoceptor density and affinity in intact mononuclear leukocytes and in membrane fractions of ten patients with essential hypertension compared with ten normotensive controls

Hypertensives	Cells		Membranes	
	B_{max}	K_d	B_{max}	K_d
MAP: 122 ± 11 Age: 52 ± 8 years $n = 10$ (4 ♀, 6 ♂)	859 ± 260	9.1 ± 7.4	812 ± 231	55.1 ± 4.6
Normotensives				
MAP: 92 ± 11 Age: 53 ± 12 $n = 10$ (3 ♀, 7 ♂)	420* ± 119	8.2 ± 6.6	930 ± 506	68.1 ± 31.0

*$p < 0.01$
Figures displayed are means ± SD in each case. B_{max}, maximum no. of binding sites per cell; K_d, dissociation constants; MAP, mean arterial blood pressure

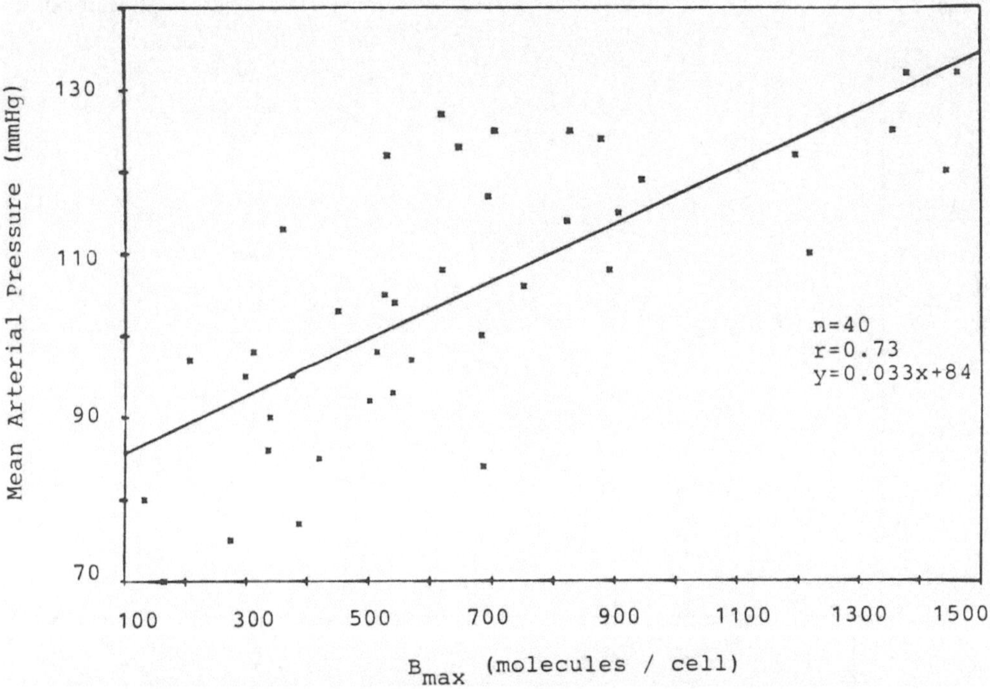

Fig. 2. Correlation between mean arterial blood pressure (mmHg) and β_2-adrenoceptor density (molecules/cell) in intact mononuclear leukocytes of 40 untreated patients and subjects

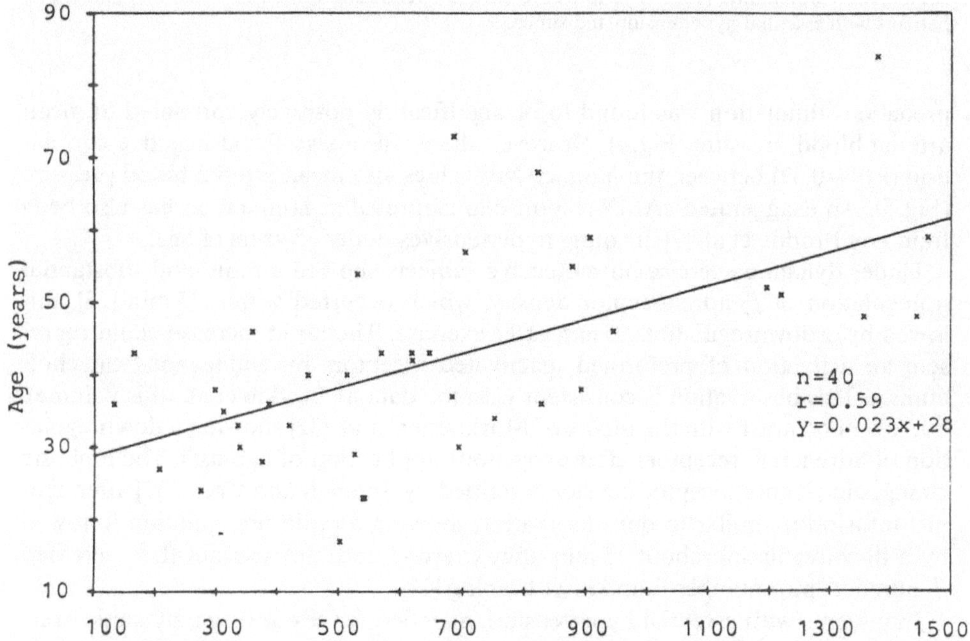

Fig. 3. Correlation between age (years) and β_2-adrenoceptor density (molecules/cell) in intact mononuclear leukocytes of 40 untreated patients and subjects

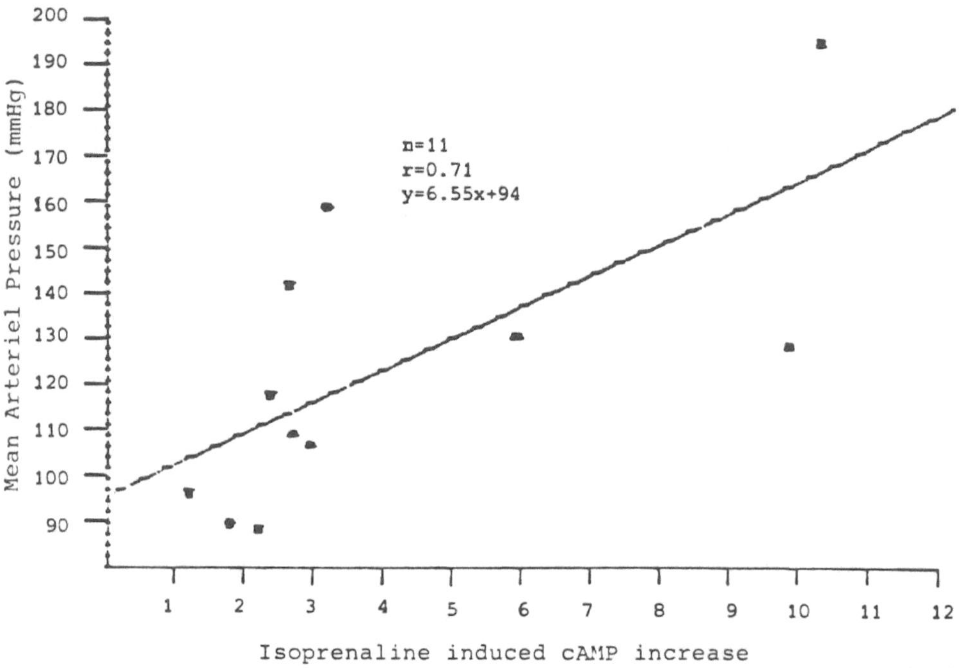

Fig. 4. Correlation between mean arterial blood pressure (mmHg) and intracellular (mononuclear leukocytes) isoprenaline (10^{-4} M) induced cAMP concentration (pmol/10^6 cells) in 11 untreated patients with essential hypertension and subjects

prenaline stimulation was found to be significantly positively correlated to mean arterial blood pressure (Fig. 4). However, there was a significant negative correlation ($r = -0.69$) between the *basal* cAMP values and mean arterial blood pressure (Fig. 5). An exaggerated cAMP response to isoprenaline stimulation has also been found by Brodde et al. [9] in young hypertensives under 45 years of age.

Under dynamic exercise normotensive subjects showed a rapid and substantial upregulation of β_2-adrenoceptor density, which occurred within 15 min [25], followed by a downregulation 15 min after exercise. The rapid increase could represent an activation of preformed inactivated receptors by endogenous catecholamines. This observation is consistent with the data of Brodde et al. (this volume), but it is in contrast with the report of Murkherjee et al. [32] showing a downregulation of adrenergic receptors after exogenous application of agonists. The biphasic changes in β_2-adrenoceptor density described by Tohmeh and Cryer [38] after agonist infusion is similar to our observation showing a rapid upregulation followed by a downregulation about 15 min after exercise and may explain the decreased β_2-adrenoceptor number found after training [11].

In patients with essential hypertension, matched for sex and age, dynamic exercise resulted in only a modest and nonsignificant upregulation of β_2-adrenoceptors (Table 4). In a recent study, we could demonstrate that an acute beta blockade with atenolol leads to normalization of the β_2-adrenoceptor-adenylate cyclase-cAMP system under dynamic stress [27]. Seven patients with essential hypertension

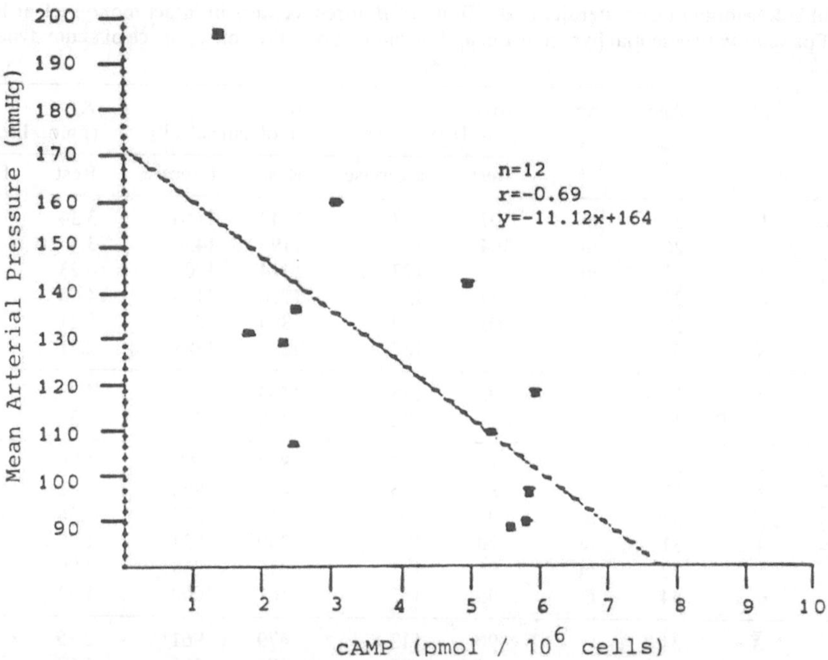

Fig. 5. Correlation between mean arterial blood pressure (mmHg) and basal cAMP concentrations (pmol/10^6 cells) in mononuclear leukocytes of 12 patients with essential hypertension and subjects

showed a significant upregulation of β-adrenoceptors 2 h after 100 mg atenolol, which was accompanied by a significant increase in basal and isoprenaline-stimulated cAMP concentrations.

Antihypertensive Therapy

Beta-blocking agents without intrinsic sympathetic activity (ISA) induce an increase of β_2-adrenoceptors on mononuclear leukocytes after long-term application [1] and after acute administration in patients with essential hypertension [27], whereas pindolol, which has ISA, results in downregulation [30]. The upregulation under propranolol [1] leads to an adrenergic hypersensitivity, which is the molecular basis for the withdrawal syndrome occurring after it is abruptly discontinued. This demonstrates how lymphocytic β_2-adrenoceptors can serve as a marker of adrenergic sensitivity and therapeutic efficiency. We were also able to demonstrate β_2-adrenoceptor upregulation with atenolol (no ISA) and downregulation with acebutolol (with ISA) [24] (Table 5).

Long-term diuretic therapy with hydrochlorothiazide was found to result in a β_2-adrenoceptor downregulation in patients with essential hypertension [26]. The decreased receptor number results in an adrenergic hyposensitivity, which could ex-

Table 4. Modulation of density and affinity of β-adrenoceptors in intact mononuclear leukocytes of patients with essential hypertension and normotensives as a consequence of acute dynamic exercise[a]

	No.	Age	Sex	MAP (mmHg)		B_{max} (molecules/cell)		K_d (pmol/liter)	
				Rest	Exercise	Rest	Exercise	Rest	Exercise
Hypertensives	1	24	m	107	137	1142	1146	3.34	2.63
	2	26	m	104	135	1195	1434	3.46	2.45
	3	23	m	96	127	1774	1909	6.23	3.84
	4	27	m	112	132	1778	2170	4.63	3.79
	5	39	m	103	149	894	1244	5.21	5.52
	6	50	f	127	187	1881	1888	2.51	2.07
	$\bar{X}$	31.5		108	145	1444	1632	4.23	3.38
	$\pm SD$	10.7		11	22	416	414	1.38	1.27
Normotensives	1	24	m	89	115	812	1.313	1.96	1.75
	2	27	m	82	85	430	860	4.22	6.34
	3	33	m	91	107	313	823	5.36	11.88
	4	31	m	90	108	340	831	1.65	2.90
	5	32	m	91	111	415	938	1.90	2.51
	6	44	f	95	153	561	1002	1.43	1.50
	$\bar{X}$	31.8		90	113	479	961*	2.75	4.48
	$\pm SD$	6.9		4.3	22	185	186	1.63	4.02

MAP, mean arterial blood pressure; B_{max}, maximum no. of binding sites per cell; K_d, dissociation constant. Figures given for B_{max} and K_d and for age of patients are means.
[a] 50–200 W for 15 min on a bicycle.
*$p < 0.01$.

Table 5. Modulation of density and affinity of β-adrenoceptors in intact mononuclear leukocytes of patients with essential hypertension and normotensives as a consequence of antihypertensive therapy with various drugs

Drug (dosage in mg)	Patients n	Age (years)	Duration (months)	MAP (mmHg)	B_{max} (molecules/cell)		K_d (mmol/l)	
					Before	After	Before	After
Atenolol (89)	9	53.4 ± 5.1	9.9 ±5.7	−15.7 ±10.9	941 ±463	2078* ±1671	8.1 ±5.7	16.2 ±18.4
Acebutolol (200)	5	36.6 ±13.7	1.2 ±0.8	−12.8 ± 8.1	1284 ±825	315* ±309	7.3 ±5.7	3.8 ±1.8
Hydrochloro-thiazide (50)	10	±49 ±5.4	±7.1 ±7.3	−14.6 ± 6.4	798 ±188	478 ±133	6.1 ±2.8	5.2 ±2.8

MAP, mean arterial blood pressure; B_{max}, maximum no. of binding sites per cell; K_d dissociation constant.
Figures given for dosages, age of patients, duration of treatment, B_{max}, K_d, and changes in MAP are means ± SD.
* $p < 0.01$.

plain the attenuated pressor effect of vasoactive agents after long-term treatment [4] contributing to the antihypertensive mechanism of diuretics (Table 5).

Conclusions

Determination of lymphocytic β_2-adrenoceptor-adenylate cyclase-cAMP system can serve as a marker of adrenergic sensitivity [13, 26] and allow the role of adrenergic mechanisms in hypertension and its therapy to be studied. The findings obtained in essential hypertension and antihypertensive therapy show that the regulation of the β_2-adrenoceptor-adenylate cyclase-cAMP system of mononuclear leukocytes is altered. If this does represent a generalized defect in adrenoceptor regulation in essential hypertension, this change in adrenergic sensitivity may be important in the pathogenesis of essential hypertension.

Summary

Alterations in the activity or sensitivity of the sympathico-adrenergic system are considered to be important in the genesis and maintenance of essential hypertension. Measurements of the catecholamine-binding sites (adrenoceptors) using radioligand binding techniques in about 20 studies on hypertensive rats, although showing some alterations in the number of adrenoceptors in myocardium, blood vessels, kidney, and brain, provided conflicting findings whose relevance in man remains uncertain.

A system easily accessible for clinical investigation in cardiovascular diseases and their therapy, e.g., in hypertension, is the human lymphocytic β_2-adrenoceptor-adenylate cyclase-cAMP system.

In patients with essential hypertension, the β_2-adrenoceptor density of mononuclear leukocytes has been found to be significantly increased, but the affinity of the β_2-adrenoceptor is unchanged. Adrenoceptor density is the same in men and women and increases with age. In normotensives, dynamic stress leads to a rapid and substantial increase of β_2-adrenoceptor density; in hypertensives it results in only a modest increase of receptor density. Mean arterial blood pressure is positively correlated to both β_2-adrenoceptor density and intracellular cAMP concentration after isoprenaline stimulation. There is a significant negative correlation between mean arterial blood pressure and basal cAMP concentration.

These findings, which demonstrate an altered regulation of the β_2-adrenoceptor-adenylate cyclase-cAMP system in mononuclear leukocytes in essential hypertension, may represent a generalized defect in adrenoceptor regulation and sensitivity.

References

1. Aarons RD, Nies AS, Gal J, Hegstrand LR, Molinoff PB (1980) Elevation of β-adrenergic receptor density in human lymphocytes after propranolol administration. J Clin Invest 65: 949-957
2. Abrass IB, Scarpace PJ (1981) Human lymphocyte beta-adrenergic receptors are unaltered with age. J Gerontol 36: 298-301
3. Adler-Graschinsky E, Langer SZ (1975) Possible role of a β-adrenoceptor in the regulation of noradrenergic release by nerve stimulation through a positive feed-back mechanism. Br J Pharmacol 53: 43-50
4. Aleksandrow D, Wysznacka W, Gejewski J (1959) Influence of chlorothiazide upon arterial responsiveness to norepinephrine in hypertensive subjects. N Engl J Med 261: 1052-1055
5. Bhalla RC, Sharma RV, Ramanathan SR (1980) Ontogenetic development of isoproterenol subsensitivity of myocardial adenylate cyclase and β-adrenergic receptors in spontaneously hypertensive rats. Biochim Biophys Acta 632: 497-506
6. Blumenthal SJ, McConnaughey MM, Iams SG (1982) Myocardial adrenergic receptors and adenylate cyclase in the developing spontaneous hypertensive rat. Clin Exp Hypertension 6: 883-901
7. Boon NA, Elliot JM, Davies CL, Conway FJ, Grahame-Smith DG, Sleight P (1983) Platelet alpha-adrenoceptors in borderline and established essential hypertension. Clin Sci 64: 265
8. Brodde OE, Prywarra A, Anlauf M, Daul A, Bock KD (1983) Increased number of β_2-adrenoceptors in circulating lymphocytes of patients with essential hypertension. J Hypertension 1 [Suppl 2]: 262-266
9. Brodde OE, Stuka N, Demuth V, Fesel R, Bergerhausen J, Daul A, Bock KD (1985) Alpha- and beta-adrenoceptors in circulating blood cells of essential hypertensive patients: increased receptor density and responsiveness. Clin Exp Hypertension A7: 1135-1150
10. Bruschi G, Orlandini G, Pavarani C, Spaggiari M, Tacinell L, Cavatorta A (1984) Lymphocytic beta-adrenoceptor abnormality in primary hypertension. IRCS Med Sci 12: 461-462
11. Butler J, O'Brien M, O'Malley K, Kelly JG (1982) Relationship of β-adrenoceptor density to fitness in athletes. Nature 298: 60-62
12. Doyle V, O'Malley K, Kelly JG, (1982) Human lymphocyte β-adrenoceptor density in relation of age and hypertension. J Cardvasc Pharmacol 4: 738-740
13. Fowler MB, Bristow MR, Laser JA, Ginsburg R, Scott LB, Schroeder JS (1984) Beta blocker therapy in severe heart failure: improvement related to beta$_1$-adrenergic receptor up regulation? Circulation 70 (2): 112
14. Kafka MS, Lake CR, Gullner HG, Tallman JF, Bartter FC, Fujita T (1979) Adrenergic receptor function is different in male and female patients with essential hypertension. Clin Exp Hypertension 1: 613-627
15. Kobayashi H, Wada A, Izumi F, Magnoni MS, Trabucchi M (1985) Alpha-adrenergic receptors in cerebral microvessels of normotensive and spontaneously hypertensive rats. Circ Res 56: 402-409
16. Landmann R, Bittinger H, Bühler FR (1981) High affinity beta$_2$-adrenergic receptors in mononuclear leukocytes: similar density in young and old normal subjects. Life Sci 29: 1761-1771
17. Landmann R, Bürgisser E, Bühler FR (1983) Human lymphocytes as a model for beta-adrenergic receptors in clinical investigation. J Rec Res 3: 71-88
18. Langer SZ (1980) Presynaptic regulation of the release of catecholamines. Pharmacol Rev 32: 337-363
19. Limas C, Limas CJ (1978) Reduced number of β-adrenergic receptors in the myocardium of spontaneously hypertensive rats. Biochem Biophys Res Commun 83: 710-714
20. Limas CJ, Limas C (1979) Decreased number of beta-adrenergic receptors in hypertensive vessels. Biochim Biophys Acta 582: 533-536
21. Majewski H, Rand MJ (1981) An interaction between prejunctional alpha-adrenoceptors and prejunctional β-adrenoceptors. Eur J Pharmacol 69: 493-498
22. Majewski H, Tung LH, Rand MJ (1982) Adrenaline activation of prejunctional β-adrenoceptors and hypertension. J Cardiovasc Pharmacol 4: 99-106
23. Middeke M, Remien J, Block LH, Kirzinger S, Landrock A, Holzgreve H (1983) Beta$_2$-adreno-

ceptor density on membranes and on intact mononuclear cells in essential hypertension. Res Exp Med 183: 227-232
24. Middeke M, Remien J, Holzgreve H (1984a) Antihypertensive Therapie und β-Adrenozeptordichte. Verh Dtsch Ges Inn Med 90: 752-754
25. Middeke M, Remien J, Holzgreve H (1984b) The influence of sex, age, blood pressure, and physical stress on β_2-adrenoceptor density of mononuclear cells. J Hypertension 2: 261-264
26. Middeke M, Remien J, Kirzinger S, Holzgreve H (1985) Adrenergic hyposensitivity during long-term diuretic therapy - a possible explanation for the antihypertensive effect of diuretics? Eur J Pharmacol 109: 401-403
27. Middeke M, Kirzinger S, Remien J, Krahl B, Holzgreve H (1986) An altered acute regulation of the β-adrenoceptor-adenylatecyclase-cAMP system in patients with essential hypertension at rest and under exercise. Clin Exp Hypertension A8: 135-136
28. Minuth M, Jakobs KH (1983) Alpha$_2$-adrenoceptors in platelets of spontaneously hypertensive rats. Naunyn-Schmiedebergs Arch Pharmacol 322: 98-103
29. Mochizuki M, Ogawa K (1984) Increase of cardiac β-adrenergic receptors in young spontaneously hypertensive rats. Jpn Heart J 25: 411-423
30. Molinoff PB, Aarons RD, Nies AS, Gerber JG, Wolfe BB, Goens MB (1982) Effects of pindolol and propranolol on β-adrenergic receptors on human lymphocytes. Br J Pharmacol 13: 365
31. Motulsky HJ, O'Connor DT, Insel P (1983) Platelet alpha$_2$-adrenergic receptors in treated and untreated essential hypertension. Clin Sci 64: 265-272
32. Mukherjee A, Caron MG, Lefkowitz RJ (1975) Catecholamine induced subsensitivity of adenylate cyclase associated with loss of β-adrenergic binding sites. Proc Natl Acad Sci USA 72: 1945-1949
33. Mukherjee A, Graham RM, Sagalowsky AI, Pettinger W, McCoy KE (1980) Myocardial beta-adrenergic receptors in the stroke prone spontaneously hypertensive rat. J Mol Cell Cardiol 12: 1263-1272
34. Palermo A, Constantini C, Mara G, Libretti A (1981) Role of the sympathetic nervous system in spontaneous hypertensive rats: changes in central adrenoceptors and plasma catecholamine levels. Clin Sci 61: 195-198
35. Roan Y, Galant SP (1981) The ontogeny of neutrophil beta-adrenergic receptors. Clin Res 29: 144 A (Abstract)
36. Robberecht P, Winan J, Chatelain P, Poloczek J, Camus J, De Neefan P, Christopher J (1981) Comparison of β-adrenergic receptors and the adenylate cyclase system with muscarinic receptors and guanylate cyclase activities in the heart of spontaneously rats. Biochem Pharmacol 30: 385-387
37. Schocken DD, Roth GS (1977) Reduced β-adrenergic receptor concentrations in ageing man. Nature 267: 856-858
38. Tohmeh JF, Cryer PE (1980) Biphasic adrenergic modulation of β-adrenergic receptors in man. J Clin Invest 65: 836-840
39. Woodcock EA, Funder JW, Johnston CI (1979) Decreased cardiac β-adrenergic receptors in deoxycorticosterone-salt and renal hypertensive rats. Circ Res 45: 560-565
40. Woodcock EA, Olsson CA, Johnston CI (1980) Reduced vascular beta-adrenergic receptors in deoxycorticosterone hypertensive rats. Biochem Pharmacol 29: 1465-1469
41. Woodcock EA, Johnston CI (1980) Changes in tissue alpha- and beta-adrenergic receptors in renal hypertension in the rat. Hypertension 2: 156-161
42. Yamada S, Ishima T, Tomita T, Hayashi M, Hayashi E (1982) Increased renal β-adrenoceptors in stroke prone spontaneously hypertensive rats. Eur J Pharmacol 83: 149-150
43. Yamada S, Ishima T, Tomita T, Hayashi M, Okada T, Hayashi E (1984) Alterations in cardiac alpha and beta adrenoceptors during the development of spontaneous hypertension. J Pharmacol Exp Ther 228: 454-460

Discussion

Skrabal: You must be asked this question often. I thought that beta receptors caused vasodilatation. How do you account for a positive correlation between blood pressure and beta receptors on the one hand and the fact that patients with high blood pressure often have reduced beta-adrenergic sensitivity and unopposed norepinephrine alpha tone on the other?

Middeke: The first question. You mean the postsynaptic $beta_2$ receptors which mediate vasodilation. The answer has already been indicated by Dr. Göthert this morning: that is really only one side of the coin. One must also consider the presynaptic $beta_2$ receptors, which increase neurotransmitter release via a positive feedback mechanism.

Brodde: I think we must make a distinction between $beta_2$ and $beta_1$ receptors. $Beta_2$ vasodilation plays a much lesser role than is repeatedly claimed. The depressed responsiveness of beta-adrenergic receptors, which Fritz Bühler, for example, showed very nicely, is isoproterenol-stimulated tachycardia; and in humans that is 90% mediated by $beta_1$ receptors. We also found that in spontaneously hypertensive rats after 5 and after 10 weeks - as Dr. Borchert showed us this morning - $beta_2$ receptors play no functional role in cardiac contractility. If they play a role at all, then only as presynaptic $beta_2$ receptors. That is a speculation which cannot be substantiated at the moment. But the $beta_2$ receptors in spontaneously hypertensive rats were markedly higher than in normotensive WKY, while the $beta_1$ receptors decreased with rising blood pressure.

Göthert: I'd like to comment on and supplement Dr. Middeke's answer with regard to $beta_2$ receptors. I said earlier that in a very well-studied synapse between a peripheral sympathetic neuron and a smooth vascular muscle in the human saphenous vein $beta_2$ receptors are present both presynaptically and postsynaptically. Again we find vasodilatory $beta_2$ receptors and liberation-increasing $beta_2$ receptors. A very elegant experiment was carried out by Kutter: He showed that the net effect of the administration of isoprenaline when you induce electrical stimulation of the sympathetic nerves in this vessel is enhanced contraction of the vessel, although dilation was induced in the vessel by isolated stimulation of $beta_2$ receptors. It may therefore be said, at least for this synapse, that the presynaptic $beta_2$ adrenoceptors predominate over the postsynaptic $beta_2$ adrenoceptors in functional importance. And I must also qualify this. You pointed out correctly that these positive effects can be mediated in the heart by presynaptic $beta_2$ receptors. The only problem is that so far no one has proved that increased numbers of presynaptic $beta_2$ adrenoceptors are present in spontaneously hypertensive rats. That is extremely difficult to accomplish in the binding state. It's practically impossible. One could only do it functionally, and it has unfortunately been shown time and time again functionally that the sensitivity of presynaptic beta adrenoceptors in hypertensive rats is like that of Wistar Kyoto control rats. But perhaps the right model was not used. Usually large-capacity vessels were studied, and these events certainly take place at the arteriole level, which at present is extraordinarily inaccessible to experiment.

Koella: In the determinations of, say, the plasma norepinephrine level or receptor sensitivity, has the time of day ever been taken into account as a factor?

Middeke: Dr. Remien is in the process of studying this question: Circadian rhythm, for example, of the $beta_2$ receptors in man. As I understand the findings so far, it may be assumed that the receptor density is certainly not constant around the clock. There are differences. Dr. Lemmer has already studied this aspect in rats. In humans there is one finding: asthmatics have marked differences in receptor density between day and night. Otherwise I don't know of any published study that has adequately investigated the circadian rhythms of adrenergic receptors in man.

Koella: You could also take the converse approach and try to determine whether hypertensives differ from normotensives in that they have different circadian rhythms in amplitude, for example, or, as is more likely, in phase.

Middeke: I assume it will be found that hypertensives differ both in amplitude and in phase from normotensives.

Philipp: On the basis of the circadian rhythms known to me it is important to perform every receptor measurement - in this case the catecholamines - as well as the reactivity measurement early in the morning.

Middeke: All the measurements presented were taken at the same time of day.

Lemmer: May I interject a comment? We investigated the cAMP content of the rat heart over a period of two-and-a-half years and found a wonderful circadian rhythm, which also varies seasonally, so that the comfortable feeling derived from always performing the measurements in the morning should be regarded with some skepsis. One question which Dr. Koella has already touched upon: With regard to the reactivity of the cardiovascular system to norepinephrine, Dr. Hossman, of the group led by Dollery, reported years ago that the time of day plays a crucial role in the increase of intra-arterial blood pressure. You too have pointed out intraindividual variations. To what extent can such findings be explained by such things? The study design alone might account for differences with regard to response, for example at night. Is there a nocturnal increase in hypertensives which in itself is not physiologic?

Middeke: Of course that must be taken into account. Measuring receptors is a tricky business; but it alone makes it possible to study hormone receptor interactions under various hemodynamic conditions at various times of day. For this reason I can concour with Dr. Philipp, who says the catecholamines must be measured at the same time. But you could also turn it around and say: the receptors must be measured at the same time. That has been done in part. Of course it would be optimal to measure the entire system with hemodynamic parameters, from the top down to the subcellular level.

Philipp: A start has been made on relating the reactivity directly to specific receptor changes. We are not yet so far that we can say, for example, that noradrenergic reactivity can be explained in terms of precisely defined changes of alpha receptors. About 6 years ago a coworker of ours, Dr. Friedrich, tried to demonstrate the circadian rhythm of norepinephrine reactivity in hypertensive patients. Finding none, he gave up after about 12 patients. I just wanted to say that it is certainly not a uniform finding.

Schulte: I'd be interested to know what you have found in borderline hypertensives with regard to the receptor density. Because they are in the initial phase of hypertension, borderline hypertensives are especially interesting with regard to pathogenesis. And the studies by Bühler and many other authors have shown, for example, that the sensitivity of the beta receptors in the isoprotenerol test is not different from that of normotensives. We have seen that in our own investigations. What about the beta receptor density in borderline hypertensives?

Middeke: Recently we have studied several borderline hypertensives. So far I have the impression that the receptor density is higher than in normotensives too.

Adrenoceptor Alterations in Different Tissues in Human and Animal Genetic Hypertension

G. BRUSCHI, M. E. BRUSCHI, A. CAVATORTA, and A. BORGHETTI

Istituto di Clinica Medica e Nefrologia, Università di Parma, Via Gramsci 14, 43100 Parma, Italy

Introduction

It is scarcely necessary to stress the importance of adrenoceptor regulation in arterial hypertension. In this disease an altered response to adrenergic agonists has been described in different organs, and particularly in the blood vessels [1-6]. Moreover, antiadrenergic drugs, and particularly alpha and beta blockers, are effective antihypertensive agents.

The tissue involved in blood pressure regulation, however, are not easily accessible for receptor studies in man. Therefore, either animal models are required or some demonstration has to be provided that changes in accessible tissues (e.g., blood cells) can reflect the changes occurring in nervous and cardiovascular structures.

This report describes adrenoceptor alterations in arterial muscle of spontaneously hypertensive rats (SHR: a widely used model of genetic hypertension) and in lymphocytes of both SHR and human patients. In addition, the suggestion is presented that receptor defects can be part of a more general alteration of cellular function in hypertension.

Methods

The methods used have generally been described in detail in previous reports [5-7]. Briefly, adrenoceptors were investigated with binding techniques, using rapid filtration to separate bound from free ligand. Ligands used were (±) or (−)-^{125}I-iodocyanopindolol for beta adrenoceptors, both in lymphocytes [7] and in isolated arterial myocytes [8]. ^{125}I-HEAT was used for alpha$_1$ adrenoceptors [6].

Isolated arterial smooth muscle cells (IASMC) were obtained from rat aorta with a collagenase-elastase treatment [8, 9]. Some difficulties encountered in binding studies of beta adrenoceptors in these cells are described elsewhere [9].

The spontaneously hypertensive rats (SHR) used in this study belonged to the Okamoto-Aoki strain, and Wistar-Kyoto (WKY) normotensive rats were used as the most appropriate controls. The origin of these rats and some of their characteristics have been reported elsewhere [10], as have the criteria used for diagnosis of essential hypertension in humans and for selection of patients used in this and other studies [7, 11].

New Aspects in Hypertension: Adrenoceptors
M. Middeke and H. Holzgreve (Eds.)
Springer-Verlag Berlin Heidelberg New York 1986

Results

Isolated Arterial Smooth Muscle Cells

Figure 1 illustrates the number (as sites per cell) and density (as sites/μm^2 surface area) of beta adrenoceptors in isolated arterial smooth muscle cells (IASMC) of WKY and SHR as a function of age. Two observations can be made. The first is that either the number or the density of beta adrenoceptors declines with age in both hypertensive and normotensive rats; as the animals grow and become adult, the number of adrenoceptors in their arterial cells decreases markedly. The second observation is that this age-related process is more evident in SHR than in controls. Rats with genetic hypertension have a lower density of beta adrenoceptors at any age, and the age-related trend is merely more evident in SHR.

Figure 2 shows the density and affinity *(K_d)* of alpha$_1$ postsynaptic adrenoceptors in IASMC at two different ages in SHR and WKY. Alpha$_1$ adrenoceptor density is increased during development in normotensive animals, while their affinity is decreased (K_d increased). In the SHR, on the contrary, the number of alpha$_1$ adrenoceptors is rather decreased during development, while their affinity decreases less than in normotensive animals. The effect of these changes is difficult to predict. One could infer that the effect should not be prominent insofar as alpha receptors per se are concerned. In fact, in WKY a decrease in density is balanced by a decrease in affinity, while in SHR changes in neither density nor affinity are significant.

If we consider the whole adrenoceptor pattern in arterial cells, i.e., the alpha:beta ratio (Fig. 3), however, we observe two facts: a) the alpha:beta ratio increases

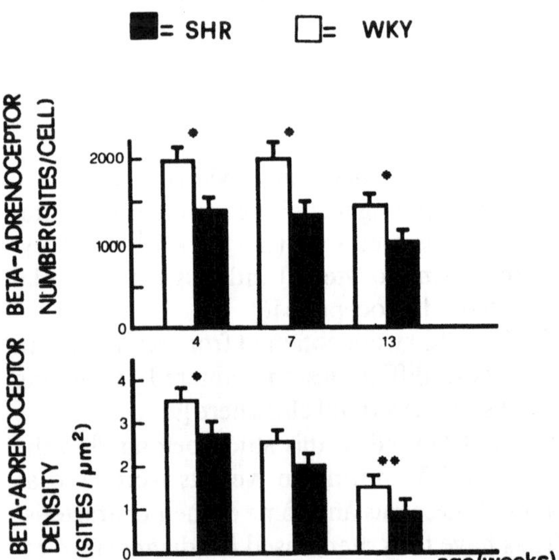

Fig. 1. Beta adrenoceptor number *(upper panel)* and density *(lower panel)* in isolated arterial myocytes of SHR and WKY rats at different ages. Density is referred to unit surface area, which was calculated from cell volume [8]. $*p < 0.05$ in statistical comparison of SHR vs WKY

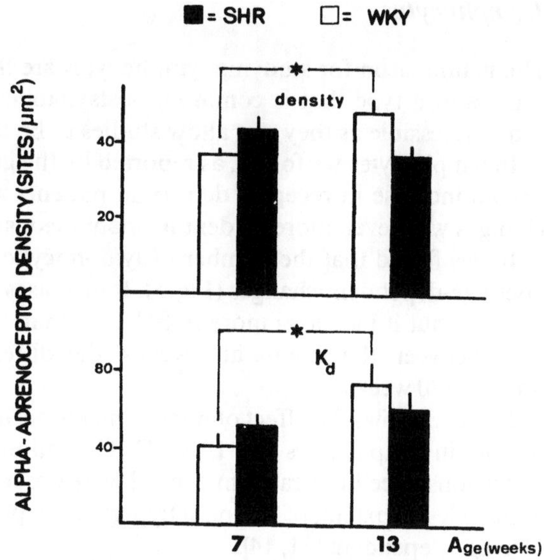

Fig. 2. Density and affinity *(K_d)* of alpha$_1$ adrenoceptors in isolated arterial smooth muscle cells of SHR and WKY at different ages. *$p < 0.05$ for the difference in WKY at different ages

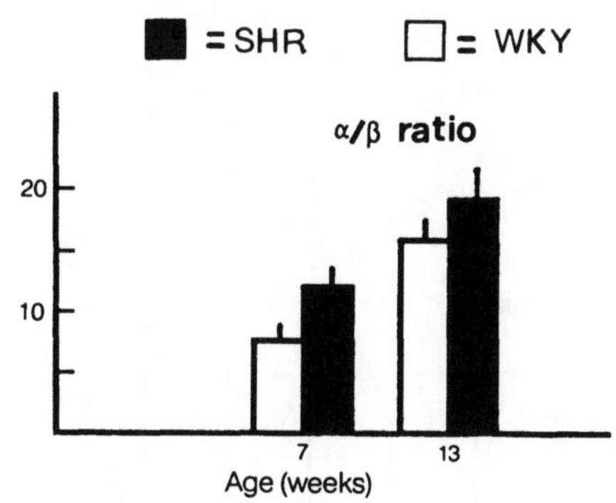

Fig. 3. Alpha:beta adrenoceptor density ratio in IASMC of SHR and WKY rats at two different ages

with age in normotensive rats; b) the alpha:beta ratio is higher at different ages in hypertensive rats. If we recall that alpha adrenoceptors mediate vasoconstriction while beta adrenoceptors mediate vasodilatation, we can find here a basis for an increased 'reactivity' in SHR [1-6]. During this age interval (7-20 weeks), the systolic blood pressure of normotensive rats increases from 90 to about 120 mmHg, while that of SHR increases to about 160 mmHg [10].

It is interesting to compare these data with pharmacologic information about an increased vasoconstrictory response of rat aorta to catecholamines during the ageing process and exaggerated vasoconstrictory responses to norepinephrine in SHR. Dilatation induced by isoproterneol similarly decreases with age, particularly in SHR [1-6].

Lymphocytes

The main reason for studying lymphocytes are that: (a) they possess $beta_2$ adrenoceptors of a type that is common, postsynaptically, to many tissues; (b) lymphocytes, accessible as they are, allow studies to be carried out in man.

In lymphocytes we found, as reported by the groups of Middeke and Brodde [12, 13], an increase in receptor density in patients with essential hypertension. These changes were even more evident in spontaneously hypertensive rats (Fig. 4).

It was found that the number of lymphocytic beta adrenoceptors (LBA) undergoes age-dependent changes (Fig. 5). It increases in normotensive rats during development, but it increases more in SHR, so that, while there is no significant difference between the strains at 6 weeks, the difference is very significant in adult animals (20 weeks).

Figure 6 shows the effect of increasing intracellular calcium on beta adrenoceptor density in lymphocytes and IASMC. The rationale for these experiments was that alterations of cellular calcium control were observed in lymphocytes of SHR and, to a much lesser extent, of essential hypertensive patients. This calcium abnormality is also age-dependent [11, 14].

An increase of intracellular calcium was induced by incubating the cells in physiological salt solutions containing two concentrations of free Ca^{2+} (1 μ*M* and

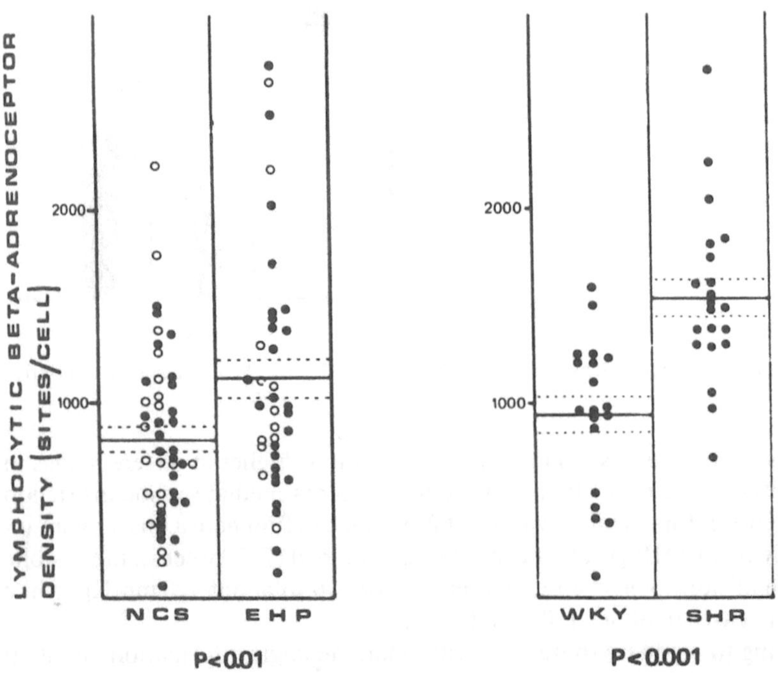

Fig. 4. Lymphocytic beta adrenoceptor density in human essential and rat spontaneous hypertension. Essential hypertensive patients *(EHP)* are compared with normotensive control subjects *(NCS)*, and spontaneously hypertensive rats *(SHR)* are compared with WKY controls. In humans, (○) and (●) denote the measurements performed on supine and standing subjects, respectively

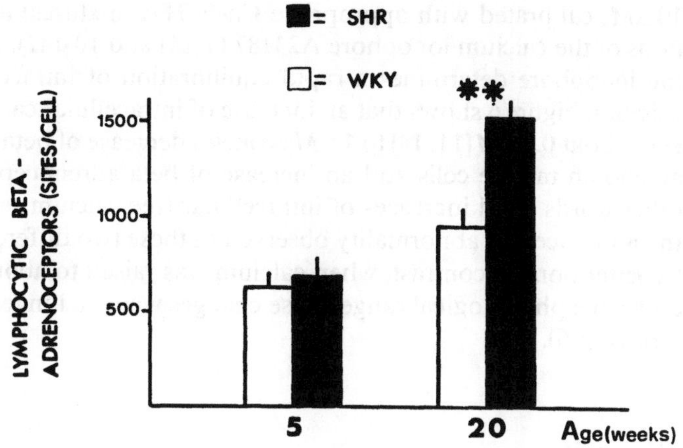

Fig. 5. LBA density in SHR and WKY at two different ages. *$p < 0.01$ of the SHR – WKY difference

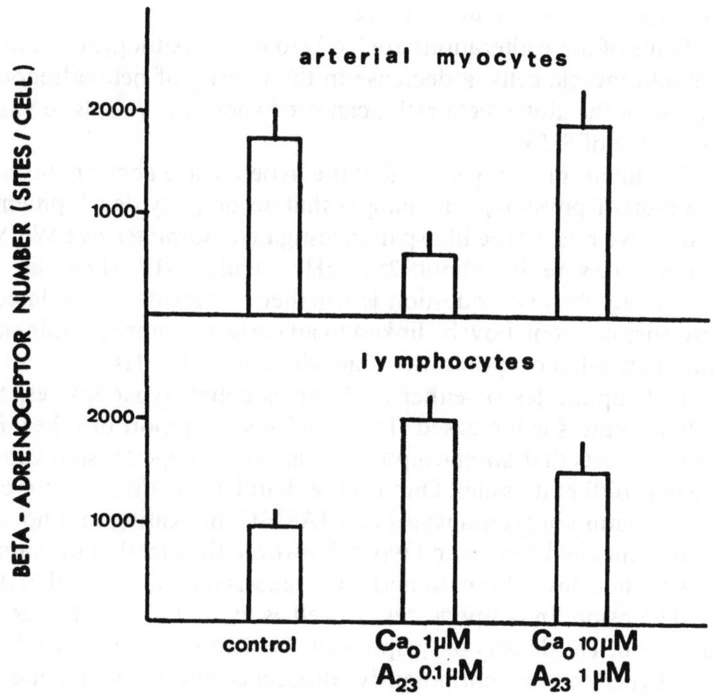

Fig. 6. Effect of increasing intracellular calcium in lymphocytes and arterial myocytes of 18-week-old WKY rats. *Left columns:* control lymphocytes, no treatment. *Center columns:* lymphocytes were exposed in vitro to the Ca ionophore A23187 in the presence of 1 μ*M* extracellular calcium. This Ca concentration was determined with Ca-EGTA mixtures. This ionophore concentration is sufficient to equilibrate extracellular and intracellular calcium. *Right columns:* Same procedure as in center, but concentrations of both ionophore and extracellular calcium were raised to about 10 μ*M*. The normal concentration of intracellular free Ca^{2+} in inact lymphocytes of these animals is about 0.1 μ*M*

10 μM; calibrated with appropriate Ca-EGTA mixtures) and different concentrations of the calcium ionophore A23187 (1 μM and 10 μM). At these concentrations, the ionophore determines a rapid equilibration of intracellular and extracellular calcium. Figure 6 shows that an increase of intracellular calcium from a normal level of about 0.1 μM [11, 14] to 1 μM evokes a decrease of beta adrenoceptors in arterial smooth muscle cells and an increase of beta adrenoceptors in lymphocytes. In other words, mild increases of intracellular free calcium reproduce to some extent the adrenoceptor abnormality observed in these two different cell types in primary hypertension. In contrast, when calcium was raised to about 10 μM, a level clearly above the physiological range, these changes were no longer expressed in either cell type (Fig. 6).

Discussion

This report demonstrates that in genetic hypertension, adrenoceptor alterations occur in tissues as different as vascular smooth muscle and blood lymphocytes and in different species like man and rat.

Some of these alterations are likely to have a pathogenetic implication. In arterial smooth muscle cells, a decrease in the density of beta adrenoceptors, with an increase of the alpha:beta ratio, can predispose the vessels to vasoconstriction early in the life of SHR.

It is interesting to observe that the hypertensive abnormalities appear as an exaggeration of physiological changes that accompany development and aging in normotensive rats. In the life span investigated, normotensive WKY rats increase their blood pressure by about 25 mmHg, while SHR show an increase of about 50 mmHg. An open question is whether this greater age-related increase in blood pressure can somehow be linked to an early and more prominent increase in the alpha:beta adrenoceptor ratio of arterial muscle in SHR.

In lymphocytes of either SHR or essential hypertensives, the density of beta adrenoceptors is increased. This confirms the report of other investigators [12, 13] and suggests that adrenoceptor alterations in hypertension can be widespread, involving different tissues. On the other hand, beta adrenoceptor changes have an opposite nature in lymphocytes and IASMC, indicating that no simple uniform pattern occurs in different cell types. However, the fact that the same defect was found in lymphocytes of humans and rats suggests that it is related to the nature of genetic hypertension. In lymphocytes, as well as in arterial muscle, age-related trends were observed. The density of lymphocytic beta adrenoceptors (LBA) increases with age. The hypertensive – normotensive difference also is age-dependent; the tendency of adult SHR to have increased LBA densities might be considered as an exaggeration of the normal trend of LBA to increase with age.

Questions arise about the mechanism of these changes that cannot be answered at present. Our previous finding that the control of intracellular free calcium is altered in lymphocytes of SHR [14] prompted us to study the effect of raising cytoplasmic calcium on the adrenoceptors of lymphocytes and arterial smooth muscle cells. It was found that increasing intracellular Ca^{2+} to 1 μM reproduced, in both cell types, the changes associated with hypertension. However, when intracellular Ca^{2+} was raised to about 10 μM, these changes were no longer apparent. Hence, a relationship between intracellular calcium and adrenoceptor regulation is suggested, but it seems to be a complex one.

In conclusion, adrenoceptor alterations in hypertension vary in different tissues, are age-dependent, and are probably related to other cellular abnormalities. Further work is required to clarify the relation between adrenoceptors and the pathophysiology of hypertension.

References

1. Lais LT, Brody MJ (1975) Mechanism of vascular hyperresponsiveness in the spontaneously hypertensive rat. Circ Res 36-37 [Suppl 1]: 1216-1221
2. Asano M, Aoki K, Matsuda T (1982) Reduced beta adrenoceptor interaction of norepinephrine enhance contraction in the femoral artery from spontaneously hypertensive rats. J Pharmacol Exp Ther 223 (1): 207-214
3. Cohen ML, Berkowitz BA (1975) Decreased vascular relaxation in hypertension. J Pharmacol Exp Ther 196 (2): 396-406
4. Cheng JB, Shibata S (1982) Vascular relaxation in the spontaneously hypertensive rat. J Cardiovasc Pharmacol 3: 1126-1132
5. Fleisch JH, Maling HM, Brodie BB (1970) Beta-receptor activity in aorta. Circ Res 26: 151-161
6. Toal CB, Leenen FHH (1984) Blood pressure responsiveness to isoproterenol during the development of hypertension in conscious, spontaneously hypertensive rats. Blood Vessels 21: 252-256
7. Bruschi G, Orlandini G, Pavarani C, Spaggiari M, Tacinelli L, Cavatorta A (1984) Lymphocytic beta-adrenoceptor abnormality in primary hypertension. IRCS Med Sci (Biochem) 12: 461-462
8. Bruschi G, Spaggiari M, Tacinelli L, Bruschi ME, Caroppo M, Cavatorta A (1984) Regulation of arterial adrenoceptors during hypertension development in spontaneously hypertensive rats. J Hypertension 2 [Suppl 3]: 89-93
9. Bruschi G, Spaggiari M, Tacinelli L, Bruschi ME, Caroppo M, Gandolfi SA, Cavatorta A (1986) Interaction of beta-adrenergic antagonists with local anesthetic acceptor sites. Arch Int Pharmacodyn Ther (in press)
10. Bruschi G, Minari M, Bruschi ME, Tacinelli L, Milani B, Cavatorta A, Borghetti A (1986) Similarities of essential and spontaneous hypertension: volume and number of blood cells. Hypertension (in press)
11. Bruschi G, Bruschi ME, Caroppo M, Orlandini G, Spaggiari M, Cavatorta A (1985) Cytoplasmic free (Ca^{2+}) is increased in the platelets of spontaneously hypertensive rats and essential hypertensive patients. Clin Sci 68: 179-184
12. Middeke M, Remien J, Block LH, Kirzinger S, Landrock A, Holzgreve H (1983) $Beta_2$-adrenoceptor density on menbranes and on intact mononuclear cells in essential hypertension. Res Exp Med 183: 227-232
13. Brodde OE, Prywarra A, Anlauf M, Daul A, Bock KD (1983) Increased number of $beta_2$-adrenoceptors in circulating lymphocytes of patients with essential hypertension. J Hypertension 1 [Suppl 2]: 263-266
14. Bruschi G, Bruschi ME, Caroppo M, Orlandini G, Pavarani C, Cavatorta C (1984) Intracellular free (Ca^{2+}) in circulating lymphocytes of spontaneously hypertensive rats. Life Sci 35: 535-542

Discussion

Brodde: First of all, congratulations on your fine data on arterial smooth muscle cells. As long as one looks at lymphocytes on the one hand and changes of beta receptors and solid tissues on the other, it appears that lymphocytes do reflect some changes in solid tissues. Molinoff, for example, has shown that propranolol increases $beta_2$ receptors in lymphocytes, heart and lung; in some tissues, however, such as arterial smooth muscle, the changes are different. In rats you can study a lot of different tissues - unlike me; I am studying human beings. Do you have any idea what the real meaning of lymphocyte $beta_2$ receptor changes in the hypertensive rats is, for instance?

Bruschi: All I can say is that if one would just once reconcile these findings one could claim that perhaps beta adrenoceptors in lymphocytes are more similar to presynaptic $beta_2$ adrenoceptors than adrenoceptors in smooth muscles, when we talk only about postsynaptic adrenoceptors. My impression, which is just a feeling and not a conclusion, is that they have something to do with the solid cell. For example, in isolated smooth muscle cells the cell was just isolated from the whole body. You can see this change for many hours. I think it has something to do with the inside of the cell rather than with the overall regulation of adrenergic tone or circulation.

Neyses: I really appreciated your work on the alteration of the receptor number in lymphocytes and also in arterial myocytes in response to calcium changes. The only problem I have now is that even at micromolar calcium levels intracellular free calcium is always at quite a high level. And we may even be activating protease or killing the cell. So although it does not have a potential in regulation, I think we should provide some information on the viability of the cells and intracellular protease.

Bruschi: Yes, of course. This information is not complete. But as far as calcium levels are concerned, we think that 1 μM is not an excessive level. I mean, we were cautious about the point of creating two different levels: one that physiologically was high, but clearly in the range of physiological excitation, and another one which was clearly unphysiological.

Neyses: I appreciated that. But as we will hear later, I think that the physiological level of calcium in lymphocytes as measured by the Quin method, for example, is around 100 n*M*, which is about a tenth of the concentration you implied. You are still quite high with regard to myocytes, but not with regard to lymphocytes.

Bruschi: I completely agree with you, but perhaps you missed a point in my presentation. I showed the basal values of platelet and lymphocyte calcium, which was of course around 100 n*M*, at least in normotensive animals. But I wanted to show that if you increase that level to whatever is comparable to what you obtain with stimulation, let's say thrombin in platelets, they really go up to 1 μM during stimulation, and I wanted to indicate that level and what happened with the receptors.

Koehler: I have only a short question. You were using A23187 to increase the calcium concentration in your cell system. My question is: Which concentration did you use as a solvent? I assume you were using DMSO? Did you investigate whether DMSO by itself produce any effect in the system?

Bruschi: I used either ethanol or DMSO and, of course, I tried it with the solvent alone. The data, which are not extensive but which are quite reproducible, indicate that there is no difference with 1.5% DMSO.

Koehler: I think that this is very high. Because at the rather high concentration of A23 187 you were using, you have to use a rather high concentration of DMSO ...

Bruschi: As I told you, there was 1.5% DMSO in the solvent and I saw no change in the receptors, while with ethanol in the same range, I think about 2% ethanol, there was a slight change in the receptors.

Koehler: ... because I would expect some aberration in the membrane structure with either DMSO or ethanol.

Bruschi: I see your point. I am not sure, actually, that 1% DMSO creates problems by itself. I am not aware of evidence of this.

Alpha$_2$ Adrenoceptor – Mediated Alteration of Contractile Systems

L. H. Block

Kantonsspital, Departement für Innere Medizin, Petersgraben 4, 4031 Basel, Switzerland

Introduction

A number of investigations have been performed to evaluate the mechanism of action of adrenaline; however, thus far its end function, i.e., activation of contractile protein(s), has not been demonstrated. Alpha adrenergic agonists have been shown to stimulate the concentration of intracellular free calcium [1–4]. More specifically, there is evidence for a calcium-gating function of adrenaline [5]. In view of the ability of various agents to cause transmembrane signals leading to the activation of contractile proteins by stimulation of the mobilization of intracellular calcium, the possible effects of adrenaline on the structural and functional properties of biological membranes was studied by using the fluorescent probe 1-anillinonaphtalene-8-sulfonic acid (ANS) [6]. In addition, the calcium-stimulated, phospholipid-dependent phosphorylation of the light chain of myosin was investigated. As a representative target for the action of adrenaline, human platelets were chosen, since they contain the pharmacologically relevant components: alpha$_2$ adrenergic receptors, contractile proteins, mitochondria, and dense bodies for storage of intracellular calcium.

Materials and Methods

Isolation and preparation of human platelets, activation of endogeneous phosphorylation, SDS-polyacrylamide gel electrophoretic analysis of platelet lysates, autoradiography, isolation of calcium-dependent protein kinase C from human platelets, enzyme assays, and assays for lipid metabolism were performed as described previously [7].

Results

One way to determine possible changes in the structural and functional properties of biological membranes as the first step of adrenaline action is the use of fluorescent probes. Molecules like ANS are nearly fluorescent in aqueous solution but be-

New Aspects in Hypertension: Adrenoceptors
M. Middeke and H. Holzgreve (Eds.)
Springer-Verlag Berlin Heidelberg New York 1986

come highly fluorescent upon binding, e.g., to cell proteins [6]. Thus, increased fluorescence has been correlated with binding of the probe to hydrophilic sites of the proteins and was interpreted as a change in their native conformation [6]. To evaluate whether (−)-adrenaline can affect the conformation of platelet membrane proteins, they were incubated with the hormone in the presence of ANS under various conditions. As depicted in Fig. 1, fluorescence intensities increased as a function of increasing concentrations of (−)-adrenaline. This effect was inhibited in the presence of the alpha$_2$ antagonist yohimbine.

We next studied the effect of the hormone of ^{32}P incorporation into specific platelet protein. Following incubation of intact platelets for 1 min with (−)-adrenaline, there was a significant increase in the phosphorylation of two proteins with apparent molecular weights of 20000 (the light chain of myosin), and of 40000 (a protein with so far unknown function) (Fig. 2).

The (−)-adrenaline-dependent phosphorylation of the two proteins was time-dependent, reaching maximum values at 1 min of incubation. Longer periods of incubation did not result in further increments of ^{32}P incorporation. The phosphorylation induced by adrenaline was inhibited by simultaneous addition of either PGE$_1$ (Fig. 2c) and/or yohimbine (data not shown).

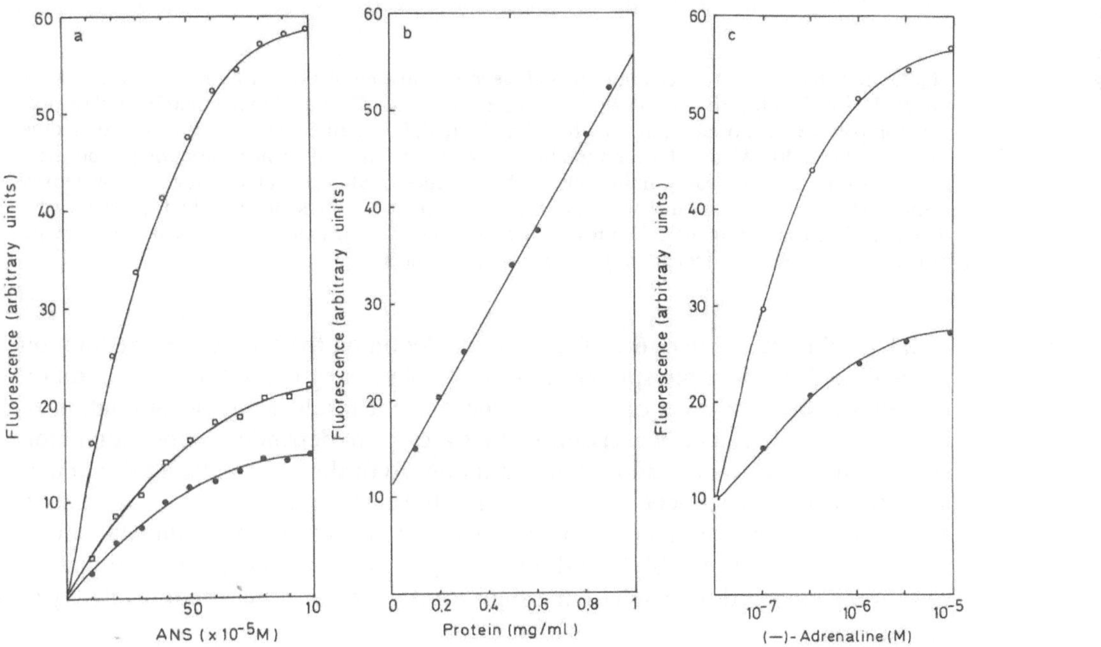

Fig. 1a–c. Effects of ANS and (−)-adrenaline on fluorescence intensities. **a** Variations of fluorescence as a function of increasing concentrations in the presence of constant amounts of platelet membrane protein (0.2 mg) (●——●), plus (−)-adrenaline 1 μ*M* (○——○), plus yohimbine 0.1 μ*M* (□——□); **b** as a function of increasing amounts of protein at constant concentration of ANS; **c** at constant amounts of ANS and protein but increasing concentrations of (−)-adrenaline without (○——○) and with yohimbine 0.1 μ*M* (●——●). The data are representative of four independently performed experiments

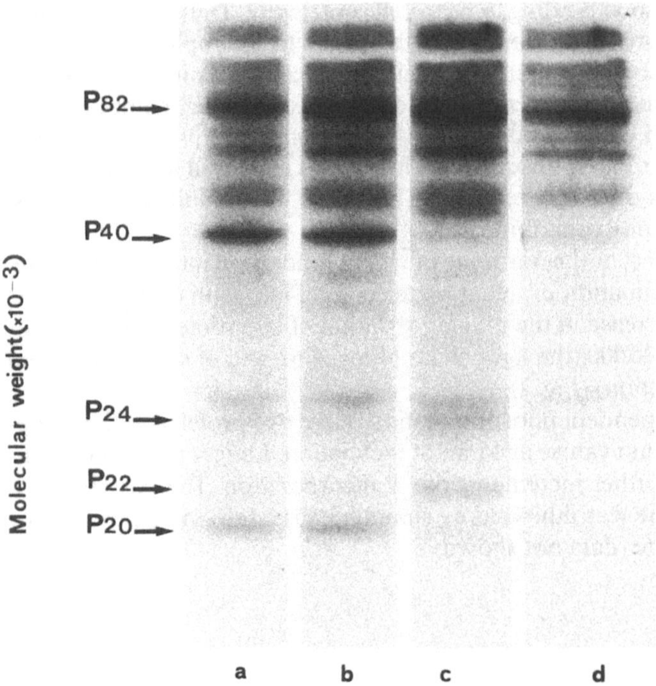

Fig. 2a-d. Effect of (−)-adrenaline on endogenous phosphorylation in human platelets. After preincubation for 1 h with (^{32}P)-phosphate (carrier free) at 23 °C, intact human platelets (90 μg protein/sample) were exposed to: **a** (−)-adrenaline 0.5 μ*M*; **b** (−)-adrenaline 1 μ*M*; **c** (−)-adrenaline 1 μ*M* plus PGE_1 10 μ*M*; and **d** incubation buffer alone, for 1 min. After the incubation period, electrophoresis on 12.5% polyacrylamide gels, in the presence of SDS, and autoradiography were performed. The apparent molecular weight of the phosphorylated bands indicated by the *arrows* were determined by calibrating the gel with standard proteins of known molecular weight. The data are representative of eight independently performed experiments [7]

Table 1 illustrates the effect of calcium depletion on the incubation medium on adrenaline-dependent phosphorylation of the platelet proteins. Since the addition of various concentrations of the hormone did not result in the accumulation of cAMP in the platelets it was assumed that a calcium-dependent phosphorylation step was involved in the action of the hormone. To further substantiate this alternative, the calcium-dependent protein kinase C, the enzyme responsible for the catalysis of this process, was isolated and stimulated under various experimental conditions. As illustrated in Table 2, addition of (−)-adrenaline plus calcium to platelet membrane preparations resulted in a significant increase in the reaction velocity of the enzyme.

Considering that phospholipid (P_I) turnover is the signal for activation of the enzyme, correspondingly rapid P_I turnover and protein phosphorylation should occur. Indeed, when platelets were stimulated with (−)-adrenaline as described above, 40000- and 20000-molecular-weight proteins became phosphorylated; the reaction was preceded by transient formation of endogeneous diacylglycol (data not shown).

Table 1. Changes in the incorporation of ^{32}P-phosphate into human platelet proteins as a function of duration of exposure to (−)-adrenaline, in the presence and absence of calcium[a]

Condition	CPM at 0	30 s	60 s	120 s	180 s	Specific proteins
Initial	380± 49	415± 36	367± 74	379± 36	390± 61	20 K protein
EGTA	374± 71	368± 41	390± 49	406± 64	374± 67	
EGTA plus (−)-adrenaline	416± 69	494± 78	526± 57	596± 80	571± 92	
(−)-adrenaline plus Ca^{2+}	512± 87	1020±154	1662±147	1664±196	1704±137	
Ca^{2+}	407± 37	547± 72	697± 62	704± 68	802± 94	
Initial	476± 47	537± 29	550± 67	597± 73	608± 80	40 K protein
EGTA	501± 72	567± 63	616± 92	609± 63	594± 72	
EGTA plus (−)-adrenaline	604± 67	807± 92	1562±216	1497±174	1592±204	
(−)-Adrenaline plus Ca^{2++}	617±114	2002±198	2496±306	2496±402	2506±316	
Ca^{2++}	509± 49	874± 63	997±103	1013±204	1097±124	

[a] After preincubation with carrier-free ^{32}P-phosphate for 1 h at 23 °C, platelets (90 µg protein/sample) were preincubated with EGTA 1 m*M*, (b) (−)-adrenaline 1 µ*M* plus EGTA, (−)-adrenaline plus $CaCl_2$ 0.5 m*M*, or $CaCl_2$ alone. At the times indicated, stop solution was added and the phosphorylation of platelets was analyzed by SDS-PAGE and autoradiography. After the protein staining pattern was recorded by spectophotometry, the gels were sliced into 2-mm sections. Each section was dissolved (with shaking) in 0.5 ml 30% hydrogen peroxide at 60 °C for 4 h. The $^{32}P_i$ content of the resulting solution was determined by liquid scintillation spectroscopy. The data represent the $^{32}P_i$ content of gel sections of the 40K and 20K regions. The results represent the mean of four independently performed experiments (±SD)

Table 2. Effects of (−)-adrenaline[a], $CaCl_2$, diolein, and yohimbine on the activation of protein kinase C

Additions			Reaction velocity (cpm)
(−)-Adrenaline	10^{-7} *M* + $CaCl_2$ 0.5 µ*M*		4800± 390
	10^{-6} *M*		10800±1370
	10^{-5} *M*		11600±1860
	10^{-5} *M*	+yohimbine 0.1 µ*M*	4960± 510
	10^{-5} *M* + diolein alone		4200± 430
$CaCl_2$	10^{-6} *M* + (−)-adrenaline 1 µ*M*		1400± 240
	10^{-5} *M*		8300± 980
	10^{-4} *M*		10600±1170
	10^{-4} *M*	+yohimbine 0.1 µ*M*	4090± 280
	10^{-4} *M* + diolein alone		1110± 160

[a] The effect of adrenaline on reaction velocity of protein kinase C was assayed by the presence of varying amounts of hormone and constant concentrations of $CaCl_2$, or fixed amounts of $CaCl_2$ and varying amounts of hormone, in the absence and presence of yohimbine and in the presence of constant amounts of platelet membrane (20 µg/ml) and diolein (2.4 µg/ml). The results are the means of five independently performed experiments ± SD

Discussion

The data indicate a specific increase in fluorescence of ANS on the addition of adrenaline. These changes do not seem to lead to modification of the hydrophobicity of the sites to which ANS binds, as judged by the constancy of the relative fluorescence intensities, but rather due to an increase in the ANS binding sites which presumably become affected during the interaction of the hormone and the alpha$_2$ receptors expressed on platelet membranes. An increase in fluorescence intensities of ANS has been interpreted as being suggestive of a change in a conformation of proteins [6]. It may therefore be suggested that the first step of the action of adrenaline leads to conformational changes in membrane proteins subsequent to binding to the alpha$_2$ receptors. This initial event could explain why the anchored calcium-stimulated, phospholipid-dependent protein kinase C can be activated on the addition of the hormone.

The argument that the P_I turnover can only be stimulated by alpha$_1$ adrenergic agents can no longer be considered true, for the following reasons: Various reports have shown that the phospholipid turnover can be stimulated by virtually any type of tissue stimulated by a variety of extracellular messengers [2]. The fact that the receptors in platelets are alpha$_2$ in type, and the observation that the action of adrenaline can be inhibited by the specific alpha$_2$ antagonist yohimbine, indicate that the P_I turnover can not only be ascribed to alpha$_1$ but also to alpha$_2$ receptors. Moreover, possible effects of adrenaline on phospholipid metabolism have already been indicated by previous observations [8-10], and the production of phosphatylinositol as the primary event during alpha-adrenergic activation was reported. However, one cannot formally exclude the possibility that there may be a stimulation of a variety of factors (e.g., ADP) during adrenaline action causing stimulation of P_I turnover.

Our studies on the effect of calcium depletion in the incubation medium during the action of adrenaline indicate a calcium-dependent phosphorylation step during the action of the hormone. The results indicate further that adrenaline stimulates protein kinase C and that membrane constituents (including phospholipids), diolein, and calcium play a cooperative role in the stimulation of the activity of the enzyme. This is strenghtened by experiments using various acidic phospholipids in place of platelet membrane, showing that phosphatylinositol was by far the most active membrane phospholipid as support of enzyme activation (data not shown).

Based on experimental evidence provided above, it may be concluded that adrenaline action occurs in the following sequence: Hormone binds the receptor leading to conformational changes of membrane proteins resulting in the activation of membrane anchored protein kinase C. In parallel, P_I turnover is initiated, and intracellular calcium is mobilized from intracellular stores, leading to full activation of protein kinase C. Finally, the two proteins with molecular weights of about 20000 and 40000 become phosphorylated by the calcium-stimulated, phospholipid-dependent protein kinase C.

Summary

The molecular mechanism of action of adrenaline was studied by investigating structural changes in the membranes of human platelets and biochemical events leading to functional response to the hormone. The structural changes were analyzed by the use of the fluorescent probe 1-anillinonaphthalene-8-sulfonic acid (ANS), which is highly fluorescent when located in biomembranes, but not in water. Thus, in the presence of the hormone, the fluorescence of ANS was increased several-fold as a function of both (−)-adrenaline and membrane protein. Conversely, the (−)-adrenaline-induced effect was almost completely inhibited by the addition of yohimbine, suggesting that the alpha$_2$-mediated signal leads to conformational changes of platelet membrane proteins involved in signal transduction.

In human platelets, adrenaline stimulated, approximately fourfold as compared with controls, the phosphorylation of primarily two proteins with molecular weights of 20000 and 40000. Maximum phosphorylation occurred after incubation for 1 min and was inhibited by the addition of yohimbine, prostaglandin E_1, or EGTA. Phosphorylation of the two proteins was accompanied by diacylglycerol formation. The (−)-adrenaline-induced phosphorylation of proteins corresponds to the activation of a calcium-dependent protein kinase partially purified by DEAE cellulose and Sephadex G 150 column chromatography. The enzymatic activity was modulated by addition of (−)-adrenaline and $CaCl_2$, by diolein, and in the presence of membranes.

References

1. Parot RJ, Putney JW Jr (1978) Calcium fluxes in isolated acinar cells from rat parotid. J Physiol (Lond.) 281: 359-371
2. Chen JL, Babcock F, Lardy HA (1978) Norepinephrine, vasopressin, glucagon, and A23187 induced effect of calcium from an exchangeable pool in isolated rat hepatocytes. Proc Natl Acad Sci USA 75: 2234-2238
3. Miller BE, Nelson DL (1977) Calcium fluxes in isolated acinar cells from rat parotid. J Biol Chem 252: 3629-3636
4. Erne P, Bühler FR, Affolter H, Bürgisser E (1983) Excitatory and inhibitory modulation of intracellular free calcium in human platelets by hormones and drugs. Eur J Pharmacol 91: 331-332
5. Owen NE, Feinberg H, Le Breton GL (1980) Epinephrine induces Ca^{2++} uptake in human blood platelets. Am J Physiol 239: H483-H488
6. Azzi A (1974) The use of fluorescent probes for the study of membranes. Methods Enzymol 32: 234-257
7. Block LH, Jaschke H, Erne P, Bolli P, Bühler FR (1985) (−)-Adrenaline-induced, calcium-dependent phosphorylation of protein in human platelets. J Clin Invest 75: 1600-1607
8. Michell RH (1975) Inositol phospholipids and cell surface receptor function. Biochim Biophys Acta 451: 81-147
9. Michell RH, Jones LM (1974) Enhanced phosphatidylinositol labelling in rat parotid fragments exposed to alpha-adrenergic stimulation. Biochem J 138: 47-52
10. Jones LM, Michell RH (1975) Relationship of calcium to receptor-controlled stimulation of phosphatidylinositol turnover. Biochem J 148: 479-485

Discussion

Philipp: Could you explain again in a few sentences the main differences between normotensives and patients with essential hypertension, for example with respect to concentrations of protein kinase C?

Block: As far as I can tell, there is practically no difference - in the enzyme concentrations present in platelets but rather in its reaction velocity. It is interesting to note in this context that 2 years ago Meyer found differences in the formation of phosphatidylinositol derivatives and metabolites in the platelets of spontaneously hypertensive rats.

Jakob: In your representation you suggested that $alpha_2$ receptors are involved in PI turnover. In none of the cells so far investigated is that the case. In all of the studies conducted to date by other groups, including those on platelets, that is not the case and only you claim otherwise. My question is therefore: How can you exclude the possibility that the effects which you see with epinephrine are not of an indirect nature, that is, caused by ADP, thromboxane, or the like?

Block: That is not true, if I may correct you. There are several studies which show just the opposite. I'd like to go into your question briefly. One conclusive experiment is the incubation with yohimbine, which clearly shows that phosphorylation, which is $alpha_2$-dependent, is blocked in the presence of yohimbine.

Jacob: I disagree. That is not correct. You're doing something with the receptor that may lead to the release of some substance or another from platelets, which then induces phosphorylation.

Block: I admit that is an interesting speculation, that e.g. ADP may be involved in the activity of adrenaline leading to phosphorylation of platelet proteins. I can not exclude that possibility.

Beta Adrenoceptor Changes in Hypertension Induced by Dynamic Exercise*

O.-E. BRODDE

Universitätsklinikum Essen, Biochem. Forschungslabor der Medizinischen Klinik und Poliklinik, Abteilung für Nieren- und Hochdruckkranke, Hufelandstr. 55, 4300 Essen 1, FRG

Introduction

During the last decade, radioligand binding studies have greatly advanced our knowledge of the molecular pharmacology of β-adrenoceptors. With this technique, it has become increasingly apparent that the tissue concentration of β-adrenoceptors is not a fixed number but is rather dynamically regulated by a variety of drugs, hormones, pathological and physiological conditions [14, 16, 19, 20, 24]. In vitro and in vivo studies have shown that in numerous tissues, long-term exposure to β-adrenergic agonists results in an impaired β-adrenergic function. This reduced responsiveness of β-adrenoceptors was consistently found to be due to decreased receptor density and/or to a diminished activity of the adenylate cyclase-cAMP system.

To study such alterations in β-adrenoceptor function in man, circulating lymphocytes containing a homogeneous population of β_2-adrenoceptors [2, 13, 31] coupled in an excitatory manner to the adenylate cyclase [1, 5] are frequently used. We have recently demonstrated [6] that in man the β-adrenoceptor density in circulating lymphocytes is significantly correlated with the corresponding β-adrenoceptor density and responsiveness (evaluated as positive inotropic responses to isoprenaline) in the right atrial appendages obtained from the same subjects. These results, therefore, strongly support the view that changes in β-adrenoceptors in circulating lymphocytes mirror changes which might occur in solid tissues (at least in the heart) of the human being.

As mentioned above, it is now generally accepted that a long-term increase in the activity of the sympathetic nervous system leads to a reduced tissue responsiveness to β-adrenergic stimulation. *Acute* stimulation of the sympathetic activity, however, seems to affect β-adrenoceptor density in a rather different manner, since it has been shown that in healthy volunteers, dynamic exercise (vigorous stimulus of the sympathetic activity) leads to a rapid increase of lymphocyte β_2-adrenoceptor density [3, 10, 17]. This is, therefore, a suitable model to study the acute regulation of β-adrenoceptors in man.

In essential hypertension, the activity of the sympathetic nervous system seems to be altered [11, 12, 30]. Thus, it was of interest to investigate whether acute regulation

* This work was supported by the *Landesamt für Forschung Nordrhein-Westfalen* and the SANDOZ *Stiftung für Therapeutische Forschung.*

New Aspects in Hypertension: Adrenoceptors
M. Middeke and H. Holzgreve (Eds.)
Springer-Verlag Berlin Heidelberg New York 1986

of β-adrenoceptors might be impaired in essential hypertension. For this purpose the effects of dynamic exercise (15 min on a bicycle at 80% of maximum heart rate) on lymphocyte β_2-adrenoceptor density (assessed by (−) [^{125}I] iodocyanopindolol (ICYP) binding) and responsiveness (assessed as 10 μ*M* (−)-isoprenaline-induced increases in the intracellular level of lymphocyte cAMP) were determined in ten normotensive volunteers and compared with those in ten patients with essential hypertension.

Subjects and Methods

Ten male normotensive (P_{diast} <90 mmHg) volunteers (mean age: 26.5 ± 2.2 (19–45) years; mean blood pressure: 119.9 ± 2.6/79.1 ± 2.9 mmHg) and ten patients with essential hypertension (P_{diast} >95 mmHg; seven males, three females; mean age: 42.1 ± 2.7 (30–57) years; mean blood pressure: 161 ± 10/103 ± 9 mmHg) participated in the study after having given informed written consent. The experimental protocol (Fig. 1) was the same as described elsewhere [3]. Briefly: The exercise was performed on a bicycle ergometer (Bosch, Berlin, FRG) in the supine position, starting with an initial work load of 50 W. The workload was increased by 25 W every 2 min until 80% of the maximum heart rate (calculated by the formula: 200 − age beats/min) was reached. The final work load (usually 100–150 W) was kept constant until a total exercising time of 15 min was reached. Immediately before exercise, at the end of exercise, and 1 h after exercise (indicated by the arrows in Fig. 1) 30 ml heparinized blood (500 I.U./10 ml blood) for determination of lymphocyte β_2-adrenoceptor density and lymphocyte cAMP content and 10 ml ice-cold EDTA blood for determination of plasma catecholamines were taken. Blood pressure and heart rate were recorded automatically by means of a Tonomed (Speidel und Keller, Jungingen, FRG) and an electrocardiogram.

(−)-ICYP binding to lymphocyte β_2-adrenoceptors and determination of the effects of 10 μ*M* (−)-isoprenaline on lymphocyte cAMP content was performed es-

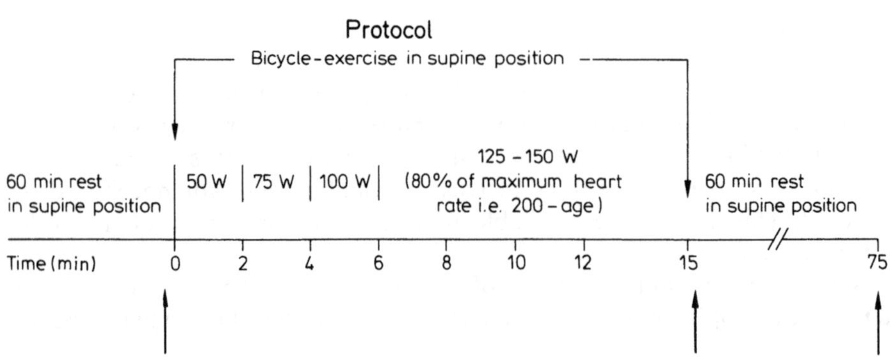

Fig. 1. Experimental protocol. Blood samples: 30 ml heparinized blood (for β-adrenoceptor density and cAMP content in lymphocytes); 10 ml EDTA blood (for plasma catecholamines). Blood pressure and heart rate measured automatically with a Tonomed

sentially as recently described [7]. Plasma catecholamines were assessed by an HPLC method with electrochemical detection.

The experimental data given in the text and figures are expressed as means ± SEM of n experiments. The significance of differences was estimated by Student's t-test; a P value smaller than 0.05 was considered to be significant.

Results

Dynamic exercise (80% of maximum heart rate for 15 min) led in the normotensive control group to a significant increase in systolic blood pressure from 119.9 ± 2.6 to 183 ± 5 mmHg ($n = 10$), which was accompanied by a two- to threefold increase in the concentration of plasma catecholamines (Fig. 2). At the end of the exercise test, lymphocyte β_2-adrenoceptor density was increased by about 100%, while the K_d values for affinity of ICYP to the β_2-adrenoceptors were not significantly changed (Fig. 2). The lymphocyte responsiveness to β-adrenoceptor stimulation followed these changes in β_2-adrenoceptor density, since the increase in lymphocyte cyclic

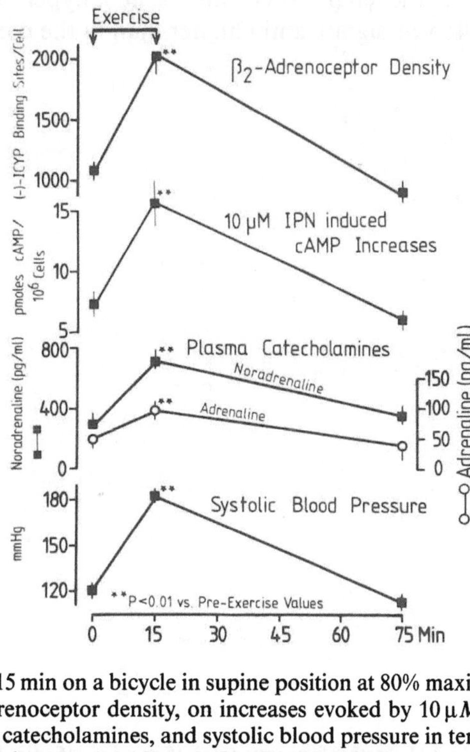

Fig. 2. Changes, induced by dynamic exercise (15 min on a bicycle in supine position at 80% maximum heart rate), induced in lymphocyte β_2-adrenoceptor density, on increases evoked by 10 μM (−)-isoprenaline in lymphocyte cAMP, plasma catecholamines, and systolic blood pressure in ten male normotensive volunteers. *Ordinate (top* to *bottom):* lymphocyte β_2-adrenoceptor density assessed by Scatchard analysis [22] of ICYP binding (ICYP binding sites/cell); lymphocyte cAMP increases evoked by 10 μM (−)-isoprenaline (pmol cAMP/10^6 cells); plasma noradrenaline (*left,* ■——■) and plasma adrenaline (*right,* O——O) (pg/ml); systolic blood pressure (mmHg). *Abscissa:* time in min

AMP content induced by 10 μ*M* isoprenaline was also exaggerated (Fig. 2). One hour after exercise, β_2-adrenoceptor density, systolic blood pressure, plasma catecholamines, and isoprenaline-induced increases of lymphocyte cAMP content had decreased to values identical to, or slightly below, pre-exercise values.

Pretreatment of the volunteers with the nonselective β-adrenoceptor antagonist propranolol (5 mg i.v. 45 min prior to exercise) did not affect basal β_2-adrenoceptor density, isoprenaline-induced cAMP increases, blood pressure, or plasma catecholamines (Fig. 3). However, in the presence of propranolol, the effects of dynamic exercise on lymphocyte β_2-adrenoceptor density and cAMP responses to isoprenaline stimulation were significantly suppressed (Fig. 3). Pretreatment of the volunteers with the highly selective β_1-adrenoceptor antagonist bisoprolol [23, 28] (2.5 mg i.v. 30 min prior to exercise), however, did not affect dynamic-exercise-induced increases of lymphocyte β_2-adrenoceptor density and responsiveness (Fig. 4). On the other hand, the same concentration of bisoprolol abolished the isoprenaline-induced increases of plasma renin activity in healthy volunteers (data not shown), which in the human being is mediated by intrarenal β_1-adrenoceptor stimulation [27, 29]. This indicates that the concentration of bisoprolol used in the present experiments was sufficient to completely antagonize β_1-adrenoceptor-mediated effects.

In the ten patients with essential hypertension, lymphocyte β_2-adrenoceptor density was significantly higher than in the controls (Fig. 5); the same held true for the

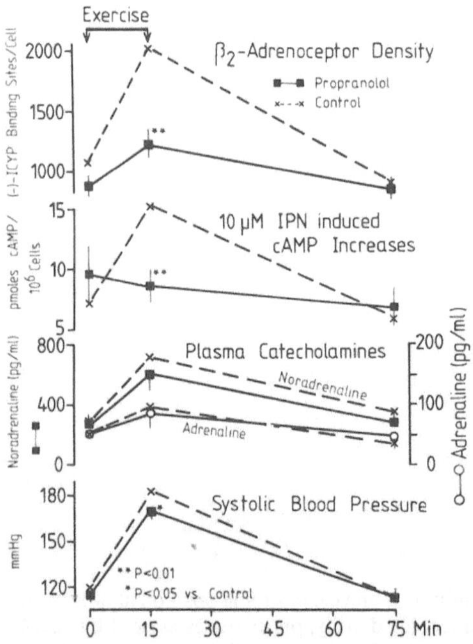

Fig. 3. Effects of propranolol (5 mg i.v. 45 min before exercise) on dynamic-exercise-induced changes in lymphocyte β_2-adrenoceptor density, on increases evoked by 10 μ*M* (−)-isoprenaline in lymphocyte cAMP and on plasma catecholamines, and systolic blood pressure in ten male normotensive volunteers. For details see legend to Fig. 2. For comparison, the control responses in the absence of propranolol from Fig. 2 are given in *broken lines*

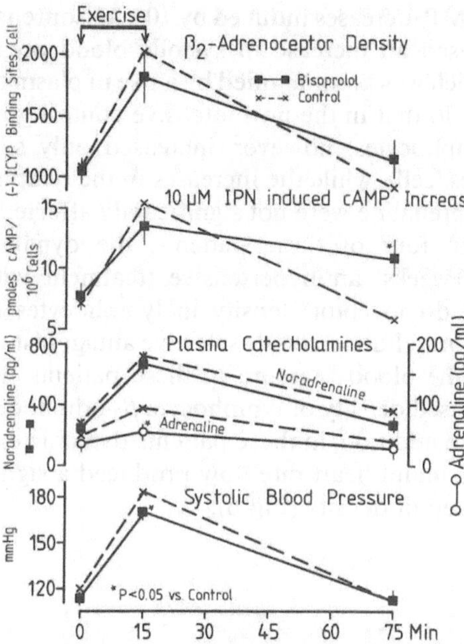

Fig. 4. Effects of bisoprolol (2.5 mg i.v. 30 min prior to exercise) on dynamic-exercise-induced changes of lymphocyte β_2-adrenoceptor density, increases evoked by 10 µM(−)-isoprenaline in cAMP, and plasma catecholamines and systolic blood pressure in ten male normotensive volunteers. For details see legend to Fig. 2. For comparison, the control responses in the absence of bisoprolol from Fig. 2 are given in *broken lines*

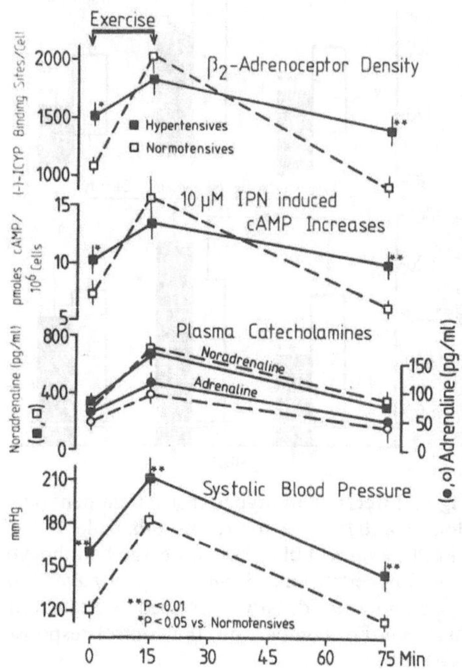

Fig. 5. Dynamic-exercise-induced changes in lymphocyte β_2-adrenoceptor density, cAMP increases evoked by 10 µM(−)-isoprenaline, plasma catecholamines, and systolic blood pressure in ten patients with essential hypertension. For details see legend to Fig. 2. For comparison, the control responses in normotensive volunteers from Fig. 2 are given in *broken lines* and *open symbols*

cAMP increases induced by 10 μM isoprenaline. In these patients, dynamic exercise caused an increase in systolic blood pressure from 161±10 to 210±13 mmHg, which was accompanied by a rise in plasma catecholamine concentrations very similar to that in the normotensive control group (Fig. 5). β_2-Adrenoceptor density in lymphocytes, however, increased only slightly (up to 1859±154 ICYP binding sites/cell), while the increases in the lymphocyte cAMP content induced by 10 μM isoprenaline were not significantly affected by the dynamic exercise (Fig. 5).

In four of these patients, the dynamic exercise test was repeated after a 4-6 weeks' antihypertensive treatment with agents which do not *directly* affect β_2-adrenoceptor density in lymphocytes (the diuretics hydrochlorothiazide and chlorthalidone, the β_1-selective antagonist *without* ISA atenolol). The normalization of the blood pressure in these patients was accompanied by a significantly decreased density of lymphocyte β_2-adrenoceptors (Fig. 6).

In addition, in these patients dynamic exercise for 15 min on a bicycle at 80% of maximum heart rate now produced a significantly increased lymphocyte β_2-adrenoceptor density (Fig. 6).

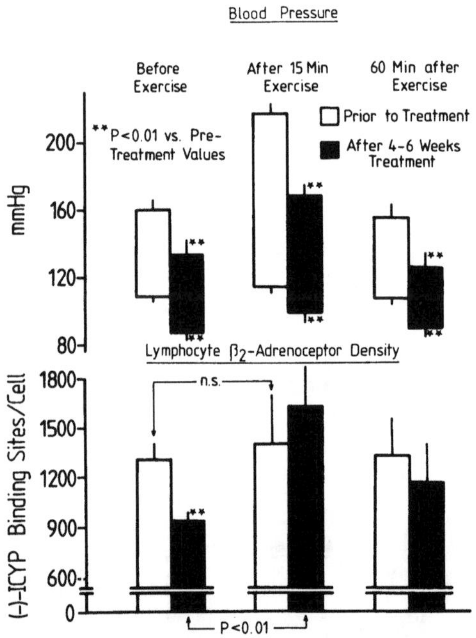

Fig. 6. Effects of antihypertensive treatment (atenolol: 1-2 × 50 mg/d and/or diuretics: chlorthalidone 1 × 100 mg, or hydrochlorothiazide 1-2 × 25 mg/d) for 4-6 weeks on dynamic-exercise-induced changes of blood pressure and lymphocyte β_2-adrenoceptor density in four patients with essential hypertension. *Ordinate: (upper panel)* blood pressure in mmHG; *lower panel:* lymphocyte β_2-adrenoceptor density - assessed by Scatchard-analysis [23] of ICYP binding - in ICYP binding sites/cell. For comparison, the control responses before antihypertensive treatment are given in *open columns*

Discussion

Acute stimulation of the sympathetic nervous activity by dynamic exercise on a bicycle leads to a rapid increase of β_2-adrenoceptor density in lymphocytes of healthy volunteers; concomitantly, the increase in the intracellular level of lymphocyte cAMP induced by isoprenaline 10 μM is exacerbated (cf. Fig. 2) [3, 10, 17]. The mechanism of these acute changes of lymphocyte β_2-adrenoceptor density and responsiveness is not completely understood at present. However, similar effects of acute increases in lymphocyte β_2-adrenoceptor density have been previously observed during infusion of adrenaline or isoprenaline in man [26]. In addition, Strittmatter et al. [25] have shown in rat reticulocyte ghosts that stimulation of β-adrenoceptors increases enzymatic methylation of phospholipids and that phospholipid methylation may unmask "cryptic" β-adrenoceptors, resulting in an increased receptor density. Thus, the dynamic-exercise-induced β_2-adrenoceptor alterations might be caused by the increase in endogenous catecholamines via β-adrenoceptor stimulation. This assumption is supported by the fact that pretreatment of the volunteers with propranolol (5 mg i.v. 45 min before exercise) markedly attenuated dynamic-exercise-induced lymphocyte β_2-adrenoceptor increases.

The highly selective β_1-adrenoceptor antagonist bisoprolol (2.5 mg i.v. 30 min before exercise), on the other hand, had no effect on dynamic-exercise-induced changes in lymphocyte β_2-adrenoceptors (cf. Fig. 4), although this concentration was sufficient to antagonize β_2-adrenoceptor-mediated effects, as demonstrated by the complete inhibition of isoprenaline-induced increases in plasma renin activity. These results are, therefore, compatible with the view that the β_2-adrenoceptor involved in dynamic-exercise-induced lymphocyte β_2-adrenoceptor alterations is of the β_2 subtype.

In the patients with essential hypertension, the density and responsiveness of lymphocyte β_2-adrenoceptors was significantly higher than in the controls, in accordance with recently reported data from several laboratories [4, 8, 9, 15, 17]. In these patients, however, dynamic exercise produced only a small intensification of lymphocyte β_2-adrenoceptor density and isoprenaline-induced cAMP increases, although the rise in plasma catecholamines was very similar to that in the normotensive controls (cf. Fig. 5). As discussed above, exercise-induced changes in lymphocyte β_2-adrenoceptors might be caused by endogenous catecholamines through a β_2-adrenoceptor-dependent process. The blunted effect of dynamic exercise in essential hypertensive patients on β_2-adrenoceptor density favors the idea, therefore, that in essential hypertension the acute regulation of the β-adrenoceptor-adenylate-cyclase system is impaired.

In the present study normalization of the blood pressure in four of the hypertensive patients by antihypertensive treatment was accompanied by a reduction in the density of lymphocyte β_2-adrenoceptors to values which were not significantly different from those in an age-matched normotensive control (Fig. 6; [21]). A similar reduction of the increased density of lymphocyte β_2-adrenoceptors in patients with essential hypertension has also been observed by Middeke et al. [14] after long-term antihypertensive treatment with hydrochlorothiazide and by Daul et al. (this volume) after antihypertensive therapy with nifedipine and hydergine. In addition, as shown in Fig. 6, after normalization of blood pressure and lymphocyte β_2-adrenoceptor density, dynamic exercise now produced in these patients - in contrast to the effects in untreated patients - significant increases in lymphocyte β_2-adrenoceptor density indicating that the impairment of the acute regulation of β-adrenoceptors seems to corrected. These results strongly support the view that in essential hypertension the increase in lymphocyte β_2-adrenoceptor density is directly related to the elevated blood pressure. It cannot, however, be decided from the present experiments whether the increased β_2-adrenoceptor density is the cause or the effect of the elevation in blood pressure in essential hypertension.

Summary

In patients with essential hypertension, lymphocyte β_2-adrenoceptor density and responsiveness is increased. To gain further insight into β_2-adrenoceptor alterations in essential hypertension, the effects of acute stimulation of the sympathetic activity on lymphocyte β_2-adrenoceptor density (assessed by (−)[^{125}I]iodocyanopindolol (ICYP) binding) and responsiveness (cAMP responses to 10 μ*M* isoprenaline stimulation) were investigated in ten normotensive ($P_{diast} < 90$ mmHg) volunteers and in ten patients with essential hypertension ($P_{diast} > 95$ mmHg). In the control group, dynamic exercise on a bicycle for 15 min (80% of maximum heart rate) caused an almost 100% increase in lymphocyte β_2-adrenoceptor density; this rise was accompanied by a significant increase in β_2-adrenoceptor responsiveness since 10 μ*M* (−)-isoprenaline produced after exercise significant greater increases in the intracellular level of cAMP. Pretreatment of the volunteers with propranolol (5 mg i.v. 45 min prior to exercise) completely abolished exercise-induced β_2-adrenoceptor alterations, while pretreatment with the selective β_1-adrenoceptor antagonist bisoprolol (2.5 mg i.v. 30 min prior to exercise) had no effect, indicating that the exercise-induced increase in lymphocyte β_2-adrenoceptors is mediated by β_2-adrenoceptor stimulation. In the ten patients with essential hypertension, however, dynamic exercise caused only a slight, 25% increase in lymphocyte β_2-adrenoceptor density and in isoprenaline-induced cAMP increases. Four of these patients were treated with antihypertensive agents which do not *directly* affect β_2-adrenoceptor density in lymphocytes (diuretics and/or the β_1-selective antagonist *without* ISA atenolol). In these patients, normalization of blood pressure was accompanied by a significant reduction in lymphocyte β_2-adrenoceptor density; in addition, after normalization of blood pressure, dynamic exercise for 15 min produced significant increases of lymphocyte β_2-adrenoceptor density, which were very similar to those in healthy controls. These results indicate that in patients with essential hypertension (a) the acute regulation of the β-adrenoceptor/adenylate cyclase system is impaired and (b) the increased density of lymphocyte β_2-adrenoceptors is linked to the elevated blood pressure. Whether this increased β_2-adrenoceptor density is cause or effect of the elevation of blood pressure remains to be elucidated.

References

1. Bourne HR, Melmon L (1971) Adenyl cyclase in human leukocytes: evidence for activation by separate β-adrenergic and prostaglandin receptors. J Pharmacol Exp Ther 178: 1-7
2. Brodde OE, Engel G, Hoyer D, Bock KD, Weber F (1981) The β-adrenergic receptor in human lymphocytes: subclassification by the use of a new radio-ligand, $(\pm)$-^{125}iodocyanopindolol. Life Sci 29: 2189-2198
3. Brodde OE, Daul A, O'Hara N (1984) β-Adrenoceptor changes in human lymphocytes, induced by dynamic exercise. Naunyn-Schmiedebergs Arch Pharmacol 325: 190-192 Erratum: Naunyn-Schmiedebergs Arch Pharmacol 328: 362
4. Brodde OE, Prywarra A, Daul A, Anlauf M, Bock KD (1984) Correlation between lymphocyte β_2-adrenoceptor density and mean arterial blood pressure: elevated β-adrenoceptors in essential hypertension. J Cardiovasc Pharmacol 6: 678-682
5. Brodde OE, Daul A, O'Hara N, Khalifa AM (1985) Properties of α- and β-adrenoceptors in circulating blood cells of patients with essential hypertension. J Cardiovasc Pharmacol 7 [Suppl 6]: 162-167
6. Brodde OE, Kretsch R, Ikezono K, Zerkowski HR, Reidemeister JC (1985) Human β-adrenoceptors: relation of myocardial and lymphocyte β-adrenoceptor density. Science 231: 1584-1585 (1986)
7. Brodde OE, Brinkmann M, Schemuth R, O'Hara N, Daul A (1985) Terbutaline-induced desensitization of human lymphocyte β_2-adrenoceptors. Accelerated restoration of β-adrenoceptor responsiveness by prednisone and ketotifen. J Clin Invest 76: 1096-1101
8. Brodde OE, Stuka N, Demuth V, Fesel R, Bergerhausen J, Daul A, Bock KD (1985) Alpha- and beta-adrenoceptors in circulating blood cells of essential hypertensive patients: increased receptor density and responsiveness. Clin Exp Hypertension A7: 1135-1150
9. Bruschi G, Orlandini G, Pavarini C, Spaggiari M, Tacinelli L, Cavatorta A (1984) Lymphocytic beta-adrenoceptor abnormality in primary hypertension. IRCS Med Sci 12: 461-462
10. Butler J, Kelly JG, O'Malley K, Pidgeon F (1983) β-Adrenoceptor adaption to acute exercise. J Physiol (Lond) 344: 113-118
11. De Champlain J (1978) The contribution of the sympathetic nervous system to arterial hypertension. Can J Physiol Pharmacol 56: 341-353
12. Folkow B (1982) Physiological aspects of primary hypertension. Physiol Rev 62: 347-504
13. Galant SP, Underwood S, Duriseti L, Insel PA (1978) Characterization of high affinity β_2-adrenergic receptor binding of $(-)$-^{3}H-dihydroalprenolol to human polymorphonuclear cell particulates. J Lab Clin Med 92: 613-618
14. Hoffman BB, Lefkowitz RJ (1980) Radioligand binding studies of adrenergic receptors: new insights into molecular and physiological regulation. Annu Rev Pharmacol Toxicol 20: 581-608
15. Landmann R, Bürgisser E, Bühler FR (1983) Human lymphocytes as a model for beta-adrenergic receptors in clinical investigation. J Recept Res 3: 71-88
16. Lefkowitz RJ (1982) Clinical physiology of adrenergic receptor regulation. Am J Physiol 243: E43-E47
17. Middeke M, Remien J, Holzgreve H (1984) The influence of sex, age, blood pressure and physical stress on β_2-adrenoceptor density in mononuclear cells. J Hypertension 2: 261-264
18. Middeke M, Remien J, Kirzinger S, Holzgreve H (1985) Adrenergic hyposensitivity during long-term diuretic therapy - a possible explanation for the antihypertensive effect of diuretics? Eur J Pharmacol 109: 401-403
19. Motulsky HJ, Insel PA (1982) Adrenergic receptors in man. Direct identification, physiologic regulation and clinical alterations. N Engl J Med 307: 18-28
20. Nahorski SR, Barnett DB (1982) Biochemical assessment of adrenoceptor function and regulation: new directions and clinical relevance. Clin Sci 63: 97-105
21. O'Hara N, Daul AE, Fesel R, Siekmann U, Brodde OE (1985) Different mechanisms underlying reduced β_2-adrenoceptor responsiveness in lymphocytes from neonates and old subjects. Mech Ageing Dev 31: 115-122
22. Scatchard G (1949) The attraction of proteins for small molecules and ions. Ann NY Acad Sci 51: 660-672
23. Schliep HJ, Harting J (1984) β_1-Selectivity of bisoprolol, a new β-adrenoceptor antagonist, in anesthetized dogs and guinea pigs. J Cardiovasc Pharmacol 6: 1156-1160

24. Stiles GL, Caron MG, Lefkowitz RJ (1984) β-Adrenergic receptors: biochemical mechanisms of physiological regulation. Physiol Rev 64: 661–743
25. Strittmatter WJ, Hirata F, Axelrod J (1981) Regulation of the β-adrenergic receptor by methylation of membrane phospholipids. Adv Cyclic Nucleotide Res 14: 83–91
26. Tohmeh JF, Cryer PE (1980) Biphasic adrenergic modulation of β-adrenergic receptors in man: agonist-induced early increment and late decrement in β-adrenergic receptor number. J Clin Invest 65: 836–840
27. Vanhees L, Fagard R, Hespel P, Lijnen P, Amery A (1985) Renin release: β_1- or β_2-receptor mediated? N Engl J Med 312: 123–124
28. Wang XL, Brinkmann M, Brodde OE (1985) Selective labelling of β_1-adrenoceptors in rabbit lung membranes by (−)-^{3}H-bisoprolol. Eur J Pharmacol 114: 157–165
29. Weber F, Brodde OE, Anlauf M, Bock KD (1983) Subclassification of human beta-adrenergic receptors mediating renin release. Clin Exp Hypertension A5: 225–238
30. Weber MA, Drayer JIM (1982) The sympathetic nervous system in primary hypertension. Miner Electrolyte Metab 7: 57–66
31. Williams LT, Snyderman R, Lefkowitz RJ (1976) Identification of beta-adrenergic receptors in human lymphocytes by (−)-^{3}H-alprenolol binding. J Clin Invest 57: 149–155

Discussion

Fritschka: Did you also measure aggregation during exercise?

Brodde: We only measured beta adrenoceptors.

Fritschka: You showed that aggregation is age-dependent, and I would be interested to know whether perhaps that changes during exercise.

Brodde: We did exercise only with beta and aggregation only with alpha.

Fritschka: Through what mechanism do diuretics cause a change in the beta receptors?

Brodde: I said that the increased receptor density must somehow be related to blood pressure. The receptors also decrease with blood pressure. Which is the chicken and which the egg? It always boils down to the same question. I'm afraid I can't say.

Göthert: You showed very nicely that the increase of beta$_2$ adrenoceptors in lymphocytes has something to do with an activation of beta$_2$ adrenoceptors. At the same time you showed that catecholamine levels increase. That was much more impressive with norepinephrine. All in all, in absolute terms you found only a very slight increase in the order of 30%–40%.

Brodde: For epinephrine?

Göthert: Yes.

Brodde: 100%.

Göthert: 100%. But I mean in absolute terms it was very slight.

Brodde: I beg your pardon?

Göthert: In one case you had increases of 30, 40, 50 pg, but in the other case 300 pg. I wonder whether it should not after all be regarded as a slight flaw. One would have actually expected norepinephrine to increase by much more. And then all these inactivation possibilities Dr. Philipp mentioned before are irrelevant, because they come directly from the adrenal medulla.

Brodde: As usual, you've touched the sore point. It is, in fact, a bit difficult to explain why 100 pg of epinephrine, or 100 ng per ml, should produce an increase in beta receptors. First, our findings strongly indicate that it is a beta-adrenergic-mediated effect. If it is a beta-adrenergic effect, it's a beta$_2$ effect. It is also pretty clear - at least that's how I would interpret it - that it must be epinephrine, because the concentration of norepinephrine is too low. I think we should consider one thing: Even if Dr. Wellstein protests, we still do not know for certain whether the concentrations needed in vivo really correspond to those in vitro. There is a very impressive experiment by Dr. Franklin, which is now some 10 years old. He grew cell cultures in the presence and in the absence of isoprenaline and was able to show that when 1 pg per ml of IPN is added the medium produces about 50% fewer beta receptors than when no isoprenaline is present. And that's the same concentration. You know that isoprenaline has a K_i in the high-affinity state of 10 nmol. A picogram does not suffice. What I mean is that it is very difficult to determine the in vivo concentration. Nor do we know how local the concentrations are.

Of course I cannot answer this delicate question satisfactorily, but I hope I have at least given an example showing that it is likely that the mechanism plays a role. Another question is what role cortisone plays. We cannot answer that, but we certainly should not forget it, especially since we have shown that receptors which are downregulated, owing to terbutaline or in asthmatics, for example, can readily be upregulated with cortisone.

Middeke: Does thrombocytosis also occur during exertion? The reason I ask is that there was once some discussion to the effect that the increase in receptors might be due to a change in the subpopulations of lymphocytes under stress. You have now shown that lymphocytosis also occurs during a beta blockade under stress. This is an argument against the claim that the increase in lymphocytic beta receptors under stress is due to a change of the subpopulations.

Brodde: Well, the experiments were performed because we in Essen are simply too stupid to measure B and T cells during exercise. Actually the most elegant proof would be to show that it is due to a B and T cell shift, since the B cells have more receptors than the T cells. As for the platelets, they too increase a little, but not nearly as strongly. I also wanted to point out with regard to the platelets: we checked precisely, in a Coulter counter, whether platelets have even a minute trace of contamination by white blood cells.

Krawietz: You measured the beta receptors in the platelets with Iodopindolol. Is that identical to Iodohydroxypindolol?

Brodde: No. Iodopindolol is an iodinated pindolol. What you're thinking of is iodohydroxybenzylpindolol.

Krawietz: That forms unspecific alpha receptor binding. Is that possibility excluded?

Brodde: That is excluded because we have yohimbine in it. I'd like to say something else. You have to use pindolol. If you try it with IodoCYP on platelets it won't work.

Krawietz: A second question. You referred to the results of Dr. Middeke. Dr. Middeke also showed the difficulty involved in measuring lymphocytes, a relatively strong interindividual variation. You have a very low interindividual variation of no more than 10%.

Brodde: I am not of your opinion there. If you recall the fourth slide, I showed that the beta receptors in the lymphocytes of neonates vary from 200 to 1300. In our hypertensives the variation of the SEM was 11%. The hypertensives - I can tell you exactly - had from 900 to 2400 binding sites.

Unidentified: Following up Dr. Göthert's question about whether the catecholamines are sufficient for the beta receptors on lymphocytes to alter either with age or hypertension or under stress. In all the studies only the peripheral beta receptors are measured. What about the central beta receptors? Are they now excluded as mechanisms for the action of the antihypertensive drugs. That is most unlikely in humans, yet should we completely forget them?

Brodde: We certainly should not forget them, but we all know that it is difficult to make any statement about central beta receptors and antihypertensive drugs. The famous example that is always cited is that a stronly hydrophilic beta blocker like timolol lowers blood pressure very well, although it does not pass the blood-brain barrier.

Unidentified: Of course it does.

Brodde: Yes, but in concentrations that are far from sufficient. Just an example. What I mean is that it still appears very difficult to determine any role of central beta receptors in blood pressure regulation.

Unidentified: Very simple. For me the $beta_2$ receptor is simply a receptor that is essentially capable of mediating vasodilation. We all believe that. Could it not be a consequence of the blood pressure increase, quite independently of the catecholamines, that the receptors increase? I can't show the pathway, but with the goal of inducing vasodilation. Is it known whether a blood pressure rise induced with other substances, for example with angiotensin, also leads to $beta_2$ stimulation?

Brodde: I'd like to contradict: Your hypothesis does not account for the fact that propranolol completely abolishes the increase of beta receptors, although it does not have a great effect on the increased blood pressure. Of course that was lowered somewhat, by 10 or 14 mmHg, but not more. Bisoprolol, although it also lowers the blood pressure by 15 mmHg, has no effect during exercise. That would go against what you said.

Göthert: Just one more brief comment. I certainly agree with you, Dr. Brodde, that we still know little about the significance of central beta adrenoceptors and the development of hypertension. On the other hand, Mr. Filippo has already shown very nicely in his experiments with Feldberg's push-pull canular technique that they play a role in circulatory regulation. For example, he showed that $beta_2$ adrenoceptors occur in the posterior hypothalamus, whose stimulation with suitable agonists leads to a rise in blood pressure. And this effect can be inhibited with $beta_1$ blockers. In principle they play a role in circulatory regulation, but whether they play an important role is unknown.

Unidentified: I have a question on beta receptor determination in the human myocardium. The hearts used certainly come from the operating theater because they are diseased.

Brodde: They are from patients with coronary heart disease who receive a bypass. The cardiac tissue itself is completely intact.

Unidentified: But there are also reports that patients with heart failure have altered beta receptors in the heart, possibly also as a consequence of the pathological catecholamine levels. Have you done any research along this line?

Brodde: We received three explanted hearts from Hannover, taken from patients with end-stage congestive heart disease. We measured $beta_1$ and $beta_2$ receptors in the right and left atria, in the right and left ventricle and found drastically reduced $beta_1$ receptors and unchanged $beta_2$ receptors, unchanged $beta_2$ cyclase and drastically lowered $beta_1$ cyclase.

Effect of Fludrocortisone on Adrenoceptors and Free Intracellular Calcium in Man

E. Fritschka, A. Kribben, S. Harwig, H. Haller, T. Lenz, H. M. Thiede, M. Luedersdorf, Th. Philipp, and A. Distler

Medizinische Klinik und Poliklinik, Klinikum Steglitz, Freie Universität Berlin, 1000 Berlin 45, FRG

Introduction

The mineralocorticoid - induced blood pressure increase in normotensive man is characterized by an early rise in cardiac output during the 1st week of steroid administration and a persistent increase in total peripheral resistance (TPR), which is observed later on, when cardiac output returns to pretreatment values [1, 2]. The initial rise in cardiac output has been linked to sodium and volume retention [3, 4]. The mechanism of the persistent increase in TPR in the presence of a normal or subnormal cardiac output remains elusive. Alterations of sympathetic nervous system activity and increased passive membrane permeability for sodium have been observed in animal models of mineralocorticoid hypertension [5, 6]. The present study examined parameters of sympathetic activity and intracellular calcium concentration, which ultimately should be linked to altered cellular sodium transport [7] in normotensive volunteers, in whom a mineralocorticoid-induced blood pressure increase was evoked by oral administration of fludrocortisone.

Subjects and Methods

Eight men (mean age 24 ± 1 years) received 0.8 mg/day fludrocortisone p.o. for 6 weeks. Blood pressure measurements and blood samples were obtained at weeks 0, 1, 3 and 6, and also 3 weeks after treatment, after 30 min in a supine position at 07.30 a.m. Blood pressure was measured with a random zero sphygmomanometer on the left arm. Means of three measurements were taken. Blood samples were obtained through an indwelling cannula positioned in a forearm vein 30 min before sampling. Blood samples were assayed for platelet alpha$_2$ and lymphocyte beta$_2$-adrenoceptors. In addition, total and free calcium, sodium, potassium, plasma renin activity, and plasma cortisol were measured. Alpha$_2$ adrenoceptors were determined on platelet membranes by ^{3}H-yohimbine binding. Platelet - rich plasma was prepared from citrated blood (100 *g*, 15 min) and diluted with Tris.HCl (50 m*M* Tris, 150 mM NaCl, 20 m*M* EDTA), pH 7.35, and centrifuged at 20000 *g*. This step was repeated twice. Lysis of platelets was then performed by suspension in hypotonic Tris buffer (5 m*M* Tris, 5 m*M* EDTA), pH 7,5, and by homogenization with an Ultra-Turrax (Jahnke and Kunkel, Staufen) for 15 s. After centrifugation at 30000 *g*

New Aspects in Hypertension: Adrenoceptors
M. Middeke and H. Holzgreve (Eds.)
Springer-Verlag Berlin Heidelberg New York 1986

(4 °C) for 15 min the membranes were suspended in incubation buffer (pH 7.5) containing 50 m*M* Tris and 0.5 m*M* EDTA. Membrane suspension 150 µl was incubated in an assay volume of 250 µl containing 50 µl phentolamine in a final concentration of 10^{-5} *M* for the determination of unspecific binding. After incubation for 30 min at 25 °C in a covered shaking bath, the reaction was stopped by addition of 10 ml ice-cold incubation buffer. The membranes were then separated by rapid vacuum filtration on Whatman GF/C filters using a multifold filtration device (Millipore Corporation, Bedfort, Mass., USA). Liquid scintillation counting was then processed using a Packard Tri Carb 300 C apparatus at an efficiency of 70%.

Beta$_2$-adrenoceptors were determined on whole lymphocytes obtained from heparinized blood, diluted with equal volumes of PBS (20 ml): 20 ml of diluted blood was layered on 15 ml Ficoll-Paque (Pharmacia AB, Uppsala, Sweden). The lymphocyte band, obtained after 40 min centrifugation at 400 *g* (4 °C), was suspended in 40 ml of PBS and again centrifuged at 400 *g* (4 °C) for 10 min. This step was repeated once. The pellet was then suspended in Tris buffer (10 m*M* Tris, 150 m*M* NaCl, 0,01% ascorbic acid), pH 7.2. The suspension was then preincubated at 37 °C for 15 min. Subsequently, 150 µl cell suspension was incubated in an assay volume of 250 µl, containing 50 µl (-)- propranolol (5×10^{-6} *M*) and 50 µl ^{125}I-(-)-cyanopindolol in an assay concentration of 3-130 p*M*. Incubation time was 75 min at 37 °C. Filtration was performed as described for alpha$_2$-receptors. Counting was processed at an efficiency of 70% (Berthold apparatus, Berlin, FRG).

The protein content of the samples was determined by the Lowry method [8].

The saturation curves (12 ligand concentrations each) were analyzed by a computer-assisted non-linear regression analysis using a modified Gauss Newton iterative parameter adjustment method on a Hewlett Packard 9826 computer.

Intracellular free calcium was measured in platelets with a nondisruptive fluorescent dye technique [9, 10]. Platelet rich plasma was prepared by centrifugation of blood samples at 140 *g* for 20 min. Quin2-tetraacetoxymethyl-ester (Quin 2-AM, Sigma Inc.) was added to preincubated platelet-rich plasma (37 °C) at a final concentration of 10 µ*M*. Incubation was continued for 20 min. The platelet suspension was then gel-filtered at room temperature on a Sepharose-2B-Cl column with an elution medium containing 10 mM Hepes, 145 m*M* NaCl, 5 m*M* KCl, 1 m*M* $MgCl_2$, 0.5 m*M* Na_2PO_4 and 6 m*M* glucose (pH 7.4). The extracellular calcium concentration was restored to 1 m*M* after gel-filtration. Fluorescence of the suspension ($2-6 \times 10^7$ platelets /ml) was measured with an Aminco-Bowman spectrofluorometer in thermostated (37 °C) quartz cuvettes at 340 nm excitation and 492 nm emission wavelength. The calibration of intracellular fluorescence was processed according to Tsien and Rink [9]. Platelet shape change was excluded before and after chromatography using a Baker 810 platelet analyzer. Platelet function was tested by measurement of thrombin-induced (0.25 units/ml) changes in intracellular calcium concentration.

Plasma plasma renin activity and plasma cortisol were measured by radioimmunoassays [11, 12].

Statistical analysis included assessment of heterogeneity of data by Friedman's rank test. Consecutively, a multiple comparison was made by the Wilcoxon-Wilcox test.

Results

Mean arterial pressure (MAP) increased by 8 mmHg within the 1st week ($p<0.05$). MAP was 11 mmHg higher ($p<0.05$) than before treatment after 6 weeks of fludrocortisone medication (Table 1).

Body weight increased by 1.4 kg within the 1st week ($p<0.05$) and remained significantly elevated throughout the experimental period (Table 1).

Alpha$_2$ adrenoceptor density decreased from 220 (control) to 178 fm/mg protein (week 6, $p<0.05$), returning to baseline values (217 fm/mg protein) 3 weeks after cessation of fludrocortisone (Fig. 1). The affinity of alpha$_2$ receptors did not change during the study (Table 1).

Beta$_2$ adrenoceptor density decreased from 60 to 43 fm/mg protein ($p<0.05$) (Fig. 2). Three weeks after treatment, beta$_2$ receptor density was again 60 fm/mg protein. In contrast to alpha$_2$ receptors, the affinity of beta receptors decreased by weeks 3 and 6 ($p<0.05$; Table 1). The decrease in alpha receptor density occurred

Table 1. Effect of fludrocortisone on hemodynamic parameters, weight, adrenoceptors, electrolytes, plasma renin activity, and plasma cortisol in eight normotensive men

+/−SEM		control		week 1		week 3		week 6		control	
		mean	SEM	mean	SEM	mean	SEM	mean	SEM	mean	SEM
P_{syst}	(mmHg)	116	4	126*	5	129	6	126	5	118	3
P_{diast}	(mmHg)	76	3	83*	2	80	3	88*	3	80	2
MAP	(mmHg)	89	3	98	3	97	4	101*	4	93	2
HR	(b/min)	64	3	61	4	60	4	59	2	64	4
Weight	(kg)	75.7	2	77.1*	2	76.9*	2	76.7*	2	75.4	2
Alpha$_2$	(fm/mgP)	230	19	179*	18	162*	15	178*	14	217	19
K_d	(n*M*)	1.6	0.2	2.0	0.4	1.4	0.2	1.4	0.1	1.6	0.2
Beta$_2$	(fm/mgP)	60	3	64	8	46*	4	43*	3	60	4
K_d	(p*M*)	42	5	22*	3	16*	1	17*	2	35	5
Ca^{2+}	(m*M*)	2.3	0.02	2.2	0.02	2.3	0.02	2.3	0.02	2.2	0.02
ion. Ca^{2+}	(%)	47	2	45	1	43	1	40*	1	46	2
Ca_i^{2+}	(nmol)	99.9	8	179.5**	21	123.5	14	121.6	12	109.4	3
K^+	(m*M*)	4.09	0.09	3.69*	0.09	3.56*	0.09	3.55*	0.06	4.08	0.09
Na^+	(m*M*)	139	0.60	143*	0.80	142*	0.60	143*	0.80	141	0.80
$U_{Na^+} \cdot V$	(mmol/24h)	150	17	112*	12	133*	14	144	8	158	10
Plasma renin	($ng \cdot ml^{-1} \cdot h^{-1}$)	1.54	0.5	0.52	0.1	0.47*	0.1	0.31*	0.1	2.15	0.6
Cortisol	(n*M*)	597	30	592	31	515*	18	495	32	645	41

P_{syst}, systolic arterial pressure; P_{diast}, diastolic arterial pressure; *MAP*, mean arterial pressure; *HR*, heart rate; *alpha$_2$*, alpha$_2$ adrenoceptors on platelet membranes; *beta$_2$*, beta$_2$ adrenoceptors on whole lymphocytes; K_d, dissociation constant of adrenoceptors; Ca^{2+}_{pl}, total plasma-calcium concentration; *ion.* Ca^{2+}, ionized plasma calcium concentration (% total calcium concentration); Ca_i^{2+}, free intracellular calcium concentration of platelets; K^+, serum potassium; Na^+, serum sodium concentration; $U_{Na^+} \cdot V$; 24-h sodium excretion; *cortisol*, plasma cortisol concentration (*$p<0.05$; **$p<0.01$)

prior to the decrease in beta receptor density within 1 week, during a period of increased cardiac output. The decrease in beta receptor density was observed during the period of increased total peripheral resistance (at weeks 3 and 6).

Ionized plasma calcium decreased from 47% to 40% of total calcium by week 6 ($p < 0.05$), whereas total plasma calcium concentration was unchanged during the study (Table 1). Free intracellular platelet calcium was 99 nmol before treatment and rose significantly by week 1 to 179 nmol ($p < 0.01$). Yet during the period of increased peripheral resistance (at weeks 3 and 6), only insignificant changes of free intracellular calcium concentration vs control were noted (Table 1). The 24-h excretion of sodium was decreased by weeks 1 and 3 ($p < 0.05$), but did not differ from control values at week 6 or 3 weeks after treatment (Table 1).

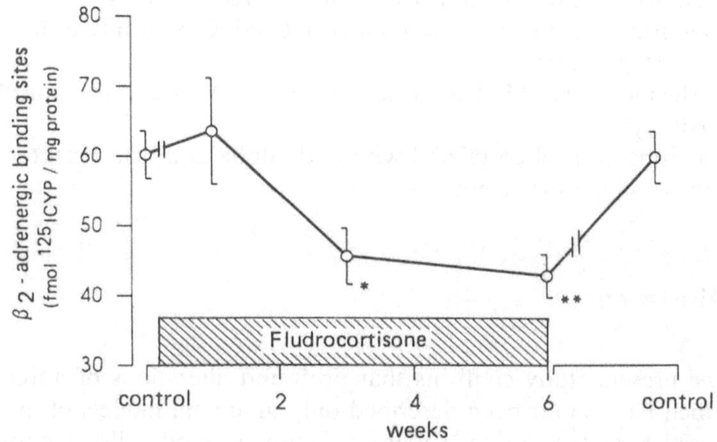

Fig. 1. Alpha$_2$-adrenoceptor density on platelet membranes during mineralocorticoid-induced blood pressure increase in normotensive man (* $p < 0.05$ vs control)

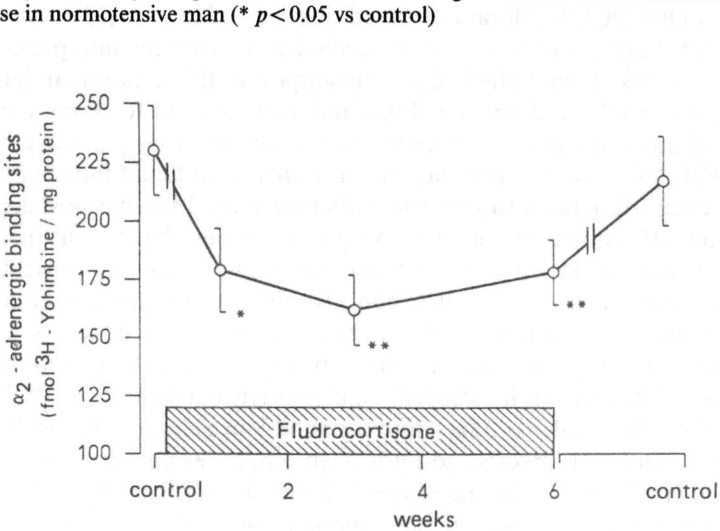

Fig. 2. Beta$_2$-adrenoceptor density on whole lymphocytes during mineralocorticoid-induced blood pressure increase in normotensive man (* $p < 0.05$ vs control)

Serum potassium was significantly decreased throughout the experimental period ($p<0.05$). Serum sodium was increased between weeks 1 and 6 ($p<0.05$) (Table 1).

Plasma renin activity decreased from 1.54 to 0.47 and 0.31 ng/ml/h (control) by weeks 3 and 6 (Table 1).

Serum cortisol was significantly decreased by week 3 only ($p<0.05$) (Table 1).

A significant negative correlation was found between $alpha_2$ receptor density and mean arterial pressure ($r=-0.47$, $p<0.05$), systolic pressure ($r=-0.50$, $p<0.01$), and diastolic pressure ($r=-0.36$, $p<0.05$) in the complete data set. An inverse correlation was found between serum sodium and $alpha_2$ receptor density ($r=-0.43$, $p<0.05$), whereas serum potassium correlated directly with alpha receptor density ($r=0.50$, $p<0.05$). A weak inverse correlation was found between serum sodium concentration and affinity of $beta_2$ receptors ($r=-0.33$, $p<0.05$). Likewise, 24-h urinary excretion of sodium correlated with affinity of $beta_2$ receptor density ($r=0.41$, $p<0.05$).

The increase in MAP after the 1st week correlated with intracellular free calcium ($r=0.7$, $p<0.05$).

Plasma cortisol correlated with both alpha and beta receptor densities ($r=0.44$ and $r=0.45$, respectively, $p<0.05$).

Discussion

The present study confirms that profound alterations of adrenoceptor densities, which have so far been described only in animal models of mineralocorticoid-induced hypertension, take place on human blood cells of normotensive subjects treated with a mineralocorticoid.

In the DOCA-salt rat decreased densities of cardiac [13], vascular [14], and renal [15] beta receptors have been described and have been interpreted as a reflection of an increased sympathetic drive. In support of this concept, an increased peripheral turnover of noradrenaline [16], a reduced capacity for noradrenaline uptake [17], and increased plasma noradrenaline concentrations [18] have been found in the DOCA-salt rat. In contrast, human mineralocorticoid-induced blood pressure increases are known to result in rather decreased plasma noradrenaline concentrations [1]. The decreased adrenoceptor densities observed in the present study are therefore unlikely to represent a downregulated state as a consequence of increased noradrenaline turnover. It is conceivable that sodium and volume retention may contribute to alterations of membrane fluidity and, hence, to decreased receptor densities and increased ion permeability. In addition, alterations of adrenoceptor density by changes in intracellular electrolyte concentration [19, 20] or direct steroid effects should also be taken into account. Since alpha receptors located at the proximal tubule [21] mediate sodium retention, a decreased renal sympathetic nervous activity [22], viz. a decreased renal $alpha_2$ receptor density could counteract sodium retention in mineralocorticoid hypertension. In this context, it is interesting to note that we also found decreased $alpha_2$ adrenoceptor densities in human patients with essential hypertension [23], suggesting that different types of arterial hypertension are linked with decreased $alpha_2$ receptor densities[1]. Since increased sodium concentrations have been found to decrease selectively high affinity binding of $alpha_2$ agonists to platelet membranes in vitro [20], it is tempting to speculate that the decreased binding of ^{3}H-yohimbine in this study is partly due to a loss of high affinity binding sites. Clearly, further studies using agonist binding are now warranted to test this hypothesis. The decrease in alpha receptor density in this study occurred early, during the period of increased cardiac output. The decreased alpha receptor density therefore could contribute at this point to the initially low peripheral resistance.

The decreased density of $beta_2$ adrenoceptors observed during the period of increased peripheral resistance could contribute to a decreased vasodilator capacity, which has also been described in the DOCA-salt hypertensive dog [24]. A decreased venous distensibility caused by decreased vascular beta receptors and abnormal vascular tissue water and ion content [25] could in addition result in a decreased postcapillary blood volume [26] described in the same model.

The decreased ionized plasma calcium levels found in this study are in line with observations in patients with primary hyperaldosteronism [27] and ind DOCA-salt rats [28] and are likely to be caused by alkalosis. The transient increase in intracellular free calcium is possibly a consequence of an increased sodium-calcium exchange, which should peak at the time of maximal sodium retention at week week 1. The functional consequences of this increase in intracellular calcium concentration are unknown, but could involve increased cardiac contractility. This is supported by the correlation between arterial pressure and intracellular free calcium concentration found in this study after 1 week of treatment. Furthermore, calcium antagonists may prevent DOCA-salt hypertension in rats. Although this action has been suggested to be partly due to inhibition of vasoconstrictor effects of vasopressin, it points to a role of intracellular calcium also in the pathogenesis of DOCA-salt hypertension [29]. In conclusion, marked changes in adrenoceptor densities and intracellular calcium occur in human mineralocorticoid-induced blood pressure increase. Both do not appear simply to reflect changes of sympathetic nervous activity, but may be viewed as the result of mineralocorticoid-induced sodium and volume retention. Altered membrane properties, causing decreased vasodilator capacity and increased membrane permeability for calcium ions, may contribute to the mineralocorticoid-induced blood pressure increase in normotensive man.

Summary

The mineralocorticoid - induced blood pressure increase in normotensive man is caused by a transient increase in cardiac output and a later persistent increase in total peripheral resistance (TPR), the mechanism of the latter being unclear. The present study examined the effect of fludrocortisone (0.8 mg/day), administered for 6 weeks to eight male volunteers, on platelet $alpha_2$, and lymphocyte $beta_2$ adreno-

[1] Sodium restriction in turn appears to increase the number of platelet $alpha_2$-adrenoceptors in salt-sensitive patients with essential hypertension [30].

ceptors, as well as on platelet intracellular free calcium measured by the quin2 method. Both alpha and beta receptor densities decreased during treatment. Alpha receptor density decreased during the period of increased cardiac output (after 1 week of steroid medication) from 222 to 178 fm/mg protein. Beta receptor density decreased later, during the period of increased TPR, from 60 to 43 fm/mg protein (week 6). Intracellular free calcium increased within 1 week from 99 to 179 nmol, returning to baseline later. The observed alterations are interpreted as indicators of decreased sympathetic activity and of altered membrane permeability for ions during mineralocorticoid-induced blood pressure increase in man. A decreased vasodilator capacity and an increased intracellular calcium concentration may contribute to the blood pressure increase in this setting.

References

1. Distler A, Philipp TH, Lueth B, Wucherer G (1979) Studies on the mechanism of mineralocorticoid-induced blood pressure increase in man. Clin Sci 57: 303s-305s
2. Wenting GJ, Man in 'T Veld AJ, Schalekamp MADH (1981) Time-course of vascular resistance changes in mineralocorticoid hypertension of man. Clin Sci 61: 97s-100s
3. Chobanian AV, Burrows BA, Hollander W (1961) Body fluid and electrolyte composition in arterial hypertension. II. Studies in mineralocorticoid hypertension. J Clin Invest 40: 416-422
4. Wenting GJ, Man in 'T Veld AJ, Derkx FHM (1982) Recurrence of hypertension in primary aldosteronism after discontinuation of spironolactone. Time course of changes in cardiac output and body fluid volumes. Clin Exp Hypertension A4 (9, 10): 1727-1748
5. Mecca TE, Lamb FS, Hall JL, Webb RC (1985) Cerebral intraventricular 6-hydroxydopamine prevents vascular changes in the mineralocorticoid hypertensive rat. (42094). Proc Soc Exp Biol Med 179: 248-253
6. Garwitz ET, Jones AW (1982) Aldosterone infusion into the rat and dose dependent changes in blood pressure and arterial ionic transport. Hypertension 4: 374-381
7. Friedman SM, Nakashima M (1978) Evidence for exchanged Na transport in hypertension induced by DOCA in the rat. Can J Physiol Pharmacol 56: 1029-1035
8. Lowry OH, Rosebrough NJ, Farr AL, Randall RJ (1951) Protein measurement with the Folin phenol reagent. J Biol Chem 193: 265-275
9. Tsien RY, Pozzan T, Rink TJ (1982) Calcium homeostasis in intact lymphocytes: cytoplasmic free calcium monitored with a new intracellular trapped fluorescent indicator. J Cell Biol 94: 325-334
10. Rink TJ, Smoth SW, Tsien RY (1982) Cytoplasmic free Ca^{++} in human platelets. Ca^{++} thresholds and Ca^{++}-independent activation for shape change and aggregation. FEBS Lett 148: 21-26
11. Haber E, Koerner T, Page LB, Kliman B, Purnode A (1969) Application of a radioimmunoassay for angiotensin I to the physiologic measurements of plasma renin activity in normal human subjects. J Clin Endocrinol Metab 29: 1349-1355
12. Oelkers W, Belkien L, Baumann J, Meyland M (1982) The effect of captopril on renin, angiotensin II, cortisol, and aldosterone during ACTH-infusion in man. Clin Exp Hypertension A4 (9, 10): 1505-1517
13. Woodcock EA, Funder JW, Johnston CI (1979) Decreased cardiac beta-adrenergic receptors in deoxycorticosterone-salt and renal hypertensive rats. Circ Res 45: 560-565
14. Woodcock EA, Olsson CA, Johnston CI (1980) Reduced vascular beta-adrenergic receptors in deoxycorticosterone-salt and renal hypertensive rats. Biochem Pharmacol 29: 1465-1468
15. Yamada S, Yamamura HI, Roeske WR (1980) Alterations in central and peripheral adrenergic receptors in deoxycorticosterone/salt hypertensive rats. Life Sci 27: 2405-2416
16. De Champlain J, Mueller RA, Axelrod J (1969) Turnover and synthesis of norepinephrine in experimental hypertension in rats. Circ Res 25: 285-291

17. Krakoff LR, Ben-Ishay D, Mekler J (1985) Reduced sympathetic neuronal uptake (uptake1) in a genetic model of deoxycorticosterone-NaCl hypertension. Proc. Soc Exp Biol Med 178: 240-245
18. Reid JL, Zivin JA, Kopin IJ (1975) Central and peripheral adrenergic mechanisms in the development of deoxycorticosterone-saline hypertension in rats. Circ Res 37: 569-579
19. Insel PA, Motulsky HJ (1984) A hypothesis linking intracellular sodium, membrane receptors, and hypertension. Life Sci 34: 1009-1013
20. Mooney JJ, Horne WC, Handin RI, Schildkraut JJ, Alexander RW (1982) Sodium inhibits both adenylate cyclase and high-affinity ^{3}H-labeled p-aminoclonidine binding to alpha2-adrenergic receptors in purified platelet membranes. Mol Pharmacol 21: 600-608
21. Di Bona GR (1978) Neural control of renal tubular sodium reabsorbtion in the dog. Fed Proc 37: 1214-1217
22. Katholi RE, Naftilan AJ, Oparil S (1980) Importance of renal sympathetic tone in the development of DOCA-salt hypertension in the rat. Hypertension 2: 266-273
23. Fritschka E, Kribben A, Hoyer J, Schudrowitsch L, Thiede HM, Distler A, Philipp T (1985) Adrenerge Rezeptoren bei Patienten mit essentieller Hypertonie. Einfluß von Alter und familiärer Belastung. Hochdruck 6: 43-44
24. Hamed AT, Lokwandala MF (1982) Impairment of neurally-mediated vasoconstriction in DOCA-salt hypertensive dogs. Clin Exp Hypertension A4 (6): 867-881
25. Pamnani MB, Overbeck HW (1976) Abnormal ion and water composition of veins and normotensive arteries in coarctation hypertension in rats. Circ Res 38: 375-380
26. Brock TA, Fleming BP, Diana JN (1981) Pre- and postcapillary vascular responses to sympathetic nerve stimulation in DOCA-hypertensive dogs. Hypertension 3: 471-478
27. Resnick LM, Laragh JL (1985) Calcium metabolism and parathyroid function in primary aldosteronism. Am J Med 78: 385-390
28. Wright GL, Rankin GD (1982) Concentrations of ionic and total calcium in plasma of four models of hypertension. Am J Physiol 243: H365-H370
29. Hall CE, Hungerford S (1983) Prevention of DOCA-salt hypertension with the calcium blocker nitrendipine. Clin Exp Hypertension A5 (5): 721-728
30. Ashida T, Tanaka T, Yokouchi M, Kuramochi M, Deguchi F, Kimura G, Kojima S, Ito K, Ikeda M (1985) Effect of dietary sodium on platelet α_2-adrenergic receptors in essential hypertension. Hypertension 7: 972-978

Discussion

Brodde: Two short questions. The first is: Does fludrocortisone have any influence on the number of B or T lymphocytes? The second is: we agreed today that a change in the K_d of a ligand towards the receptor is an extremely rare occurrence. The sites vary, but the K_d itself seldom change. This is simply a characteristic of the ligand towards the receptor. What explanation is there for your K_d changes, which, of course, can exert an immense influence on the B_{max}?

Fritschka: One example of when the K_d changes is when the intracellular sodium concentration changes. P.A. Insel, for example, suggested that the intracellular sodium concentration does not alter the receptor density but rather only the K_d of the receptors and explains on the grounds of this mechanism alone why the affinity in hypertensives is different from that of normotensives[1]. Thus, there are very controversial views as far as the K_d is concerned. Point 2: the K_d values of the alpha re-

[1] Insel PA, Motulsky HJ (1984) A hypothesis linking intracellular sodium, membrane receptors, and hypertension. Life Sci 34: 1009-1013

ceptors are not changed at all. However, the alpha receptors exhibited reduced density. As to the question regarding B and T cells, I must say that we are also in contact with the hematology department but have not yet performed any studies with subsets.

Brodde: Actually, I only wanted to know whether the B-to-T ratio is the same before and after fludrocortisone administration. In other words, is the receptor density drop a genuine decrease in receptors or does the drug, for example, kill off the B cells so that the T cells remain, which have only half as many receptors as the B cells, resulting in a drop in receptor density.

Fritschka: As far as I know, fludocortisone as a mineralocorticoid has no effect on the lymphocyte populations, in contrast to cortisone.

Lemmer: I'm not sure whether I recall correctly. I think Nakamura and Toenen found an increased turnover of norepinephrine in DOCA rats in 1962. That would fit in with your findings and your conclusion.

Fritschka: There are several studies in the literature showing that the norepinephrine turnover is increased and the uptake 1 of labeled norephinephrine is reduced [16, 17]. This means that one may assume the presence of a storage defect in the DOCA rat without increased turnover necessarily being always present. In man it is more complicated, in that in this study the norepinephrine plasma level is lowered, but the elimination of free and sulfated norephinephrine in the urine is increased, at least in the third to final weeks, so that at least in the kidney there could be increased turnover. This, in turn, would fit in well with the findings that the alpha and beta receptor densities in kidneys of the DOCA rat are reduced [15].

Bruschi: When we try to induce DOCA salt-type hypertension in rats, we find that there are rats that become hypertensive immediately and others for which you either have to increase the dose or increase the duration of treatment. In fact, there are many investigators who perform unilateral nephrectomy to obtain hypertension in all the animals. My question is, do you have the same pattern in humans? You have responders and nonresponders, and if so, do you select your patients from the responder population?

Fritschka: We did not select normotensive volunteers and we did not observe any marked difference in the rise in blood pressure in any patient. I am aware of the fact that the DOCA-salt rat is somewhat distorted. A lot of surgery has been done, and those rats drink a lot of water and take in large amounts of salt, so the comparison beween this model and the human being is rather difficult. We would conclude that the pattern in humans with respect to salt sensitivity is not entirely clear.

Daily Variations in the Beta-Adrenoceptor-Adenylate-Cyclase - cAMP-Phosphodiesterase System*

B. LEMMER and P.-H. LANG

Klinikum der J. W. Goethe Universität, Zentrum der Pharmakologie, Theodor-Stern-Kai 7, 6000 Frankfurt 70, FRG

Beta-adrenoceptor-blocking drugs are of therapeutic value in the treatment of various cardiovascular disorders, such as coronary heart disease, hypertension, and arrhythmias. However, the effects of beta-receptor blockers have been shown to vary markedly with the time of the day. In healthy volunteers and in hypertensive patients, beta-receptor blockers caused a more pronounced reduction in heart rate and blood pressure during the day (activity period for humans) than during the night (resting period) (e.g., [1-5]; for review see [6, 7]). In patients suffering from stable angina pectoris, an exercise-limited increase in heart rate and ST-segment depression varied with the time of day, independently of whether they were treated with beta-receptor blocking drugs [8]. These data indicate a circadian-phase dependency in the reactivity of the cardiovascular system. Similar results have been obtained in nocturnally active rodents. In light/dark-synchronized male rats the endogenous noradrenaline concentration in the heart did not display a circadian rhythm ([9], see Fig. 1). However, a temporal dependency was found in the turnover of this biogenic amine [9-11], demonstrating that sympathetic tone is higher in the activity period of the rats, i.e., during darkness (D), than in the resting period, i.e., during light (L) (Fig. 1). This finding goes well together with a higher heart rate of rats in the dark phase than in the light phase [12, 13]. Figure 2 shows that in conscious rats, beta receptor blockade by propranolol affected heart rate quite differently depending on the time of drug application [12, 13]. In accordance with the findings obtained in man, propranolol reduced heart rate in rats more effectively in the activity period than in the resting period: In L the maximum achievable decrease in heart rate was obtained by 10 μmol/kg. During D, however, propranolol decreased heart rate in a dosage-dependent way ([12, 13]; Fig. 2).

In man and in experimental animals, a temporal dependency in the pharmacokinetics of various drugs has been shown (see [6, 14]). In order to evaluate whether a circadian-phase dependency in the pharmacokinetics of propranolol could be responsible for the temporal dependency in the drug's effects, chronopharmacokinetic studies were performed in rats. Figure 3 shows that elimination half-lives of racemic propranolol were significantly shorter in plasma, heart, and brain when the drug was intravenously injected in D than in L [15]. Thus, it seemed unlikely that the more pronounced effect of propranolol on heart rate in D could be due to the drug's chronokinetics. However, propranolol has properties (high lipophilicity, he-

* This work was supported by grants from the *Deutsche Forschungsgemeinschaft*.

New Aspects in Hypertension: Adrenoceptors
M. Middeke and H. Holzgreve (Eds.)
Springer-Verlag Berlin Heidelberg New York 1986

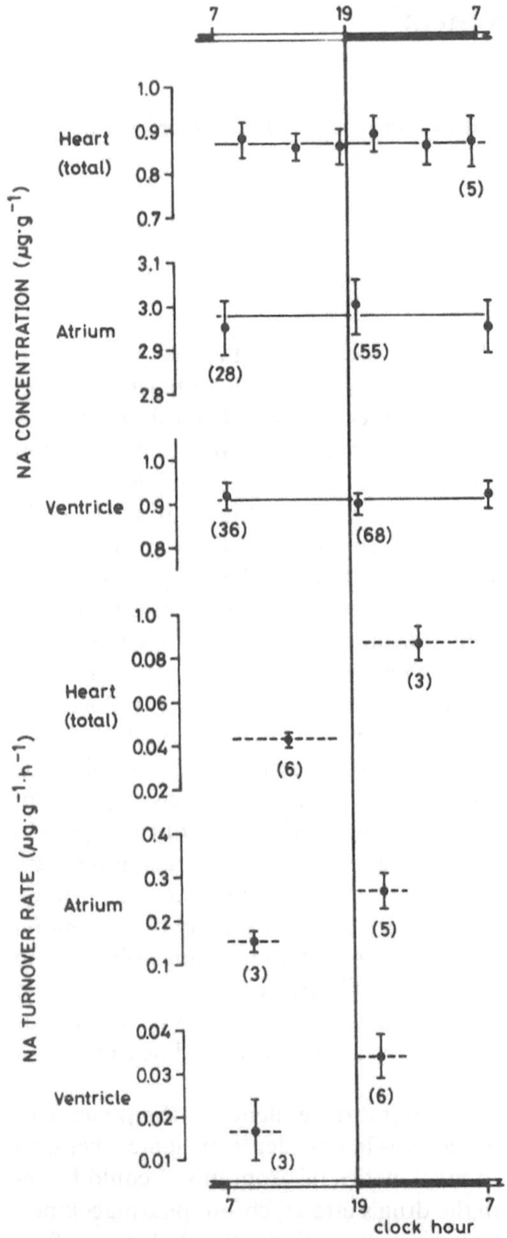

Fig. 1. Noradrenaline concentration and turnover rate in whole hearts, atria, and ventricles of light-dark-synchronized male rats at different circadian times. Lights from 7 to 19 h; *broken line* represents time period of turnover determination. [Data from 9, 11, 12]

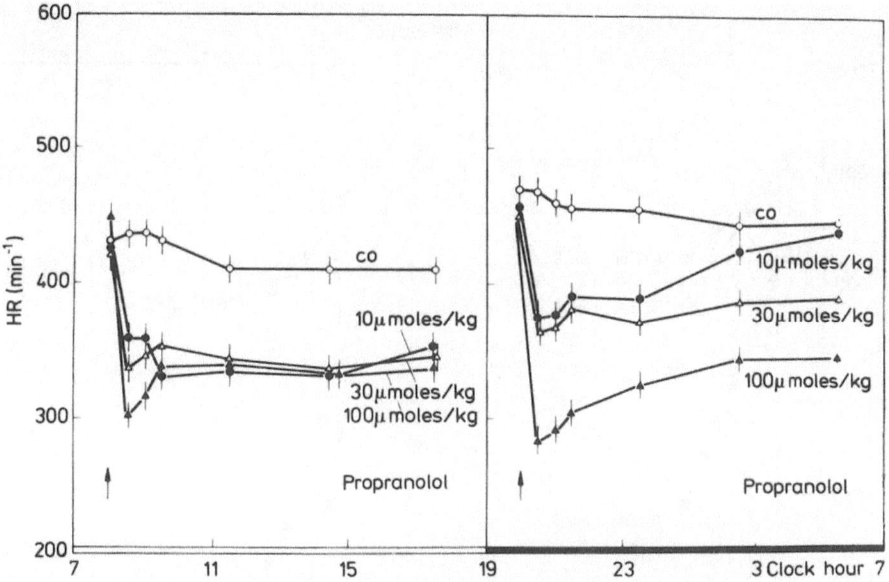

Fig. 2. Circadian-phase-dependent effects of propranolol (10–100 μmol/kg, s. c.) on heart rate of conscious rats. Propranolol was injected either at 0730 h or at 1930 h *(arrows)*. (From [13])

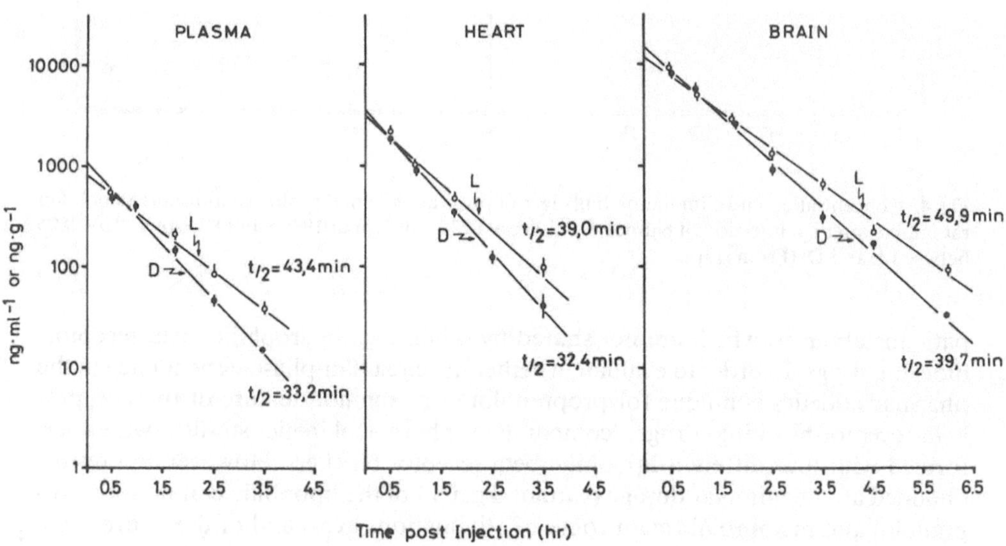

Fig. 3. Concentrations and elimination half-lives of propranolol (8.89 mg/kg i. v.) in plasma, heart and brain of rats during the light span *(L, open circles)* and the dark span *(D, closed circles)*. Significance between L and D: plasma $p < 0.005$; heart $p < 0.02$; brain $p < 0.001$. (From [15])

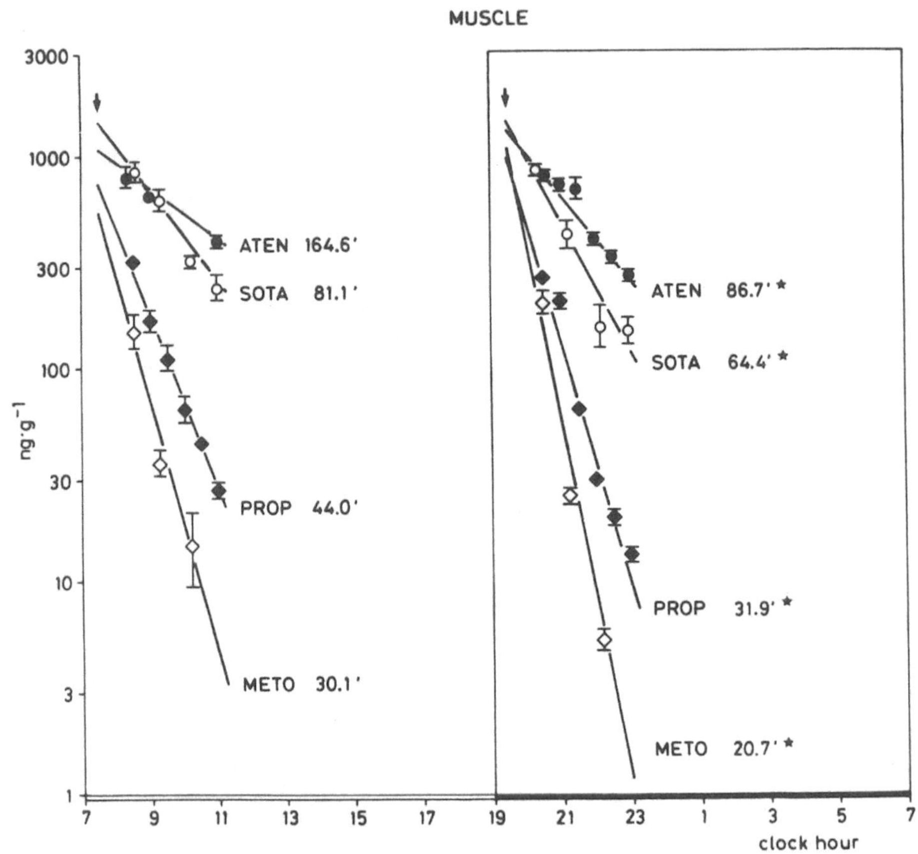

Fig. 4. Concentration and elimination half-lives of propranolol, metoprolol, sotalol, and atenolol in rat muscle after i.v. injection of 6 µmol/kg either at 0730 h in L or at 1930 h in D *(arrows)*. $*p < 0.05$ between L and D. (From [13])

patic metabolism) which are not shared by other, e.g., hydrophilic, beta-receptor-blocking drugs. In order to evaluate whether the circadian-phase dependency in the pharmacokinetics is unique for propranolol or a common feature of the group of beta-receptor-blocking drugs, comparative pharmacokinetic studies were performed with four different lipophilic beta receptor blockers. However, the results obtained after equimolar dosage (6 µmol/kg, i.v.) of the lipophilic compounds propranolol and metoprolol (main route of elimination: liver) and of the hydrophilic drugs sotalol and atenolol (main route of elimination: kidney) revealed that independently of lipophilicity and the main route of elimination, shorter half-lives of both drugs were obtained in plasma, heart, muscle, lung, and brain in D than in L [13]. Figure 4 shows the results obtained in rat muscle as one representative organ. These results clearly demonstrate that drug half-lives after single dose application were mainly due to circadian variation in drug elimination, with a higher hepatic (propranolol, metoprolol) or renal (sotalol, atenolol) elimination in the activity period of rats during D [13]. In accordance with these findings, shorter elimination half-

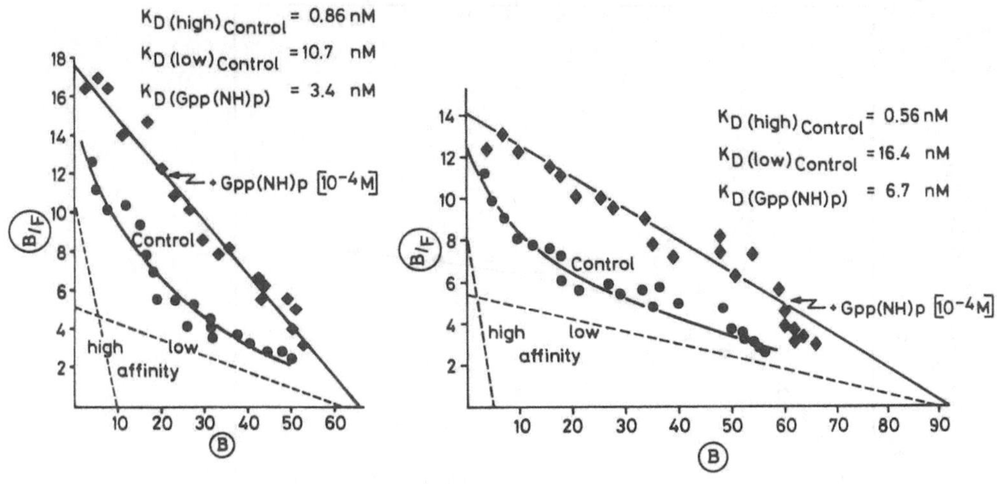

Fig. 5. Representative Scatchard plots of saturation isotherms with ^{3}H-DHA at rat heart ventricular membranes of animals killed either at 8 h in the light span *(left)* or at 20 h in the dark span *(right)*. In this experiment, total number of ^{3}H-DHA binding sites in L and D were 69.7 and 93.2 fmol/mg protein. (From [16, 17])

lives were found in the activity period of man in L than in D after oral dosing of propranolol in healthy volunteers [5].

However, though a temporal dependency in the pharmacokinetics of beta-receptor blockers has been demonstrated in animal and man, these results cannot explain the more pronounced drug effects in the activity period of the respective species. Thus, it is more likely that circadian variations in the sensitivity or reactivity of the sympathetic nervous systems may be responsible for the temporal dependency of the drugs' effects. Whereas in man there is a lack of information on daily variations at the cellular and subcellular level of the adrenergic nervous system such results have been obtained in L/D-synchronized rats.

In receptor-binding studies with the antagonist ligand ^{3}H-dihydroalprenolol [16], about 38% more beta-adrenoceptors were observed at rat heart ventricles at the onset of the dark period than at the onset of the light period [17, 18]. Figure 5 gives representative Scatchard plots of saturation isotherms of animals killed either at 8 h or at 20 h [17, 18]. In these experiments with rat heart ventricles, two specific affinity states of the beta-adrenoceptor were found using the lipophilic antagonist ligand ^{3}H-DHA and the hydrophilic ligand ^{3}H-CGP 12177 [16].

It has been proposed that the total number of binding sites identified with antagonist ligands may not be representative of the functional state of the beta-adrenoceptor. Therefore, the complete beta adrenoceptor-adenylate cyclase-cAMP-phosphodiesterase system was studied at eight different circadian times in a peripheral organ (rat heart ventricle) and in the central nervous system (rat brain without medulla oblongata, cerebellum, pineal gland) of the same animals. In these experiments, receptor-binding studies with ^{3}H-DHA were performed as described in detail elsewhere [16]. Most interestingly, in contrast to rat heart ventricles in rat brain membranes, only one specific binding site of ^{3}H-DHA was found. A representative

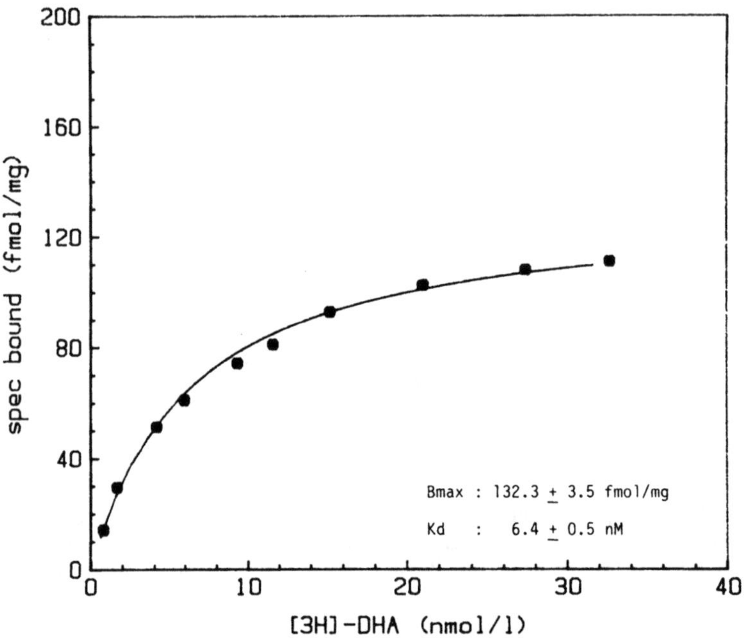

Fig. 6. Specific binding of ^{3}H-DHA to rat brain membranes. Shown is a representative example of a computerized nonlinear least-square fit of binding data

computer-assisted nonlinear least-square fit (MODFIT, see [19]) of specific ^{3}H-DHA binding to brain membranes is shown in Fig. 6. Basal cAMP content was determined by radioimmunoassay in the presence of EDTA and IBMX, the activity of unstimulated adenylate cyclase (AC) was determined in the presence of IMBX using 0.5 m*M* ATP as substrate; for phosphodiesterase (PDE) activity 0.1 m*M* cAMP was used as substrate [20, 21]. The overall significance of daily variations was tested by ANOVA, and a nonlinear least-square analysis of sine-curve fitting was applied to calculate rhythm-adjusted 24-h means, amplitude, and period of rhythms (MODFIT together with subprogram SIN, see [19]). In rat heart ventricles, specific binding of ^{3}H-DHA was studied only at one (16 n*M*) ligand concentration, whereas in brain the B_{max} and K_d values were calculated from saturation isotherms (see Fig. 6). In these studies overall significant daily variations were detected in AC, cAMP, and PDE in rat heart ventricles and in rat brain (Table 1). The rhythm-adjusted 24-h means and amplitudes are compiled in Table 1. In contrast, overall significance was not obtained in specific binding of ^{3}H-DHA to rat heart ventricles and in B_{max} values obtained in rat brain (Table 1), though significance was found between distinct time points by Neuwman-Keuls test. In Figs. 7 and 8, the rhythms of AC, cAMP, and PDE are given as percentages of the individual 24-h means for heart and brain. In rat heart (Fig. 7), peak values of PDE and AC coincided with daily minimum of cAMP in the early light phase. The peak of cAMP and the minimum of PDE occurred at onset of dark period, with AC reaching its second 24-h peak. Thus, in this experiment it looked as though the rhythm in basal cAMP content in rat heart ventricles was mainly determined by rhythmic changes of PDE activity (Fig. 7).

Table 1. Rhythm-adjusted 24-h means and amplitudes of basal beta-adrenoceptor-adenylate-cyclase-cAMP-phosphodiesterase system in rat heart ventricles and rat brain. Significance of rhythm was tested by analysis of variance (ANOVA) [Data from 20, 21]

	24-h-Mean ±SD	Amplitude ±SD	ANOVA
Heart:			
Beta-receptor spec. binding (fmol/mg)	18.8±0.2	1.0±0.3	$F(7/23)=1.41$ n.s.
Adenylate cyclase (pmol cAMP/mg/10 min)	53.3±2.3	26.9±3.3	$F(7/39)=19.92$ $p<0.0001$
cAMP (pmol/mg)	124.1±2.3	22.8±3.1	$F(7/55)=5.59$ $p<0.001$
Phosphodiesterase (nmol cAMP/mg/min)	2.2±0.08	0.7±0.1	$F(7/31)=4.89$ $p<0.001$
Brain:			
Beta-receptor			
B_{max} (fmol/mg)	105 ±2	8.6±2.5	$F(7/24)=1.76$ n.s.
K_d (nM)	5.8±0.1	0.3±0.1	$F(7/24)=0.16$ n.s.
Adenylate cyclase (nmol cAMP/mg/10 min)	3.0±0.1	1.0±0.1	$F(7/30)=5.27$ $p<0.001$
cAMP (pmol/mg)	14.4±0.8	8.7±1.2	$F(7/50)=15.14$ $p<0.0001$
Phosphodiesterase (nmol cAMP/mg/min)	28.4±0.3	3.1±0.4	$F(7/31)=3.55$ $p<0.01$

A different pattern was found in brain of the same animals (Fig. 8). In brain, 24-h rhythms were found in cAMP and AC, whereas PDE exhibited a predominant 12-h rhythm. There was no simple interrelationship between the rhythms of the three parameters. Interestingly, the peak value of cAMP in brain occurred at the end of D and onset of L, i.e., at the time of the trough value in the cardiac cAMP rhythm. The results clearly demonstrate for the first time rhythmic changes in the basal beta-receptor-AC-cAMP-PDE system of the rat heart and brain. The peak value of cAMP content in rat heart around the dark phase [12, 22] fits in well with the increased noradrenaline turnover in the activity period of the rats [9–12]. However, the present results are restricted to the basal activities of the system, which do not allow definite conclusions on the mechanisms underlying the circadian-phase dependency of the effects of drugs. Obviously, further studies, including stimulation-dependent circadian variations, are needed to allow further insight into the regulation and the possible therapeutic implications of the rhythms in the beta-receptor-AC-cAMP-PDE system.

Acknowledgement. We are grateful to Dr. A. B. Cashelin, Department of Pharmacology London and Bern, for his help in the computer-assisted nonlinear least-square fitting programs.

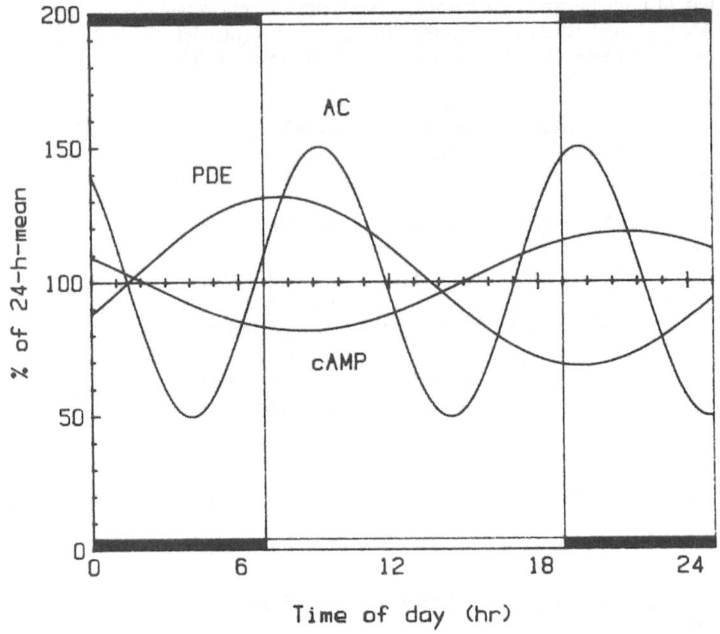

Fig. 7. Rhythms in cAMP content, adenylate cyclase *(AC)*, and phosphodiesterase *(PDE)* activities in rat heart ventricles. Curves are nonlinear least-square fitted sine curves as percentages of the corresponding 24-h mean; for absolute data see Table 1

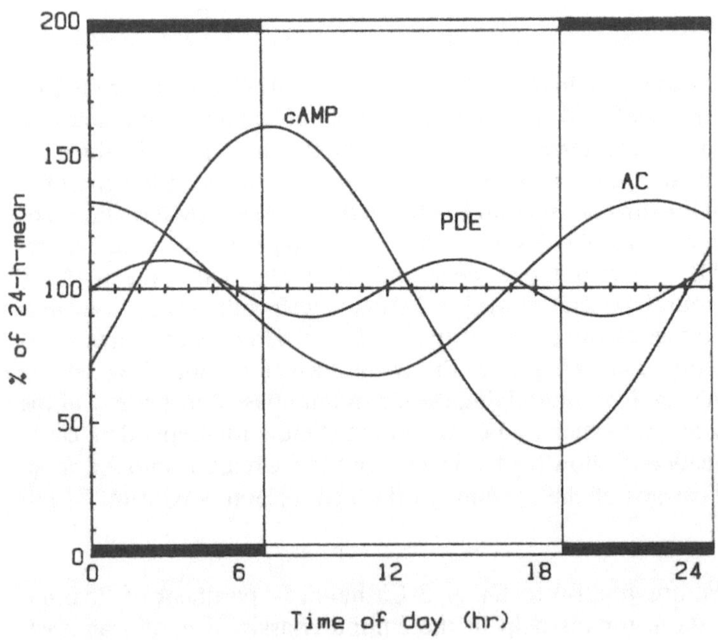

Fig. 8. Rhythms in cAMP content, adenylate cyclase *(AC)* and phosphodiesterase *(PDE)* activities in rat brain. Curves are nonlinear least-square fitted sine curves as percentages of the corresponding 24-h mean; for absolute data see Table 1

References

1. Raftery EB (1983) Eur Heart J 4: 61
2. Balasubramanian V, Mann S, Millar-Craig MW, Raftery EB (1979) Br J Clin Pharmacol 8: 955
3. Magometschnigg D, Hitzenberger G (1983) In: Magometschnigg D, Hitzenberger G (eds) Blutdruckvariabilität. Uhlen Wien, p 101
4. Mann S, Millar-Craig MW, Balasubramanian V, Raftery EB (1980) Br J Clin Pharmacol 10: 443
5. Lemmer B, Langner B (1985) Naunyn-Schmiedebergs Arch Pharmacol 329: R 60
6. Lemmer B (1984) Chronopharmakologie, 2nd edn. Wissenschaftliche Verlagsgesellschaft, Stuttgart
7. Lemmer B (1986) Annual review chronopharmacology, vol 2. Pergamon, pp 199–228
8. Joy M, Pollard CM, Nunan TO (1982) Br Heart J 48: 156
9. Lemmer B, Saller R (1974) Naunyn-Schmiedebergs Arch Pharmacol 282: 75
10. Lemmer B, Charrier A (1980) Naunyn-Schmiedebergs Arch Pharmacol 313: 205
11. Lemmer B, Weimer R (1983) Experientia 39: 998
12. Lemmer B, Bathe K, Lang PH, Neumann G, Winkler H (1983) J Am Coll Toxicol 2: 347
13. Lemmer B, Winkler H, Ohm T, Fink F (1985) Naunyn-Schmiedebergs Arch Pharmacol 330: 42
14. Reinberg A, Smolensky MH (1983) Biological rhythms and medicine. Springer, Berlin Heidelberg New York Tokyo
15. Lemmer B, Bathe K (1982) J Cardiovasc Pharmacol 4: 635
16. Lang PH, Lemmer B (1985) J Cyclic Nucleotide Res 10: 341
17. Lemmer B, Lang PH (1984) Pol J Pharmacol Pharm 36: 275
18. Lemmer B, Lang PH (1984) Chronobiol Int 1: 217
19. McIntosh JEA, McIntosh RP (1980) Mathematical modelling and computers in endocrinology. Springer, Berlin Heidelberg New York
20. Lemmer B, Lang PH, Bissinger H (1984) Naunyn-Schmiedebergs Arch Pharmacol 325: R 32
21. Lemmer B, Lang PH, Gorka Z, Schmidt S, Bärmeier H (1985) J Interdiscipl Cycle Res 16: 142
22. Lang PH, Bissinger H, Lemmer B (1985) Chronobiol Int 2: 41

Discussion

Brodde: When I see that the receptor count is little changed, that the phosphodiesterase is also not exactly subject to large fluctuations, that cAMP and cyclase diverge, then I ask myself, what have cyclase and cAMP to do with each other besides the fact that cyclase synthesizes cAMP?

Lemmer: Yes, that's exactly why we did these investigations, to find a correlation and above all to see what we are actually doing in the receptor binding studies when we measure B_{max} and K_d values. Apparently – and this was a discussion point yesterday – the B_{max} values characterize the physiological or pharmacologic state inadequately or hardly at all. The differences in the phosphodiesterase activity were relatively slight in the brain; they were markedly more pronounced in the ventricular membranes of the heart. The adenylate cyclase activity was quite high in the brain, but diurnally reduced in the cardiac ventricles, so that both the variation and the opposing phase relationship in the peripheral and central organs showed no direct correlations. I cannot answer the question at this time. I've become skeptical as to whether it is so simple that when an agonist binds to a receptor an adenylate cyclase is stimulated, cAMP rises, and then the secondary reaction takes place. Whether it is so simple when one takes into consideration the daily rhythm ...

Brodde: That was not quite my question. Let's forget about the receptors for the moment. Let's just take cyclase, the enzyme that synthesizes cAMP. I think it would be logical to say that when the activity of cyclase is high, cAMP is also high, and when it is low, cAMP is low. Yet that is not the case.

Lemmer: No it's not.

Brodde: And so I'm asking you how that can be. And what else does cyclase have to do with cAMP?

Lemmer: I cannot answer that. My only clue would be to regard the stimulability of cyclase against the background of daily rhythm. And it may very well be, as with other parameters, that when we have low basal activities response to stimulation is perhaps high; when we have high basal activities the stimulation potential is much lower. I expect to find a rhythm, but we must investigate the stimulability. That appears to be crucial.

Middeke: Do you think it is possible that you perhaps do not measure the fluctuations of receptor density in cardiac muscle cells adequately with your assays? Might it be possible, if you take another radioligand, that these parallel fluctuations you find in adenylate cyclase and in phosphodiesterase are also to be found in the receptor density?

Lemmer: It is true; I said that purely for the sake of work economy we measured only the specific binding at one concentration in the cardiac ventricles in this study. In a previous one we had two affinity states, we had 24 ^{3}H-DHA concentrations, and at each time four saturation experiments. That's quite a bit of work. In retrospect it was perhaps a mistake to use only one ^{3}H-DHA concentration in the study on heart membranes. But we performed complete saturation experiments in the brain membranes, and the variation in B_{max} was not exactly overwhelming. Nor is it significant, whereas all the other parameters are highly significant. A rhythm is certainly present, but it is not very impressive.

Krawietz: Again with regard to the stimulability of adenylate cyclase. I can perhaps complement what was said with our own findings. We found a high basal activity in hypothyroidism, for example, as opposed to hyperthyroidism – a markedly lower percentage stimulability as measured in terms of the adenylate cyclase activity in rat heart muscle cells. That might point in the same direction.

Lemmer: That's what I would expect, because all the parameters are governed by a certain pattern; even if you look at the blood pressure the magnitude of the drop in blood pressure and heart rate is not independent of the initial state. It is for this reason that we performed these basal studies, in order to see whether any rhythms exist in basal activities and then to draw conclusions regarding stimulability, because stimulability is not directly correlated to the level of the initial state, as you yourself can confirm.

Kolloch: Your point of departure was the varying efficacy of beta-receptor blockers as a function of the time of day. And now you're trying to establish a relationship with the activity of the two systems you described. The problem remains, when you look at the diurnal blood pressure curve, that the efficacy of the beta-blockers is apparently dependent on the initial blood pressure values. In other words, at times of day at which the blood pressure is very high the effect is also stronger, and at night when the blood pressure is relatively low the antihypertensive effect is also less.

And this is true not only of the beta blockers. My question is, therefore, to what extent does a relationship really exist here between the antihypertensive efficacy of beta blockers and the described activity changes of these systems?

Lemmer: The relationship is certainly, as you correctly pointed out, between the sympathetic tone and the blockade of the beta-receptors by the beta-receptor blockers. When this is varied the effect is also varied. Actually, we would have been more interested in how it looks at the cellular or subcellular level. The sympathetic tone in itself is not sufficient to allow conclusions, and at present I am still in a state of confusion, as you see, because we expected variations but not such weird correlations in the peripheral and central organs. The next step is to determine whether a different dominance of alpha- or beta-receptors is responsible for the early-morning increase, which is not prevented by beta-blockers.

Göthert: You really do frighten us pharmacologists, and you frighten us even more when you mention, as you did this afternoon, that besides these diurnal fluctuations there are also seasonal fluctuations. Now you haven't mentioned them at all. Does seasonal fluctuation mean that these individual curves are flatter or steeper, or do completely new rhythms arise? And a second question with regard to what we said yesterday about humans: Have you tried to measure diurnal rhythms in the receptor density of human blood cells, for instance? That would be an important aspect for us pharmacologists, because we might have to adapt our rhythms to those of the rats. I don't know when we'd have to work. That was my second question.

Lemmer: As to the second part of the second question, you can adapt simply by keeping the rats in the dark during the day. My working group has not concerned itself with peripheral cells, and I would therefore prefer to make no statements about them. However, rhythms have been shown in blood cell cultures by Ashkenasi in Jerusalem, for example, so that I would also expect that there. As to the first part of your question, we also found seasonal variations in the heart ventricle membrane (I left that out here). But I can't discern any system in it. I would have to carry out a new experiment every 2 months, which I haven't done so far. But there are shifts, both in amplitude and in absolute values. The relationship of the maxima is also different. Actually, that doesn't surprise me at all, because in several studies, including epidemiological studies, in England, for example, the seasonal blood pressure under the influence of placebo, diuretics, and beta receptor blockers has been investigated. And it was found with all three therapeutic forms that the blood pressure is always higher - with or without therapy - in the winter and lower in the summer months.

Haehn: I just have a short comment on Mr Brodde's question right at the beginning. The interesting thing about these chronopharmacological experiments is that we are investigating an overall biological system. And I believe we must change our way of thinking and not simply conclude from a high activity of an enzyme that the product of this enzyme reaction is also high. We must also check whether the substrate concentration for this enzyme is even available at the appropriate time of day for large quantities of the product to be produced.

Lemmer: Thank you again.

Hypotensive Effect of β-Adrenoceptor Blockers

B. N. C. Prichard and F. Bompart

Department of Clinical Pharmacology, University College London and The Middlesex Hospital Medical School, The Rayne Institute, 5 University Street, London WC1E 655, England

Introduction

Pronethalol was the first beta adrenoceptor blocking drug to be used in the treatment of hypertension (Prichard 1964), Pronethalol was withdrawn because of its tumour-producing action in mice (Paget 1963), but the use of propranolol in hypertension was reported soon after (Prichard and Gillam 1964). These drugs were only slowly accepted in the treatment of hypertension. This was possibly because beta receptor antagonists inhibit cardiac contraction and this was considered to be an undesirable effect. The consequent increase in peripheral resistance from acute beta-adrenergic blockade from propranolol also seemed disadvantageous. Additionally, the antihypertensive effect had not been described in animals, and the mechanism of this action was unknown. Another reason for this slow acceptance of beta-adrenergic blockade was the use of inadequate doses, so that the full hypotensive effect was often delayed. Early investigators tended to fix doses at suboptimal levels, despite original reports (Prichard and Gillam 1964, 1966) emphasizing the importance of variable dosage regimens. The misgivings about dosage arose from erroneous concepts of complete beta adrenoceptor blockade. A relatively small dose of propranolol had been observed to block the effect of isoprenaline, which had previously caused a maximal tachycardia. Considerably larger doses are needed to produce maximum inhibition of exercise-induced tachycardia or even the supine or standing resting heart rate (Boakes et al. 1973), and the same is true for other beta-adrenergic blocking drugs, such as oxprenolol (Taylor and Meeran 1973a). It is these higher doses that are sometimes needed to give the full antihypertensive effect that could be achieved from beta-adrenergic blockade. It was also felt that large doses had a "direct depressing action" ("quinidine-like effect"; "membrane action"; "local anaesthetic effect") on the heart in man. A membrane action is seen with large doses in animals (Fitzgerald 1972) and does cause depression of myocardial function independently of beta-adrenergic blockade. It has no relevance to the treatment of hypertension, however, and is certainly not responsible for the haemodynamic effects of beta-adrenergic blocking drugs, since no significant membrane activity occurs with clinically effective doses of beta blocking drugs (Waal-Manning 1970; Prichard and Boakes 1977). It is inhibition of sympathetic activity per se that produces the negative inotropic and chronotropic effect on the heart in man. The use of the term "negative inotropic effect" might be best avoided, but if applied to beta

New Aspects in Hypertension: Adrenoceptors
M. Middeke and H. Holzgreve (Eds.)
Springer-Verlag Berlin Heidelberg New York 1986

adrenoreceptor blocking drugs it should be regarded as referring to their sympathetic blocking effect.

The use of beta-adrenergic blocking drugs in hypertension is their principal therapeutic application, and drugs with and without the associated properties of beta$_1$ selectivity, intrinsic sympathomimetic effect (ISA) or partial agonist activity (PAA) or coexistent alpha-adrenergic blockade have been found to be effective.

Haemodynamic Effects of Beta-Adrenergic Blocking Drugs

The full assessment of beta adrenoceptor blockade (McDevitt 1977) requires a measure of the inhibition of endogenous sympathetic activity. The greater the level of endogenous sympathetic activity, the more sensitive is the test for beta-adrenergic blockade. The supine resting heart rate is the result of a low sympathetic tone, vagal tone predominating, while on standing there is a modest increase in sympathetic tone. Even these low levels of sympathetic activity are sufficient for it to be possible to demonstrate a dose-response relationship with a beta adrenoceptor antagonist that does not possess partial agonist activity (Prichard and Gillam 1971). However, as levels of exercise are increased toward the maximum there is an increased discrimination for beta-adrenergic blockade (McDevitt 1977).

The administration of intravenous propranolol reduces heart rate, cardiac output, peripheral resistance increases, and there is thus little effect on resting blood pressure (Shinebourne et al. 1967; Ulrych et al. 1968). The cardiac output and heart rate are reduced to a similar degree after acute and long-term drug administration (Tarazi and Dustan 1972; Gibson 1974), but there is usually some delay in the falls of blood pressure and peripheral resistance declines (Tarazi and Dustan 1972; Hansson 1973; Ablad et al. 1976). Other beta-adrenergic blocking drugs that do not possess intrinsic sympathomimetic activity show similar results; sotalol (Svedmyr et al. 1970), nadolol (Textor et al. 1982), and timolol (Dunn et al. 1978; Franciosa et al. 1973).

The beta-adrenergic blocking agents with intrinsic sympathomimetic activity (ISA) at rest give less of a fall in resting heart rate than those not having this property (Prichard et al. 1970a; McDevitt et al. 1977; Svendsen et al. 1979; Taylor et al. 1982a; Aellig 1983; Kostis et al. 1982). At modest levels of exercise heart rates may be similar for drugs with and without ISA, but at high levels of exercise drugs with ISA at maximum dosage produce less of a reduction in exercise tachycardia (McDevitt 1977; McDevitt et al. 1977; Carruthers 1982). Exercise tachycardia with a beta-adrenergic blocking drug without ISA is a result of vagal de-inhibition, whereas the possession of partial agonist activity supplies some modest sympathetic stimulus to further increase the heart rate. It should be noted that this difference between drugs with and without ISA may only be seen at maximum blocking dosage, and doses below maximum may not demonstrate this difference.

Changes in the heart rate after the administration of beta-adrenergic blocking drugs usually parallel alterations in cardiac output (Gibson 1977). There is evidence that these drugs, which possess ISA when given at low levels of sympathetic activity, eg., during rest, result in less of a reduction in cardiac ouput. This has been observed for pindolol (Svendsen et al. 1979; Velasco et al. 1982), practolol (Svendsen et al. 1979; Taylor et al. 1982a; Man in 'T Veld and Schalekamp 1982), and oxprenolol (Grandjean and Rivier 1968; Taylor et al. 1982a). In association with the absence of a decline in cardiac output with beta-adrenergic blocking drugs with intrinsic sympathomimetic activity, such as pindolol (Velasco et al. 1982), peripheral resistance does not increase, as it does with drugs without this property, but may even fall. Additionally, pindolol has some direct peripheral β_2 adrenoceptor-mediated vasodilator activity (Chang et al. 1985). In spite of some suggestions to the contrary (Gibson 1977), it appears that non-ISA cardioselective drugs produce a similar fall in cardiac output to non-ISA nonselective agents (Man In't Veld and Schalekamp 1982; van Herwaarden et al. 1979).

The dual action of alpha and beta adrenoceptor inhibition (e.g. labetalol) produces different responses from those of beta blockade alone. Blood pressure is reduced acutely after oral or intravenous administration (Richards and Prichard 1979). Cardiac output at rest shows little change after labetalol (Koch 1976; Edwards and Raftery 1976; Mehta and Cohn 1977). At high levels of exercise there is some reduction of cardiac output (Edwards and Raftery 1976), but in patients with ischaemic disease changes have been found to be less than after propranolol (Silke et al. 1982).

Classification of Beta-Adrenergic Blocking Drugs

The beta-adrenoceptor blocking drugs may be subdivided according to various associated properties, those which are non-selective and those which have a selective action on the $beta_1$ receptors, and further division into those which in addition possess alpha receptor blocking properties. They may be subdivided into various groups according to the presence or absence of intrinsic sympathomimetic activity and membrane activity (Fitzgerald 1972; Prichard 1978).

Non-Selective Beta-Adrenergic Blocking Drugs (Division I)

Group I

These drugs have both a membrane-stabilizing action and intrinsic sympathomimetic activity.

A comparison of oxprenolol showed it produced a similar antihypertensive effect to propranolol, practolol, tolamolol and metoprolol (Davidson et al. 1976). This was also true when oxprenolol was compared with propranolol in combination with a diuretic (Gavras et al. 1979). Many other studies have confirmed the effect of oxprenolol in hypertension (Leisham et al. 1970; Tuckman et al. 1972; Andersson et al. 1976a; Materson et al. 1976a; Waal-Manning 1976; Franciosa et al. 1979), an efficacy that has also been demonstrated with 24-h monitoring of blood pressure (Millar-Craig et al. 1981).

An additional member of this group is alprenolol, which is also an effective antihypertensive drug (Furberg and Michaelson 1969; Tibblin and Ablad 1969; Bengtsson 1972; Morgan et al. 1974; Nik-Akhthar et al. 1975; Hartikainen and Heikkila 1976), as is a further example of this group, penbutolol (Cangiano et al. 1979; Lund-Johansen 1979; Heel et al. 1981). More recently, a further non-selective beta-adrenergic blocking drug with membrane-stabilizing activity and partial agonist effect, indendolol, has been found to lower the blood pressure (Sega et al. 1983).

Group II

These beta-adrenergic blocking agents have membrane activity but no intrinsic sympathomimetic action.

Propranolol. The value of beta receptor blocking agents in hypertension was established with studies with propranolol (Prichard and Gillam 1964, 1966, 1969; Frohlich et al. 1968; Karlberg and Hornkuist 1971; Zackarias et al. 1972; Veterans Administration 1977). Propranolol was found to give similar overall control of blood pressure to that obtained with bethanidine, guanethidine and methyldopa (Prichard and Gillam 1969; Prichard et al. 1970b; Zacharias et al. 1972). Some investigators who found less favourable responses of blood pressure to propranolol (Humphreys and Delvin 1968; Waal-Manning 1966) used maximum doses lower than the average dose of 400–500 mg/day used by Prichard and Gillam (1969), who in addition, unlike the investigators finding poor results, used a diuretic in more than half their patients. Zacharias et al. (1972) found a larger proportion of their 311 patients achieved satisfactory blood pressure control than they usually observed with other antihypertensive drugs. A within-patient, randomized comparison of bethanidine, methyldopa and propranolol (Prichard et al. 1976) confirmed that the three drugs are of similar efficacy and that propranolol does not produce postural or exercise hypotension. In severe and moderately severe hypertensives an average dose of propranolol is 400–500 mg/day, with about half the patients needing a diuretic in addition. In a few instances the addition of other hypotensive agents may be required. A total requirement of 1 g propranolol or more daily is occasionally needed, but a few patients only need 40–80 mg/day. Variation in dosage is not unusual for antihypertensive drugs; beta-adrenergic blocking drugs have now been subjected to careful pharmacokinetic studies, and it appears that the principal reason, at least for dosage variation of propranolol, is difference in systemic absorption, which can vary over 20-fold (Shand 1976), mainly due to variation in hepatic metabolism. In earlier studies propranolol was given three or four times a day, but administration twice (Hansson et al. 1971) or even once daily (Wilson et al. 1976) is often effective. Now a slow-release form of propranolol has been developed (Mc Ainsh et al. 1978), which can be given once daily for hypertension (Floras et al. 1982).

Group III

The members of this group have partial agonist activity but no significant membrane activity.

Pindolol is the most potent beta adrenoceptor blocker in general use. It is effective in the treatment of hypertension (Morgan et al. 1972; Feltham et al. 1972; Waal-

Manning and Simpson 1974), and some studies have found it similar in efficacy to propranolol (Laver et al. 1974) and other beta-adrenergic blocking drugs (Hartikainen and Heikkila 1976). Likewise, Gonasun (1982) reported that pindolol was similar in blood pressure control to propranolol, hydrochlorothiazide, methyldopa and chlorthalidone. Similarly, Doyle (1983) found pindolol gave similar control of the blood pressure to the calcium antagonist verapamil in mild and moderate hypertension. Pindolol may be given once daily (Wilson et al. 1976).

Carteolol is a more recently described member of this group. It is highly potent and has an exceptionally long duration of action (Stoll et al. 1981) and has been found effective in hypertension (Saraste et al. 1982). *Bopindolol* is similar (Aellig 1985) and has been found to be similarly effective to pindolol and atenolol in lowering the blood pressure (Schiess et al. 1984).

Group IV

Beta-adrenoceptor blocking drugs in this group have no intrinsic sympathomimetic effect or significant membrane activity.

Sotalol has been found to be equally effective an antihypertensive drug as propranolol (Berglund 1977); it appears to have the same efficacy as methyldopa (Prichard and Boakes 1974) and can be given on a once-daily basis (Mann et al. 1981).

Timolol lowers the blood pressure (Morgan et al. 1974; Alcocer et al. 1975; Brogden et al. 1975; Lohmoller and Frohlich 1975; Lund-Johansen 1976a; Castenfors 1977); in mild hypertension most effect was seen with 20 mg daily, only a marginal further effect being achieved with a dose of 60 mg/day (Simon et al. 1978). In a double-blind factorial trial (Chalmers et al. 1976) there was an additive effect with the combination of timolol (10 mg t.d.s.) and hydrochlorothiazide (50 mg daily).

Nadolol is another member of this group. It has a half-life of about 24 h and a prolonged duration of action, and has been shown to be effective in hypertension (Heel et al. 1980; Duchin et al. 1980; Wilcox and Hampton 1982). There has been some suggestion that nadolol, in contrast to other beta-adrenergic blocking drugs, may increase renal blood flow (Hollenberg et al. 1979; Textor et al. 1982). However, Mueller et al. (1983) could not find any difference in the effect of atenolol and nadolol on renal function in patients with renal impairment. Also, in elderly patients, O'Malley et al. (1983) found that cardioselective drugs appeared to reduce renal blood flow less than drugs.

Beta$_1$ ("Cardioselective") Beta-Adrenergic Blocking Drugs (Division II)

Group I

These drugs possess intrinsic sympathomimetic activity and membrane activity.

Acebutolol has been found effective in hypertension (Letac et al. 1974), with progressively increasing effects seen with 400 mg, 600 mg, and 1200 mg daily (Hansson et al. 1977). It is as effective twice daily as once daily (Ogilvie et al. 1983).

Group II

These drugs have intrinsic sympathomimetic action but no membrane activity.

Practolol lowers the blood pressure (Leishman et al. 1970; Prichard et al. 1971), but unfortunately also induces serious adverse reactions involving the eyes and skin, and a sclerosing peritonitis. Practolol is no longer used in the treatment of hypertension.

Group III

These drugs have neither ISA nor membrane activity.

Atenolol is an effective antihypertensive drug (Hansson et al. 1975; Lund-Johansen 1976b; Douglas-Jones and Cruickshank 1976; Zacharias et al. 1977). Some studies show it to be more effective than bendrofluazide (Petrie et al. 1975; Fagard et al. 1976). Scott et al. (1982) found in nine patients that while 3 weeks of 100 mg atenolol a day gave a greater fall in blood pressure, the difference from 50 mg/day was not significant. The effect of atenolol 100 mg at 24 h after drug administration was greater than metoprolol 100 mg or 200 mg of a sustained-release preparation. Intra-arterial monitoring of blood pressure for 24 h confirms that atenolol can be given once daily (Floras et al. 1982).

A comparative study of atenolol with oxprenolol, propranolol and pindolol given in variable dosage revealed similar degrees of control of the blood pressure, but the diastolic pressures on atenolol were lower during isometric (hand grip) exercise and mental arithmetic (Waal-Manning 1979). In a fixed dose comparison, atenolol (100 mg/day) was found to be more effective than methyldopa (250 mg t.d.s.) (Kristensen et al. 1981). In a similar study in 37 patients, atenolol 100 mg/day was found to be similar to methyldopa 250 mg or 500 mg t.d.s. (Magnani et al. 1981). Atenolol has been found capable of producing a useful reduction of the blood pressure in the acute control of severe hypertension (Bannan and Beevers 1981).

It appears that *metoprolol* (Bengtsson et al. 1975; Hansson et al. 1977) at doses of 50 mg t.d.s. ($n=15$) or 100 mg t.d.s. ($n=8$) is equivalent in its antihypertensive effect to propranolol 40 mg t.d.s. and 80 mg t.d.s. respectively, in mildly hypertensive women (Bengtsson 1976). Davidson et al. (1976) found metoprolol was about 1.4 times as potent as propranolol. It is equieffective to methyldopa in the treatment of mild and moderate high blood pressure (Bergstrand et al. 1976). While metoprolol once daily controlled blood pressure as effectively as a three times daily regimen, fluctuations in plasma concentration were greater and there was less consistent control of exercise tachycardia (Reybrouck et al. 1978). With the sustained release preparation of metoprolol control of blood pressure was similar at 24 h and at 2 h after administration, but exercising systolic blood pressure and heart rate tended to be higher at 24 h after administration (Comerford and Besterman 1982).

A more recently introduced drug in this group, *betaxolol* (Giudicelli et al. 1980), is effective in mild and moderate hypertension at doses of 20 and 40 mg (Salonen and Palminteri 1982).

Beta Adrenergic Blocking Drugs with Alpha Adrenoreceptor Blocking or Vasodilator Properties (Division III)

Labetalol, at present the only drug with beta and alpha receptor blocking properties that is widely available (Richards and Prichard 1979), has been extensively evaluated in hypertension (Andersson et al. 1976b; Balasubramanian et al. 1979; Bolli et al. 1976; Edwards and Raftery 1976; Gomez and Phillips 1980; Hansson and Hanel 1976; Kane et al. 1979; New Zealand Study 1979; Prichard and Boakes 1976; Takeda et al. 1982; Waal-Manning and Simpson 1982). Studies in severe hypertension indicate that labetalol is a powerful drug (Dargie et al. 1976; Hauger-Klevene 1981; Kristensen and Petersen 1980; Williams et al. 1979). Double-blind trials of labetalol versus placebo have confirmed its antihypertensive effect (Bolli et al. 1976; Carre et al. 1982; Frick and Porsti 1976; Kane et al. 1976; Larochelle et al. 1980). There is no evidence of tolerance developing with long-term administration in studies lasting up to 6 years (Prichard et al. 1979), 5 years (Kane et al. 1979), and an average of 57 months (Waal-Manning and Simpson 1982). The acute use of labetalol controls the blood pressure of severely hypertensive patients (Trust et al. 1976; Ronne-Rasmussen et al. 1976; Lechi et al. 1981; Joekes and Thompson 1976; Brown et al. 1977; Cumming et al. 1979; Papademetriou et al. 1982; Dal-Palu et al. 1982; Agabiti-Rosei et al. 1982).

Medroxalol is a drug that also possesses both beta- and alpha-adrenergic blocking properties, but probably in addition a vasodilator effect mediated by beta$_2$-adrenergic stimulation (Dage et al. 1981, 1983) Its beta and alpha blocking properties have been confirmed in man (Jaillon et al. 1982), and it is an effective drug in hypertension (Schechter et al. 1982).

Recently several drugs have been evaluated that possess beta-adrenergic blocking plus vasodilator activity. *Prizidolol* (Lund-Johansen and Omvik 1982) has been extensively evaluated, but this drug has been withdrawn because of animal toxicity. *Bucindolol* (Deitchman et al. 1983; Malini et al. 1983) and *carvedilol* (von Mollendorff et al. 1981; Meyer-Sabellek et al. 1983) and other similar drugs are at present in an early stage of evaluation.

Beta-Adrenergic Blocking Drugs in Combination with Other Drugs

Diuretics

Since the earliest evaluation of beta adrenoceptor blocking drugs they have been used in combination with a variety of other drugs to treat more resistant cases. The beta adrenoceptor blocking drugs have been combined with diuretics since the earliest studies. In contrast to beta-adrenergic blockers, diuretics and aldosterone antagonists, being volume-depleting agents, work best in low-renin hypertension (Karlberg et al. 1976). It is therefore quite logical to add a diuretic for patients responding inadequately to a beta-adrenergic blocker alone.

Approximately equal numbers of patients were found to need a diuretic in addition with propranolol and with previous therapy with the then generally used drugs, methyldopa and adrenergic neurone-inhibitory drugs (Prichard and Gillam 1969; Prichard et al. 1976). Beta adrenoceptor blocking drugs, besides exerting an additive antihypertensive effect (Morganti et al. 1979), may also partially antagonize the hypokalaemic effect of diuretics (Castenfors 1977). The sum of the individual falls in blood pressure may not be as great as that seen when the beta-adrenergic blocking drug or the diuretic is given alone (Bateman et al. 1979). Usually a small dose of the diuretic suffices: 12.5 mg hydrochlorothiazide was found as effective as larger doses when added to acebutolol 400 mg (MacGregor et al. 1983).

Vasodilating Drugs

When the vasodilators are used alone in the treatment of hypertension they often cause an unacceptable tachycardia (Ablad 1963; Sannerstedt et al. 1972), which is particularly undesirable in patients with ischaemic heart disease. Sodium and fluid retention and side effects such as headaches, nervousness and gastrointestinal disturbances may also occur (Gilmore et al. 1970; Kincaid-Smith et al. 1975). Beta-adrenergic blocking agents inhibit the vasodilator-induced tachycardia and the increases in plasma renin activity, which may be important in the combined antihypertensive regimen (Pettinger and Keeton 1975).

The doses of beta-adrenergic blocker should also be large enough to inhibit the reflex sympathetic activity caused by the vasodilator (Hansson et al. 1971; Ibsen et al. 1978; Aenishanslin et al. 1972; Tuckman et al. 1972, 1973; Zacest et al. 1972; Siitonen et al. 1974; Freeman and Knight 1975; Sannerstedt et al. 1972; Persson 1975; Dahr 1972; Wilcox and Mitchell 1977; Wilburn et al. 1975; Gottlieb et al. 1972; Pettinger and Mitchell 1973; Dormois et al. 1975).

Minoxidil is a powerful vasodilator. However, because of its potential for fluid retention and hirsutism its role is limited exclusively to severe, refractory hypertension and it should not be given to women. Patients with severe hypertension poorly controlled by such drugs as propranolol responded to the addition of minoxidil (Ryan et al. 1975; Mutterperl et al. 1976). Patients with severe hypertension with a poor response to propranolol (475 mg/day) and other drugs responded to minoxidil (mean dose 33 mg/day) with a fall in mean blood pressure from 144 to 108 mmHg, and this was maintained for up to 25 months (Wilburn et al. 1975): fluid retention responded to frusemide at doses up to 578 mg/day.

Nifedipine combines well with propranolol (Pedersen et al. 1980; Cain et al. 1983). In the absence of LV dysfunction or A–V nodal disease oral verapamil may be combined relatively safely with propranolol for the treatment of hypertension, and the combination is highly efficacious (Buhler et al. 1983; McInnes et al. 1985).

The drugs which inhibit the enzyme that converts inactive angiotensin I to the powerful vasoconstrictor angiotensin II are effective in the treatment of hypertension. Such agents include captopril, enalapril and lisinopril. In addition to ACE inhibition, captopril may lower blood pressure by affecting the kinin and prostaglandin system (Pickering et al. 1982).

Because propranolol may lower blood pressure, at least partly, by inhibiting the renin-angiotensin system, it seemed possible that combining propranolol with an

ACE inhibitor would not result in a further fall in blood pressure, as has been suggested by some (Drayer et al. 1982, Ferguson et al. 1983, Huang et al. 1980, and MacGregor et al. 1982).

In contrast, other investigators do show an additive effect when captopril and propranolol are combined (Frithz et al. 1982, Hammond et al. 1979, Havelka et al. 1982, Seto et al. 1980, Lederle et al. 1980, Pickering et al. 1982, Leonetti et al. 1982). Staessen et al. (1983) found that in 15 poor responders to captopril propranolol was highly effective in lowering blood pressure when added to captopril if the plasma renin activity was high, while thiazides had an excellent additive effect if the plasma renin activity was low on captopril.

Drugs Inhibiting the Innervation of the Alpha Adrenoreceptor

The $alpha_1$ adrenoreceptor blocking drug prazosin has been used in combination with beta-adrenergic blockade (Stokes and Weber 1974; Kincaid-Smith et al. 1975; Marshall et al. 1977). Stokes et al. (1982) reported a series of 171 patients treated with prazosin in combination with various beta-adrenergic blocking drugs. Labetalol, which has alpha and beta adrenoreceptor blocking activity, has become established in the treatment of hypertension (see above). The combination of beta-adrenergic blocking drugs such as propranolol with either methyldopa or a sympathetic inhibitor like bethanidine has at least an additive effect or even a potentiating action, but there is a tendency for some postural and exercise hypotension to occur, which propranolol alone does not induce (Day and Prichard 1971; Prichard 1976). Similar additive effects are seen with oxprenolol and guanethidine (Pearson et al. 1976) and atenolol and methyldopa (Webster et al. 1977; Wilson et al. 1977).

Possible Modes of Action

It is clear that beta adrenoceptor blocking drugs lower the blood pressure as a result of their beta receptor blocking action. There is a fall in blood pressure regardless of the presence or absence of the associated properties, and the membrane-active non-beta-blocking isomers are without antihypertensive effect (Waal-Manning 1970; Prichard and Boakes 1977). A number of attempts have been made to explain the hypotensive effect of beta-adrenergic blocking drugs, including a direct action on the central nervous system, adrenergic neurone blocking, anti-renin activity, an increase of vasodilator prostaglandins, effects secondary to reduced cardiac output, and resetting of baroreceptors secondary to reduced pressor peaks to various pressor stimuli from the reduction in cardiac activity consequent to beta blockade. However, the exact mode of action remains unclear (Prichard and Owens 1983; Cruickshank, this volume). It may be that in some patients one of the many effects may be of overriding importance. An anti-renin effect may be important in certain cases at low dosage, but other mechanisms may be involved with higher dose levels (Hollifield et al. 1976).

Place in Hypertension

The beta adrenoceptor-blocking drugs are used as first-choice drugs for hypertension, but care is required in patient selection. These drugs should be avoided in heart failure, as such patients are crucially dependent on sympathetic drive (Prichard and Owens 1983), and in patients with asthma, as they are sensitive to inhibition of adrenergic drive to bronchial smooth muscle and even cardioselective drugs are liable to cause a significant increase in airways obstruction (Decalmer et al. 1978). Beta-adrenergic blocking drugs are also likely to increase heart block and worsen Raynaud's phenomenon (Marshall et al. 1976; Gokal et al. 1979).

It does not seem to be possible to predict reliably which patients will respond successfully to beta-adrenergic blocking drugs. Bühler et al. (1972, 1975) have suggested that renin levels are important and perhaps the basis for the suggestion that older patients respond less is that renin concentrations fall with age (Bühler et al. 1975, 1978), other authors have not found quite such a clear relationship, however (Hollifield et al. 1976; Bravo et al. 1975; Leonetti et al. 1975; Morgan et al. 1975; Amery et al. 1976). Hollifield et al. 1976 found that even patients with low renin responded if the dose of propranolol was increased up to 960 mg a day.

It has also been observed that beta adrenoceptor sensitivity, as shown by a reduced response to isoprenaline, declines with age (Vestal et al. 1979; Dillon et al. 1980; Wilkins and Kendall 1984). However, it appears that beta-adrenergic blocking drugs are effective and useful in the elderly (Wikstrand and Berglund 1982; O'Malley et al. 1983), and some workers consider them specifically indicated (Amery 1982).

There is not a clear relationship between initial cardiac output and response to beta-adrenergic blocking drugs (Birkenhäger et al. 1971; Tarazi and Dustan 1972; Hansson et al. 1974) or age, in contrast to the findings of Bühler et al. (1975), or blood volume (Birkenhäger et al. 1971; Hansson et al. 1974). Measurements of peripheral resistance, urinary adrenaline and noradrenaline (Hansson et al. 1974; Meekers et al. 1975), aldosterone (Hansson et al. 1974) and heart rate response to isoprenaline (Hansson et al. 1974; Simon et al. 1978) have no value in predicting response to beta-adrenergic blocking drugs. Distler et al. (1978), however, found a correlation between the ratio of exercise to resting plasma noradrenaline and a good response to atenolol.

Some early studies indicated that black patients generally did not respond so well to beta-adrenergic blocking drugs (Humphreys and Delvin 1968; Richardson et al. 1968). Others have noted the restricted efficacy of propranolol in black hypertensives and recommend its use combined with a diuretic (Grell 1983; Obel 1983). Most black hypertensives have a low plasma renin activity, high-volume hypertension which responds best to a diuretic (Hammond et al. 1978). Plasma renin activity in black hypertensives is some 50% lower than in white hypertensives (Banks et al. 1981). Seedat et al. (1973) found that in contrast to black hypertensives, Asian (Indian) subjects responded well to propranolol (mean dose 760 mg/day). Asian hypertensives, primarily of Chinese extraction, also respond to propranolol, in doses up to 1 g/day (Cheah and Chia 1974), as is the case also with Japanese patients (Tsukiyama et al. 1982).

Comparison of Various Beta Adrenoceptor Blocking Drugs

The studies comparing propranolol with other non-selective beta blockers with no ISA, timolol (Morgan et al. 1974; Morioka et al. 1983), sotalol (Ames and Hill 1982; Pessina et al. 1983) and nadolol (Hill and Fand 1979; Lossnitzer et al. 1981) do not indicate any difference in antihypertensive efficacy.

The investigations that have compared propranolol with non-selective beta-adrenergic blockers with mild to modest ISA, i.e., alprenolol (Bengtsson 1972), penbutolol (Frick et al. 1978; Hayes 1983) and oxprenolol (Gavras et al. 1979, Materson et al. 1976a) indicate that all lower blood pressure to a similar extent. However, there are some studies that suggest alprenolol (Bergland and Hansson 1973) and oxprenolol (Veterans Administration 1981; Andersson et al. 1976) control diastolic blood pressure to a slightly lesser degree than propranolol, about 3 mmHg. Comparisons of propranolol with pindolol, which possesses moderate to high ISA, have shown similar efficacy on blood pressure (Laver et al. 1974; Gonasun 1982). The blood pressure at night falls about 20% in both normals and hypertensives. Pindolol, in contrast to propranolol, does not significantly lower nocturnal blood pressure (Floras et al. 1982). Under conditions of low sympathetic drive, such as sleep, the stimulant action of pindolol is more apparent and increases heart rate. Comparisons of non-selective beta-adrenergic blockers with no ISA, like propranolol, with $beta_1$-selective beta-adrenergic blockers without ISA, i.e. atenolol (Ravid et al. 1985; Floras et al. 1982) and metoprolol (Houben et al. 1983; Ravid et al. 1985), indicate overall similar antihypertensive effects. There are some studies to suggest that resting diastolic blood pressure is probably about 3 or 4 mmHg lower with a $beta_1$-selective agent (van Rooijen et al. 1979; Zacharias and Cowen 1977).

Value in Hypertension

Beta-adrenergic blocking drugs have several advantages in the treatment of hypertension. In common with several other drugs they lower the blood pressure to a similar degree regardless of the physiological circumstances; they probably have a cardioprotective effect; and finally, there may be a coexistent indication for treatment with beta-adrenergic blocking drugs (see below).

Response to Physiological Stimuli in Patients Treated with Beta-Adrenergic Blocking Drugs

After blood pressure has been lowered by beta-adrenergic blocking drugs, there is neither postural nor exercise hypotension (Prichard and Gillam 1969; Prichard et al. 1970b, c: Prichard 1976). Peripheral resistance increases on standing, as might be expected, since the innervation of the alpha constrictor adrenoreceptor is intact (Prichard et al. 1970c). Other evidence of normally functioning innervation of the alpha adrenoreceptor is afforded by a study of environmental temperature. A rise from 7 °C to 30 °C increases postural and exercise hypotension in patients treated with sympathetic neurone-inhibitory drugs such as bethanidine and guanethidine. This is probably because of uncompensated vasodilation in skin blood vessels. However, after propranolol the response of blood pressure to posture and exercise when environmental temperature was increased was not affected (Prichard et al. 1970b).

Cardioprotective and Vasculoprotective Effect

There is some evidence that the long-term administration of beta-adrenergic blocking drugs may exert a cardioprotective effect. There are several mechanisms by which this may occur (Prichard 1983).

Studies after acute myocardial infarction suggest that beta-adrenergic blocking drugs reduce the extent of the infarct, provided they are administered sufficiently promptly. This has been shown by means of post-infarct ST-segment mapping (Pelides et al. 1972), and monitoring of cardiac enzyme changes (Peter et al. 1978; Yusuf et al. 1980; Jurgensen et al. 1981), R wave changes (Yusuf et al. 1980), and chest pain (Andersen et al. 1979); all these parameters improve after beta adrenoreceptor blockade. Overall, trials of beta-adrenergic blocking drugs after infarction indicate that the drugs produce benefit (Baber and Lewis 1982;Hampton 1982; Lancet 1982; Rose 1982; Turi and Braunwald 1983), although as with all drugs there is a benefit: risk ratio (Breckenridge 1982). A number of the studies can be criticized on methodological grounds (Fitzgerald 1976; Hampton 1981), and there have been some negative results (Baber et al. 1980; Wilcox et al. 1980); but there have now been numerous reports indicating that beta-adrenergic blocking drugs are effective in reducing the recurrence rate of myocardial infarction (Ahlmark et al. 1974; Wilhelmsen et al. 1973; Multicentre International Study 1975; Hjalmarson et al. 1981; Norwegian Multicenter Study Group 1981; BHAT 1982; Hansteen et al. 1982; Julian et al. 1982; Taylor et al. 1982b). This evidence, together with that for an effect in acute myocardial infarction, suggests that there is a cardioprotective effect in high-risk patients following myocardial infarction, and there is some evidence that propranolol-treated patients with hypertension may have a lower incidence of myocardial infarction than those not given beta blocking drugs (Stewart 1976). In a further uncontrolled but larger study, Beevers et al. (1983), found fewer heart attacks and also strokes in hypertensive patients treated with beta-adrenergic blocking drugs than in those where similar blood pressure control was achieved with other antihypertensive drugs.

The MRC study in mild hypertension (Medical Research Council Working Party 1985) showed that smoking negated any reduction in the incidence of myocardial infarction by propranolol. In non-smokers the frequency of strokes was reduced by 47%, and in non-smoking men the frequency of coronary events was reduced by 33% by propranolol. In non-smokers all cardiovascular events were significantly fewer with propranolol than with the thiazide diuretic ($P = 0.01$). Deaths were not significantly reduced by treatment, in either smokers or non-smokers: indeed there was a trend towards a greater number of deaths in women receiving active treatment and a reverse trend for men.

Coexistent Disease

Beta-adrenergic blocking drugs are widely used in therapeutics. There are a number of conditions that respond to beta-adrenergic blocking drugs that not infrequently coexist with hypertension, such as angina pectoris, migraine, and anxiety with somatic features (Prichard and Owens 1983).

Conclusion

The use of beta-adrenergic blocking drugs in hypertension began rather slowly, but these drugs have now become first-line drugs in antihypertensive therapy. The way in which they lower the blood pressure remains a matter for debate. The effects of blocking the beta adrenoreceptor are very diverse, and more than one mechanism may be important in their antihypertensive action. It may be that in some patients one of the many effects may be of overriding importance, such as reducing plasma renin in patients with a high renin, whilst in others one of their other actions may be more important.

The beta-adrenergic blocking drugs can be used in all grades of severity of hypertension, both essential and renal, alone and in combination with diuretics, vasodilators and other agents. They control blood pressure regardless of physiological circumstances such as the effect of gravity, as reflexes dependent on alpha vasoconstrictor activity are intact. There is evidence that beta-adrenergic blocking drugs may possess a cardioprotective action. The side effects of beta-adrenergic blocking drugs can be readily ascribed to blockade of the beta-receptor; they are usually predictable and two important ones in particular, heart failure and asthma, can almost always be avoided by proper patient selection.

References

Ablad B (1963) A study of the mechanism of the haemodynamic effects of hydralazine in man. Acta Pharmacol Toxicol 20 [Suppl 1]: 1–53

Ablad B, Ljung B, Sannerstedt R (1976) Haemodynamic effects of β-adrenoceptor blockers in hypertension. Drugs 11 [Suppl 1]: 127–134

Aellig WH (1983) Clinical pharmacology of β-adrenoceptor blocking drugs possessing partial agonist activity with special reference to pindolol. J Cardiovasc Pharmacol 5: S16–S20

Aellig WH (1985) Pharmacological experiments in healthy volunteers with bopindolol, a long-acting β-adrenoceptor blocking drug with partial agonist activity. Br J Clin Pharmacol 19: 775–781

Aenishanslin W, Pestalozzi-Kerpei J, Dubach UC, Imhof PR, Turri M (1972) Antihypertensive therapy with adrenergic beta-receptor blockers and vasodilators. Eur J Clin Pharmacol 4: 177–181

Agabiti-Rosei E, Alicandri CL, Beschi M, Castellano M, Fariello R, Montini E, Muiesan ML, Romanelli G, Muiesan G (1982) The acute and chronic hypotensive effect of labetalol and the relationship with pretreatment plasma noradrenaline levels. Br J Clin Pharmacol 3 [Suppl 1]: 87s-92s

Ahlmark G, Saetre H, Korsgren M (1974) Reduction of sudden deaths after myocardial infarction. Lancet 2: 1563

Alcocer L, Aspe J, Gomez EA (1975) Anti-hypertensive effect of timolol, a new beta-blocking agent (Double-blind study). J Int Med Res 3: 1-9

Amery A (1982) High blood pressure above age 60. In Clinical hypertension and hypotension. Dekker (eds) New York, pp 327-350

Amery A, Billiet L, Boel A, Fagard R, Reybrouck T, Willems J (1976) Mechanism of hypotensive effect during beta adrenergic blockade in hypertensive patients. Haemodynamic and renin response to a new cardio-selective agent: tenormin or ICI 66082. Am Heart J 91: 634-642

Ames R, Hill P (1982) Disturbance in serum total cholesterol and lipoprotein cholesterol ratios during control of hypertension with beta-adrenoceptor blocking drugs. Clin Res 40: (abstract)

Andersen MP, Bechsgaard P, Frederiksen J, Hansen DA, Jurgensen HJ, Nielsen B, Pedersen F, Pedersen-Bjergaard O, Rasmussen SL (1979) Effect of alprenolol on mortality among patients with definite or suspected acute myocardial infarction. Lancet 2: 865-868

Andersson O, Berglund G, Bergman H, Cramer K, Fagerberg S-E, Forsberg S-A, Johnsen V, Lundkvist L, Rutle O, Sjolyst R (1976a) Antihypertensive effect and side effects of treatment with beta-blockers - a comparative study between oxprenolol and propranolol. Curr Ther Res 19: 43-50

Andersson O, Berglund G, Hansson L (1976b) Anti-hypertensive action, time of onset and effects on carbohydrate metabolism of labetalol. Br J Clin Pharmacol 3 [Suppl 3]: 757-761

Baber NS, Lewis JA (1982) Confidence in results of beta-blocker post-infarction trials. Br Med J 284: 1749-1750

Baber NS, Wainwright Evans D, Howitt G, Thomas M, Wilson C, Lewis JA, Dawes PM, Handler K, Tuson R (1980) Multicentre post-infarction trial of propranolol in 49 hospitals in the United Kingdom, Italy and Yugoslavia. Br Heart J 44: 96-100

Balasubramanian V, Mann S, Raftery EB, Millar-Craig MV, Altman D (1979) Effect of labetalol on continuous ambulatory blood pressure. Br J Clin Pharmacol 8 [Suppl 2]: 119s-123s

Banks RA, Markandu ND, Roulston JE, MacGregor GA (1981) Differing effects of sodium restriction, spironolactone, propranolol and captopril in black and white patients with hypertension. 8th scientific meeting of the International Society of Hypertension, Milan, 31 May-3 June 1981 (abstract)

Bannan LT, Beevers DG (1981) Emergency treatment of high blood pressure with oral atenolol. Br Med J 282: 1757-1758

Bateman DN, Dean CR, Mucklow JC, Bulpitt CJ, Dollery CT (1979) Atenolol and chlorthalidone in combination for hypertension. Br J Clin Pharmacol 7: 357-363

Beevers DG, Johnston JH, Larkin H, Davies P (1983) Clinical evidence that beta-adrenoceptor blockers prevent more complications than other anti-hypertensive drugs. Drugs 25 [Suppl 2]: 326-330

Bengtsson C (1972) Comparison between alprenolol and chlorthalidone as anti-hypertensive agents. Acta Med Scand 191: 433-439

Bengtsson C (1976) Comparison between metoprolol and propranolol as antihypertensive agents. Acta Med Scand 199: 71-74

Bengtsson C, Johnsson G, Regardh C-G (1975) Plasma levels and effects of metoprolol on blood pressure and heart rate in hypertensive patients after acute dose and between two doses during long-term treatment. Clin Pharmacol Ther 17: 400-408

Berglund G (1977) Anti-hypertensive effect of sotalol and propranolol: a double-blind crossover study. Curr Ther Res 21: 21-27

Berglund G, Hansson L (1973) A within-patient comparison of alprenolol and propranolol in hypertension. Acta Med Scand 193: 547-550

Bergstrand RH, Vedin JA, Wilhelmsson CE, Berglund G (1976) Comparative study of metoprolol and alpha-methyldopa in untreated essential hypertension. Eur J Clin Pharmacol 10: 375-379

Beta-Blocker Heart Attack Trial Research Group (1982) 1. Mortality results. A randomized trial of propranolol in patients with acute myocardial infarction. JAMA 247: 1707-1714

Birkenhäger WH, Krauss XH, Schalekamp MADH, Kolsters G, Kroon BJM (1971) Antihypertensive effects of propranolol. Observations on predictability. Folia Med Neerl 14: 67–71
Boakes AJ, Boeree BH, Prichard BNC (1973) Dose response studies to oxprenolol, pindolol, practolol, propranolol and sotalol on tilt, Valsalva's Manoeuvre and exercise tachycardia. Naunyn-Schmiedeberg Arch Pharmacol 279: R 42
Bolli P, Waal-Manning HJ, Wood AJ, Simpson FO (1976) Experience with labetalol in hypertension. Br J Clin Pharmacol 3 [Suppl 3]: 765–771
Bravo EL, Tarazi RC, Dustan HP, Lewis JW (1975) Dissociation between renin and arterial pressure responses to beta-adrenergic blockade in human essential hypertension. Circ Res [Suppl] I: 36–37
Breckenridge A (1982) Should every survivor of a heart attack be given a beta blocker? II. evidence from a clinical pharmacological standpoint. Br Med J 285: 37–39
Brogden RN, Speight TM, Avery GS (1975) Timolol: a preliminary report of its pharmacological properties and therapeutic efficacy in angina and hypertension. Drugs 9: 164–177
Brown JJ, Lever AF, Cumming AMM, Robertson JIS (1977) Labetalol in hypertension. Lancet 1: 1147
Bühler FR, Laragh JH, Baer L, Vaughan ED, Brunner HR (1972) Propranolol inhibition of renin secretion. A specific approach to diagnosis and treatment of renin dependent hypertensive diseases. N Engl J Med 287: 1209–1214
Bühler FR, Burkart F, Lutold BE, Kung M, Marbet G, Pfisterer M (1975) Anti-hypertensive beta blocking action as related to renin and age: a pharmacologic tool to identify pathogenic mechanisms in essential hypertension. Am J Cardiol 36: 653–669
Bühler FR, Betel O, Lutold BE (1978) Simplified and age-stratified anti-hypertensive therapy based on beta blockers. Cardiovasc Med 3: 135–140, 144–148
Bühler FR, Hulthen UL, Kiowski W, Bolli P (1983) Beta-blockers and calcium antagonists. Symposium on beta-blockers in the 1980's). Drugs 25 [Suppl 2]: 50–57
Cain ME, Martin TC, Sobel BE (1983) Calcium antagonists and beta-blockers in combination. J Cardiovasc Med 8: 485–502
Cangiano JL, Ayala JM, Boksay IJE, Martinez-Maldonado M (1979) Penbutolol: a new beta blocker in the treatment of moderate essential hypertension. J Clin Pharmacol 19: 334
Carre A-G, Bertrand ME, Libersa C-C, Lekieffre J-P (1982) Etude en double aveugle contre placébo de l'efficacité et de la tolérance du labétalol à 400 mg/j. dans l'hypertension artérielle essentielle modérée de l'adulte. Rev Med Interne III: 373–377
Carruthers SG (1982) Cardiac dose response relationships of oral and intravenous pindolol. Br J Clin Pharmacol 13: 193s–198s
Castenfors H (1977) Long-term effects of timolol and hydrochlorthiazide or hydrochlorthiazide and amiloride in essential hypertension. Eur J Clin Pharmacol 12: 97–103
Chalmers J, Horvath J, Tiller D, Bune A (1976) Effects of timolol and hyrochlorothiazide on blood pressure and plasma renin activity. Double blind factorial trial. Lancet 2: 328–331
Chang PC, van Brummelen P, Vermeij P (1985) Acute vasodilator action of pindolol in humans. Hypertension 7: 146–150
Cheah JS, Chia BL (1974) Propranolol in the treatment of hypertension of Asians. J Trop Med Hyg 77: 150–154
Comerford MB, Besterman EMM (1982) A comparison of the effects of the slow release formulations of metoprolol and oxprenolol in hypertension. Ann Clin Res 14: 27–31
Cumming AMM, Brown JJ, Fraser R, Lever AF, Morton JJ, Richards DA, Robertson JIS (1979) Blood pressure reduction by incremental infusion of labetalol in patients with severe hypertension. Br J Clin Pharmacol 8: 359–364
Dage RC, Cheng HC, Woodward JK (1981) Cardiovascular properties of medroxalol, a new antihypertensive drug. J Cardiovasc Pharmacol 3: 299–315
Dage RC, Hsieh CP, Spedding M (1983) Vasodilation by medroxalol mediated by beta-2 adrenergic receptor stimulation. J Cardiovasc Pharmacol 5: 143–150
Dahr AS (1972) Use of hydralazine and selective cardiac adrenergic blockade in therapy of essential hypertension. Circulation [Suppl] 45-46(II): 142
Dal Palu C, Pessina AC, Semplicini A, Hlede M, Morandin F, Palatini P, Sperti G, Rossi GP (1982) Intravenous labetalol in severe hypertension. Br J Clin Pharmacol 13: 97s–99s

Dargie HJ, Dollery CT, Daniel J (1976) Labetalol in resistant hypertension. Br J Clin Pharmacol 3 [Suppl 3]: 751-755

Davidson C, Thadani U, Singleton W, Taylor SH (1976) Comparison of anti-hypertensive activity of beta-blocking drugs during chronic treatment. Br Med J 2: 7-9

Day GM, Prichard BNC (1971) Hypotensive action from a combination of propranolol and other hypotensive drugs. Br J Pharmacol 41: 408P-409P

Decalmer PBS, Chatterjee SS, Cruickshank JM, Benson MK, Sterling GM (1978) Beta-blockers and asthma, Br Heart J 40: 184-189

Deitchman D, LaBudde JA, Seidehamel RJ (1983) Bucindolol New drugs annual: cardiovascular drugs. Raven, New York, pp 1-18

Dillon N, Chung S, Kelly J, O'Malley K (1980) Age and beta adrenoceptor-mediated function. Clin Pharmacol Ther 27(6): 769-772

Distler A, Keim HJ, Cordes U, Philipp T, Wolff HP (1978) Sympathetic responsiveness and anti-hypertensive effect of beta-receptor blockade in essential hypertension. Am J Med 64: 446-451

Dormois JC, Young JL, Nies AS (1975) Minoxidil in severe hypertension: value when conventional drugs have failed. Am Heart J 10: 360-368

Douglas-Jones AP, Cruickshank JM (1976). Once daily dosing with atenolol in patients with mild or moderate hypertension. Br Med J 1: 990-991

Doyle AE (1983) Comparison of beta-adrenoceptor blockers and calcium antagonists in hypertension. Hypertension 5 (II): 103-108

Drayer JIM, Weber MA, Lipson JL, Megaffin BB (1982) Differential effects of diuresis and beta-adrenoreceptor blockade during angiotensin-converting enzyme inhibition in patients with severe hypertension. J Clin Pharmacol 22: 179-186

Duchin KL, Vukovich RA, Dennick LG, Groel JT, Willard DA (1980) Effects of nadolol beta-blockade on blood pressure in hypertension. Clin Pharmacol Ther 27: 57-63

Dunn FG, De Carvalho JRG, Frohlich ED (1978) Haemodynamic, reflexive and metabolic alteration induced by acute and chronic timolol therapy in hypertensive man. Circulation 57: 140-144

Edwards RC, Raftery EB (1976) Haemodynamic effects of long-term oral labetalol. Br J Clin Pharmacol 3 [Suppl 3]: 733-736

Fagard R, Amery A, Deplaen JF, Lijnen P, Missotten A (1976) Plasma renin concentration and the hypotensive effect of bendrofluazide and of atenolol. Clin Sci Mol Med 51: 215s-217s

Feltham PM, Watson OF, Peel JS, Dunlop DJ, Turner AS (1972) Pindolol in hypertension: a double-blind trial. N Z Med J 76: 167-171

Ferguson RK, Vlasses PH, Koeffer H, Clementi RA, Koplin JR, Willcox CM (1983) Effect of captopril and propranolol, alone and in combination, on the respones to isometric and dynamic exercise in normotensive and hypertensive men. Pharmacotherapy 3: 125-130

Fitzgerald JD (1972) Beta-adrenergic blocking drugs. Present position and future developments. Acta Cardiol [Suppl] 15: 199-216

Fitzgerald JD (1976) The effect of beta-adrenoceptor antagonists on the morbidity and mortality in cardiovascular disease, Postgrad Med J 52: 770-781

Floras JS, Jones JV, Hassan MO, Sleight P (1982) Ambulatory blood pressure during once-daily randomized double-blind administration of atenolol, metoprolol, pindolol and slow release propranolol. Br Med J 285: 1387-1392

Franciosa JA, Freis ED, Conway J (1973) Antihypertensive and hemodynamic properties of the new beta adrenergic blocking agent timolol. Circulation 48: 118-124

Franciosa JA, Johnson SM, Tobian LJ (1979) Haemodynamic effects of oxprenolol and propranolol in hypertension. Clin Pharmacol Ther 26(6): 676-681

Freeman JW, Knight LW (1975) Oxprenolol and hydralazine in the treatment of hypertension. Med J Aust 1 [Suppl 1]: 12 -13

Frick MH, Porsti P (1976) Combined alpha- and beta-adrenoceptor blockade with labetalol in hypertension. Br Med J 1: 1046-1048

Frick MH, Hartikainen M, Porsti P (1978) Penbutolol, a new non-selective beta-adrenergic blocking compound in the treatment of hypertension. A comparison with propranolol. Ann Clin Res 10: 105-106

Frithz G, Aberg H, Asplund J, Aurell M, Conradsson T-B, Delin K, Herlitz H, Karlerg B, Morlin C, Nilsson OR, Ryden L, Wettre S, Ohman P (1982) Erfarenheter med captopril ensamt eller

i kombination med andra antihypertensiva lakemedel vid primar hypertoni. Opusc Med 27: 55-60
Frohlich ED, Tarazi RC, Dustan HP, Page IH (1968) The paradox of beta-adrenergic blockade in hypertension. Circulation 37: 417-423
Furberg C, Michaelson G (1969) Effect of Aptin, a beta-adrenergic blocking agent, in arterial hypertension. Acta Med Scand 186: 447-450
Gavras I, Gavras H, Sullican PC, Tifft CP, Chobanian AV, Brunner HR (1979) A comparative study of the effects of oxprenolol versus propranolol in essential hypertension. J Clin Pharmacol 19: 8-14
Gibson DG (1974) Pharmacodynamic properties of beta-adrenergic blocking drugs in man. Drugs 7: 8-38
Gibson DG (1977) Pharmacodynamic properties of beta-adrenergic blocking drugs in man. Beta-adrenoceptor blocking drugs; cardiovascular drugs, vol 2. Adis, Sidney, pp 1-40
Gilmore E, Weil JP, Chidsey C (1970) Treatment of essential hypertension with a new vasodilator in combination with beta-adrenergic blockade. N Engl J Med 282: 521-527
Giudicelli JF, Chauvin M, Thuillez C, Richer G, Bianchetti G, Gomeni R, Morselli PL (1980) Beta-adrenoceptor blocking effects and pharmacokinetics of betaxolol (SL 75212) in man. Br J Clin Pharmacol 10: 41-49
Gokal R, Dornan TL, Ledingham JGG (1979) Peripheral skin necrosis complicating beta-blockade. Br Med J 1: 721-722
Gomez G, Phillips LA (1980) Labetalol (Trandate) in hypertension: a multicentre study in general pracitice. Curr Med Res Opin 6 (10): 677-684
Gonasun LM (1982) Anti-hypertensive effects of pindolol. Am Heart J 104: 374-387
Gottlieb TB, Katz FH, Chidsey CA (1972) Combined therapy with vasodilator drugs and beta-adrenergic blockade in hypertension. A comparative study of minoxidil and hydralazine. Circulation 45: 571-582
Grandjean T, Rivier JL (1968) Cardio-circulatory effects of beta-adrenergic blockade in organic heart disease. Comparison between propranolol and CIBA 39089-Ba. Br Med J 3: 50-59
Grell GAC (1983) Hypertension in the West Indies. Postgrad Med J 59: 616-621
Hammond JJ, Kirkendall WM, Zama A, Thomas JC, Overturf ML (1978) Pindolol, propranolol and chlorthalidone in moderate hypertension. Pharmacologist 20: 189
Hammond JJ, Kirkendall M, Jacks VL (1979) Experience with captopril in the treatment of severe hypertension. Pharmacologist 21: 177
Hampton JR (1981) The use of beta blockers for the reduction of mortality after myocardial infarction. Eur Heart J 2: 259-268
Hampton JR (1982) Should every survivor of a heart attack by given a beta blocker? 1. evidence from clinical trials. Br Med J 285: 33-36
Hansson L (1973) Beta-adrenergic blockade in essential hypertension. Effects of propranolol on haemodynamic parameters and plasma renin activity. Acta Med Scand 55 [Suppl 1]: 1-40
Hansson L, Aberg H, Karlberg BE, Westerlund A (1975) Controlled study of atenolol in treatment of hypertension. Br Med J 1: 367-370
Hansson BG, Dymling JF, Hedeland H, Hulthen UL (1977) Long-term treatment of moderate hypertension with the beta-1 blocking agent metoprolol. Eur J Clin Pharmacol 11: 239-245
Hansson L, Hanel B (1976) Labetalol, a new alpha- and beta-adrenoceptor blocking agent in hypertension. Br J Clin Pharmacol 3 [Suppl 3]: 763-764
Hansson L, Olander R, Aberg H, Malmcrona R, Westerlund A (1971) Treatment of hypertension with propranolol and hydralazine. Acta Med Scand 190: 531-534
Hansson L, Zweifler AJ, Julius S, Ellis CN (1974) Propranolol therapy in essential hypertension. Observations on predictability of therapeutic response. Int J Clin Pharmacol 10: 79-89
Hansteen V, Moinichen E, Lorensten E, Anderson A, Strom O, Soiland K, Dyrbekk D, Refsum A-M, Tromsdal A, Knudsen K, Eika C, Bakken J, Smith P, Hoff PI (1982) One year's treatment with propranolol after myocardial infarction; preliminary report of Norwegian multicentre trial. Br Med J 284: 155-160
Hartikainen M, Heikkila J (1976) Twice-daily pindolol and alprenolol in essential hypertension of moderate severity. Ann Clin Res 8: 85-92
Hauger-Klevene JH (1981) Treatment of severe essential hypertension with labetalol: effect on active and inactive renin. Pharmatherapeutica 3: 46-54

Havelka J, Boerlin HJ, Studer A, Greminger P, Tenschert W, Luescher T, Siegenthaler W, Veter W, Walger P, Vetter H (1982) Long-term experience with captopril in severe hypertension. Br J Clin Pharmacol 14: 71S-76S

Hayes G (1983) Single-blind comparison of penbutolol and long-acting propranolol in general practice. Pharmatherapeutica 3: 456-463

Heel RC, Brogden GE, Speight TM, Avery GS (1980) Nadolol: review of its pharmacological properties and therapeutic efficacy in hypertension and angina pectoris. Drugs 20: 1-23

Heel RC, Brogden RN, Speight TM, Avery GS (1981) Penbutolol: a preliminary review of its pharmacological efficacy in hypertension and angina pectoris. Drugs 22: 1-25

Hill LS, Fand RS (1979) A report on the clinical efficacy of nadolol - a new long acting beta-blocker. J Ir Med Assoc 72: 522-529

Hjalmarson A, Elmfeldt D, Herlitz J, Holmberg S, Malek I, Nyberg G, Ryden L, Swedberg K, Vedin A, Waagstein F, Waldenstrom A, Waldenstrom J, Wedel H, Wilhelmsen L, Wilhelmsson C (1981) Effect on mortality of metoprolol in acute myocardial infarction. Lancet 2: 823-827

Hollenberg NK, Adams DF, McKinstry D, Williams GN, Borucki LJ, Sullivan J (1979) Beta-adrenoceptor blocking agents and the kidney: effect of nadolol and propranolol on the renal circulation. Br J Clin Pharmacol 7 [Suppl 2]: 219-226

Hollifield JW, Sherman K, Vander Zwaag R, Shand DG (1976) Proprosed mechanisms of propranolol's anti-hypertensive effect in essential hypertension. N Engl J Med 295 (2): 68-73

Houben H, Thien T, DeBoo T, Lemmens W, Binkhorst R, Van't Laar A (1983) Hemodynamic effects of isometric exercise and mental arithmetic in hypertension treated with selective and nonselective beta-blockade. Clin Pharmacol Ther 34: 164-169

Huang CM, Salomon J, Molteni A, Quintanilla A, Del Greco F (1980) Antihypertensive effect of captopril and propranolol Clin Pharmacol Ther 27: 258-259

Humphreys GS, Delvin DG (1968) Ineffectiveness of propranolol in hypertensive Jamaicans. Br Med J 2: 601-603

Ibsen H, Rasmussen K, Jensen HA, Leth A (1978) Changes in plasma volume and extracellular volume after addition of hydralazine to propranolol treatment in patients with hypertension. Acta Med Scand 203: 419-423

Jaillon P, Weissenburger J, Biour M, Cheymol G, Haegele K, Schechter PJ, Koch-Wester J (1982) Beta- and alpha-adrenoceptor antagonism by medraxolol in healthy volunteers: relationship to dose and plasma concentration. J Cardiovasc Pharmacol 4: 705-713

Joekes AM, Thompson FD (1976) Acute haemodynamic effects of labetalol and its subsequent use as an oral hypotensive agent. Br J Clin Pharmacol 3 [Suppl 3]: 789-793

Julian DG, Jackson FS, Prescott RJ, Szekely P (1982) Controlled trial of sotalol for one year after myocardial infarction. Lancet 1: 1142-1147

Jurgensen HJ, Frederiksen J, Hansen DA, Pederson-Bjergaard O (1981) Limitation of myocardial infarct size in patients less than 66 years old treated with alprenolol. Br Heart J 45: 583-588

Kane J, Gregg I, Richards DA (1976) A double-blind trial of labetalol. Br J Clin Pharmacol 3 [Suppl 3]: 737-741

Kane J, Gregg I, Stephens MDB (1979) A long-term study of labetalol in general practice. Br J Clin Pharmacol 8 [Suppl 2]: 167s-170s

Karlberg B, Hornkvist PE (1971) Propranolol in the treatment of hypertension. Opus Med 16: 296-299

Karlberg BE, Kagedal B, Tegler L, Tolagen K, Bergman B (1976) Controlled treatment of primary hypertension with propranolol and spironolactone. Am J Cardiol 37: 642-649

Kincaid-Smith P, MacDonald IM, Hua A, Laver MC, Fang P (1975) Changing concepts in the management of hypertension. Med J Aust 1: 327-332

Koch G (1976) Combined alpha- and beta-adrenoceptor blockade with oral labetalol in hypertensive patients with reference to haemodynamic effects at rest and during exercise. Br J Clin Pharmacol 3 [Suppl 3]: 729-732

Kostis JB, Frishman W, Hosler MH, Thorsen NL, Gonasun L, Weinstein J (1982) Treatment of angina pectoris with pindolol: the significance of intrinsic sympathomimetic activity of beta blockers. Am Heart J 104 (2, Pt II): 496-504

Kristensen BO, La Cour Petersen E (1980) Effects of long-term high dose labetalol on blood pressure in patients with severe hypertension resistant to previous therapy. Postgrad Med J 56 [Suppl 2]: 57-59

Kristensen BO, Brons M, Christensen CK, Geday E, Hacobsen FK, Jensen SN, Linde NC (1981) Anti-hypertensive effect of atenolol (100 mg once a day) and methyldopa (250 mg thrice a day). Acta Med Scand 209: 267-270

Lancet (1982) Long-term and short-term beta-blockade after myocardial infarction. Lancet 1: 1159-1161

Larochelle P, Hamet P, Hoffman B, Kuchel O, McKenzie J, Mitenko P, Ogilvie RI, Ruedy J (1980) Labetalol in essential hypertension. J Cardiovasc Pharmacol 2: 751-759

Laver MC, Fang P, Kincaid-Smith P (1974) Double-blind comparison of two beta-blocking drugs with previous therapy in the treatment of hypertension. Med J Aust 1: 174-176

Lechi A, Picotti GB, Covi G, Pomani S, Pedrolli E, Cesura AM, Danti G, Mattioli M (1981) Intravenous labetalol in severe hypertension: effects on blood pressure, renin activity and catecholamines. Arzneimittelforsch 33 (I) 3: 524-526

Lederle RM, Klaus D, Braun B (1980) Captopril in the treatment of essential hypertension. Dtsch Med Woschenschr 105: 1307-1312

Leishman AWD, Thirkettle JL, Allen BR, Dixon RA (1970) Controlled trial of oxprenolol and practolol in hypertension. Br Med J 4: 342-344

Leonetti G, Mayer G, Morganti A, Terzoli L, Zanchetti A, Bianchetti G, DiSalle E, Morselli PL, Chidsey CA (1975) Hypotensive and renin suppressing activities of propranolol in hypertensive patients. Clin Sci Mol Med 48: 491-499

Leonetii G, Biachini C, Terzoli L, Gradnik R, Tusa M, Bramati E, Zanchetti A (1982) Acute hypotensive and reninstimulating actions of captopril before and during treatment with a beta-blocking drug. Am J Cardiol 49: 1564-1565

Letac B, Fillastre JP, Wolf LM (1974) The treatment of essential hypertension with acebutolol (Sectral). Clin Trials J 11 [Suppl 3]: 92-95

Lohmoller G, Frohlich ED (1975) A comparison of timolol and propranolol in essential hypertension. Am Heart J 89: 437-442

Lossnitzer K, Rodatz W, Giensch E, Meine H (1981) Dose equivalence of nadolol and propranolol in hypertension. In: Gross F (ed) Royal society of medicine congress symposium series no. 37: international experience with nadolol: a long-acting beta-blocking agent. Proceedings of a symposium, Paris, 1980. Academic, London, pp 175-181

Lund-Johansen P (1976a) Haemodynamic long-term effects of timolol at rest and during exercise in essential hypertension. Acta Med Scand 199: 263-267

Lund-Johansen P (1976b) Haemodynamic long-term effects of a new beta-adrenoceptor blocking agent, atenolol (ICI 66082) in essential hypertension. Br J Clin Pharmacol 3: 445-451

Lund-Johansen P (1979) Long-term haemodynamic effects of penbutolol at rest and during exercise in essential hypertension. Eur J Clin Pharmacol 16: 149-153

Lund-Johansen P, Omvik P (1982) Prizidilol in essential hypertension: Long-term effects on plasma volume, extracellular fluid volume and central haemodynamics at rest and during exercise. J Cardiovasc Pharmacol 4: 1012-1017

MacGregor GA, Markandu ND, Banks RA, Bayliss J, Roulston JE, Jones JC (1982) Captopril in essential hypertension; contrasting effects of adding hydrochlorothiazide or propranolol. Br Med J 284: 693-696

MacGregor GA, Banks RA, Markandu ND, Bayliss J, Roulston J (1983) Lack of effect of beta-blocker on flat dose response to thiazide in hypertension: efficacy of low dose thiazide combined with beta-blocker. Br Med J 286: 1535-1538

Magnani B, Amberosioni E, Costa FV, Malini PL, Magelli C (1981) Comparison of anti-hypertensive activity of atenolol and methyldopa at rest and during exercise. Int J Clin Pharmacol Ther Toxicol 19: 440-444

Malini PL, Strocchi E, Ambrosioni E (1983) Comparison of the anti-hypertensive efficacy of bucindolol and propranolol. J Hypertension 1 [Suppl 2]: 348-350

Man In't Veld AJ, Schalekamp MADH (1982) How intrinsic sympathomimetic activity modulates the haemodynamic responses to beta-adrenoceptor antagonists. A clue to the nature of their anti-hypertensive mechanism. Br J Clin Pharmacol 13 [Suppl 2]: 245S-257S

Mann S, Millar Craig M, Balasubramanian V, Raftery EB (1981) Once daily beta-adrenoceptor blockade in hypertension: An ambulatory assessment. Br J Clin Pharmacol 12: 223-228

Marshall AJ, Roberts CJC, Barritt DW (1976) Raynaud's phenomenon as side effect of beta-blockers in hypertension. Br Med J 1: 1498-1499

Marshall AJ, Barritt DW, Pocock J, Heaton ST (1977) Evaluation of beta blockade, bendrofluazide and prazosin in severe hypertension. Lancet 1: 271-274

Materson BJ, Michael UF, Oster JR, Perez-Stable EC, Hernandez A, Smith M (1976a) Antihypertensive effects of oxprenolol and propranolol. Clin Pharmacol Ther 20: 142-151

Materson BJ, Oster JR, Michael UF, Perez-Stable EC (1976b) Anti-hypertensive effectiveness of oxprenolol administered twice daily. Clin Pharmacol Ther 19: 325-331

McAinsh J, Baber NS, Smith R, Young J (1978) Pharmacokinetic and pharmacodynamic studies with long-acting propranolol. Br J Clin Pharmacol 6: 115-121

McDevitt DG (1977) The assessment of beta-adrenoceptor blocking drugs in man. Br J Clin Pharmacol 4: 413-425

McDevitt DG, Brown CH, Carruthers SG, Shanks RG (1977) Influence of intrinsic sympathomimetic activity and cardioselectivity on beta-adrenoceptor blockade. Clin Pharmacol Ther 21: 556-566

McInnes GT, Findlay IN, Murray GD, Clelland JGF, Dargie HJ (1985) Clardiovascular responses to verapamil and propranolol in hypertensive patients. Second european meeting on hypertension, Milan, Italy, 9-12 June (abstract)

Medical Research Council Working Party (1981) Report of, on mild to moderate hypertension. Adverse reactions to bendrofluazide and propranolol for the treatment of mild hypertension. Lancet 2: 539-543

Medical Research Council Working Party (1985) MRC trial of treatment of mild hypertension: principal results. Br Med J 291: 97-104

Meekers J, Missotten A, Fagard R, Demuynck D, Harvengt C, Pas P, Billiet L, Amery A (1975) Predictive value of various parameters for the anti-hypertensive effect of the beta blocker ICI 66082(1). Arch Int Pharmacodyn Ther 213: 294-306

Mehta J, Cohn JN (1977) Haemodynamic effects of labetalol, an alpha and beta adrenergic blocking agent, in hypertensive subjects. Circulation 15: 370-375

Meyer-Sabellek WA, Schulte K-L, Thiede HM, Gotzen R (1983) Acute hypotensive response to the new anti-hypertensive agent BM 14190 in essential hypertensive patients. J Hypertension 1 [Suppl 2]: 351-352

Millar-Craig MW, Mann S, Balasubramanian V, Cashman P, Raftery EB (1981) Effects of oxprenolol on the intra-arterial blood pressure response to dynamic exercise in hypertensive men. J Cardiovasc Pharmacol 3: 468-476

Morgan TO, Louis WJ, Dawborn JK, Doyle AE (1972) The use of pindolol (Visken) in the treatment of hypertension. Med J Aust 2: 309-312

Morgan TO, Sabto J, Anavekar SN, Louis WJ, Doyle AE (1974) A comparison of beta adrenergic blocking drugs in the treatment of hypertension. Postgrad Med J 50: 253-259

Morgan TO, Roberts R, Carney SL, Louis WJ, Doyle AE (1975) Beta adrenergic receptor blocking drugs, hypertension and plasma renin. Br J Clin Pharmacol 2: 159-164

Morganti AA, Terzoli L, Salta C, Bianchini C, Leonetti G, Zanchetti AS (1979) Interactions between diuretics and propranolol in treatment of arterial hypertension. Cardiovasc Med 4: 43-52

Morioka S, Simon G, Shafer RB (1983) Cardiac effects of propranolol and timolol in hypertension: assessment by four non-invasive methods. Curr Ther Res 33: 626-638

Mueller J, Byrne MJ, Opie LH, van Schalkwyk J (1983) Renal impairment in hypertension not improved by nadolol when compared with atenolol. Drugs 25 [Suppl 2]: 146

Multicentre International Study (1975) Improvement in prognosis of myocardial infarction by long-term beta-adrenoceptor blockade using practolol. Br Med J 3: 735-740

Mutterperl RE, Diamond FB, Lowenthatl DT (1976) Long-term effects of minoxidil in the treatment of malignant hypertension in chronic renal failure. J Clin Pharmacol 16 (10): 498-509

New Zealand Hypertension Study Group (1979) A multicentre open trial of labetalol in New Zealand. Br J Clin Pharmacol 8 [Suppl 2]: 179S-182S

Nik-Akhtar B, Rashed MA, Khakpour M (1975) Effect of beta-adrenergic blocking agents (alprenolol and propranolol) in essential hypertension. Angiology 26: 339-343

Norwegian Multicentre Study Group (1981) Timolol-induced reduction in mortality and re-infarction in patients surviving acute myocardial infarction. N Engl J Med 304: 801-807

Obel AOK (1983) Practical therapeutics: the use of beta-adrenergic blocking agents in African patients. East Afr Med J 60: 592-596

Ogilvie RI, Hamet P, Kreeft JH, LaRochelle P, Marquez-Julio A (1983) Once-daily dosing of acebutolol in hypertension. J Cardiovasc Pharmacol 5: 157-161

O'Malley K, O'Callaghan WG, Laher MS, McGarry K, O'Brien E (1983) Beta-adrenoceptor blocking drugs and renal blood flow with special reference to the elderly. Drugs 25 [Suppl 2]: 103-107
Paget GE (1963) Carcinogenic action of pronethalol. Br Med J 1: 1266-1267
Papadmetriou V, Notargiacomo AD, Khatri IM, Freis ED (1982) Treatment of severe hypertension with intravenous labetalol Clin Pharmacol Ther 32 (4): 431-435
Pearson RM, Bending MR, Bulpitt CJ, George CF, Hole DR, Williams FM, Breckenridge AM (1976) Trial of combination of guanethidine and oxprenolol in hypertension. Br Med J 1: 933-936
Pedersen OL, Christensen CK, Mikkelsen E, Ramsch KD (1980) Relationship between the antihypertensive effect and steady-state plasma concentration of nifedipine given alone or in combination with a beta-adrenoceptor blocking agent. Eur J Clin Pharmacol 18: 287-293
Pelides LJ, Reid DS, Thomas M, Shillingford JP (1972) Inhibition by beta-blockade of the ST segment elevation after acute myocardial infarction in man. Cardiovasc Res 6: 295-301
Persson I (1975) Combination therapy of essential hypertension with pindolol (Visken) and hydralazine. Eur J Clin Pharmacol 9: 91-93
Pessina AC, Hlede M, Morandin F, Casiglia E, Gava R, Agnoletto V, Locatelli C, Dal Palu C (1983) Comparison of sotalol and propranolol in mild to moderate essential hypertension. Int J Clin Pharmacol Res III: 41-45
Peter T, Norris RM, Clarke ED, Heng MK, Singh BN, Williams B, Howell DR, Ambler PK (1978) Reduction of enzyme levels by propranolol after acute myocardial infarction. Circulation 57: 1091-1095
Petrie JC, Galloway DB, Webster J, Simpson WT, Lewis JA (1975) Atenolol and bendrofluazide in hypertension. Br Med J 3: 133-135
Pettinger WA, Mitchell HC (1973) Minoxidil - an alternative to nephrectomy for refractory hypertension. N Engl J Med 289: 167-171
Pickering TG, Case DB, Sullivan PA, Laragh JH (1982) Comparison of antihypertensive and hormonal effects of captopril and propranolol at rest and during exercise. Am J Cardiol 49: 1566-1568
Prichard BNC (1964) Hypotensive action of pronethalol. Br Med J 1: 1227-1228
Prichard BNC (1976) The combined effect of propranolol with bethanidine or methyldopa in hypertension. Adv Clin Pharmacol 2: 107-113
Prichard BNC (1978) Beta-adrenergic receptor blockade in hypertension, past, present and future. Br J Clin Pharmacol 5: 379-399
Prichard BNC (1983) Mechanisms of myocardial infarct prevention with beta-adrenergic blocking drugs. Drugs 25 [Suppl 2]: 295-302
Prichard BNC, Boakes AJ (1974) The use of sotalol in the treatment of hypertension. Advances in beta-adrenergic blocking therapy, sotalol, vol 4. Excerpta Medica, Amsterdam, pp 7-24
Prichard BNC, Boakes AJ (1976) Labetalol in long-term treatment of hypertension. Br J Clin Pharmacol 3: 743-750
Prichard BNC, Boakes AJ (1977) The use of beta-adrenergic blocking drugs in hypertension: a review. Curr Med Res Opin 4 [Suppl 5]: 51-76
Prichard BNC, Gillam PMS (1964) Use of propranolol (Inderal) in the treatment of hypertension. Br Med J 2: 725-727
Prichard BNC, Gillam PMS (1966) Propranolol in hypertension. Am J Cardiol 18: 387-391
Prichard BNC, Gillam PMS (1969) Treatment of hypertension with propranolol. Br Med J 1: 7-16
Prichard BNC, Gillam PMS (1971) Assessment of propranolol in angina pectoris. Clinical dose response curve and effect on electrocardiogram at rest and on exercise. Br Heart J 33: 473-480
Prichard BNC, Owens CWI (1970) Drug treatment of Hypertension. The action of intravenous oxprenolol, practolol, propranolol and sotalol on acute exercise tolerance in angina pectoris: the effect on heart rate and the electrocardiogram. Postgrad Med J 46 [Suppl Nov]: 77-85
Prichard BNC, Owens CWI (1983) Drug treatment of Hypertension. Hypertension 2nd edn. McGraw-Hill, New York, 1171-1210
Prichard BNC, Aellig WH, Richardson GA (1970a) The action of intravenous oxprenolol, practolol, propranolol and sotalol on acute exercise tolerance in angina pectoris: the effect on heart rate and the electrocardiogram. Postgrad Med J 46 [Suppl Nov]: 77-85
Prichard BNC, Gillam PMS, Graham BR (1970b) Beta receptor antagonism in hypertension; com-

parison with the effect of adrenergic neurone inhibition on cardiovascular responses. Int J Clin Pharmacol 4: 131-140
Prichard BNC, Shinebourne E, Flemming J, Hamer J (1970c) Haemodynamic studies in hypertensive patients on oral propranolol. Br Heart J 32: 236-240
Prichard BNC, Boakes AJ, Day GM (1971) Practolol in the treatment of hypertension. Postgrad Med J 47 [Suppl]: 84-91
Prichard BNC, Boakes AJ, Graham BR (1976) A within patient comparison of bethanidine, methyldopa and propranolol in the treatment of hypertension. Clin Sci Mol Med 51 [Suppl 3]: 567S-570S
Prichard BNC, Boakes AJ, Hernandez R (1979) Long term treatment of hypertension with labetalol. Br J Clin Pharmacol 8 [Suppl 2]: 171s-177s
Ravid M, Lang R, Jutrin I (1985) The relative antihypertensive potency of propranolol, oxprenolol, atenolol, and methoprolol given once daily. A double-blind, crossover, placebo-controlled study in ambulatory patients. Arch Intern Med 145: 1321-1323
Reybrouck T, Amery A, Fagard R, Jousten P, Lijnen P, Meulepas E (1978) Beta-blockers: once or three times a day. Br Med J 1: 1386-1388
Richards DA, Prichard BNC (1979) Clinical pharmacology of labetalol. Br J Clin Pharmacol 8 [Suppl 2]: 89s-93s
Richardson DW, Freund J, Gear AS, Mauck HP, Preston LW (1968) Effect of propranolol on elevated arterial blood pressure. Circulation 37: 534-542
Ronne-Rasmussen JO, Andersen GS, Bowal Jensen N, Andersson E (1976) Acute effect of intravenous labetalol in the treatment of systemic arterial hypertension. Br J Clin Pharmacol 3 [Suppl 3]: 805-808
Rose G (1982) Some conclusions (should every survivor of a heart attack be given a beta blocker?). Br Med J 285: 39-40
Ryan JR, Jain AK, McMahon FG (1975) Minoxidil treatment of severe hypertension. Curr Ther Res 17(1): 55-56
Salonen JT, Palminteri R (1982) Comparison of two doses of betaxolol and placebo in hypertension: a randomized double-blind crossover trial. Eur J Clin Pharmacol 23: 491-494
Sannerstedt R, Stenberg J, Vedin A, Wilhelmsson C, Werko L (1972) Chronic beta-adrenergic blockade in arterial hypertension. Haemodynamic influences of di-hydralazine and dynamic exercise and clinical effects of combined treatment. Am J Cardiol 29: 718-723
Saraste K, Tarkiainen A, Wennstrom J, Harkonen M, Gordin A, Sundberg S (1982) A placebo-controlled study of the effects of carteolol in hypertensive patients. Curr Ther Res 32: 189-195
Schechter PJ, Tanskanen A, Tuomilehto J, Koch-Weser J (1982) Treatment of mild and moderate hypertension with medroxalol, an alpha- and beta-adrenergic antagonist. J Cardiovasc Pharmacol 4: 955-959
Schiess W, Welzel D, Gugler R (1984) Double-blind comparison of once-daily bopindolol, pindolol and atenolol in essential hypertension. Eur J Clin Pharmacol 27: 529-534
Scott AK, Rigby JW, Webster J, Hawksworth GM, Petrie JC, Lovell HG (1982) Atenolol and metoprolol once daily in hypertension. Br Med J 284: 1514-1516
Seedat YK, Stewart-Wynne EG, Reddy J, Randeree M (1973) Experiences with beta-adrenergic blockade drugs in hypertension. S Afr Med J 47: 259-262
Sega R, Mailland F, Damiani E, Groothold G, Libretti A (1983) Indenolol in hypertension. Clin Pharmacol Ther 33: 289-293
Seto S, Aoi W, Doi Y, Matsumoto Y, Hashiba K (1980) Effect of captopril after propranolol in hypertensive man. 7th scientific meeting of the International Society of hypertension, Lousiana, (abstract)
Shand DG (1976) The pharmacokinetics of propranolol: a review. Postgrad Med J 52 [Suppl 4]: 22-25
Shinebourne E, Fleming J, Hamer J (1967) Effects of beta-adrenergic blockade during exercise in hypertensive and ischaemic heart disease. Lancet 2: 1217-1220
Siitonen L, Janne J, Keyrilainen O, Koskinen P, Leskinen O, Pitkajarvi T, Reinikainen M (1974) Hydralazine and beta-adrenergic blockade in the treatment of hypertension. Ann Clin Res 6: 341-346
Silke B, Nelson GIC, Ahuja RC, Taylor SH (1982) Comparative haemodynamic dose response effects of propranolol and labetalol in coronary heart disease. Br Heart J 48: 364-371

Simon G, Kiowski W, Julius S (1978) Anti-hypertensive and beta-adrenoceptor antagonist action of timolol. Clin Pharmacol Ther 23: 152-157
Staessen J, Fagard R, Lijnen P, Verschueren LJ, Amery A (1980) Beta-blockade during captopril treatment for hypertension. N Engl J Med 303: 1121-1122
Stewart I, McD G (1976) Compared incidence of first myocardial infarction in hypertensive patients under treatment containing propranolol or excluding beta-receptor blockade. Clin Sci Mol Med 51: 509s-511s
Stokes GS, Weber MA (1974) Prazosin: preliminary report and comparative studies with other anti-hypertensive agents. Br Med J 2: 298-300
Stokes GS, Raftos J, Lewis RG, Mitchell AS, Jeremy D, Frost GW, Thornell IR (1982) Combined use of prazosin and beta-blockers in hypertension. J Cardiovasc Pharmacol 4: s172-s175
Stoll RW, Cavanaugh JH, MacLeod CM (1981) Beta-blocking effect of single oral doses of carteolol. Clin Pharmacol Ther 30: 605-610
Svedmyr N, Malmberg R, Haggendal E (1970) The haemodynamic effects of sotalol (MJ 1999) and propranolol in man. Pharmacol Clin 2: 82-85
Svendsen TL, Hartling O, Trap-Jensen J (1979) Immediate haemodynamic effects of propranolol, practolol, pindolol, atenolol and ICI 89406 in healthy volunteers. Eur J Clin Pharmacol 15: 223-228
Takeda T, Kaneko Y, Omae T, Yoshinga K, Masuyama Y, Nukada T, Shigiya R (1982) The use of labetalol in Japan: results of multicentre clinical trials. Br J Clin Pharmacol 13 [Suppl 1]: 49s-57s
Tarazi RC, Dustan HP (1972) Beta-adrenergic blockade in hypertension. Practical and theoretical implications of long-term haemodynamic variations. Am J Cardiol 29: 633-640
Taylor SH, Meeran MK (1973a) Different effects of adrenergic beta-receptor blockade on heart rate response to mental stress, catecholamines, and exercise. Br Heart J 4: 257-259
Taylor SH, Meeran MK (1973b) The cardiovascular response to some environmental stresses and their modification by oxprenolol. In: Burley, Frier, Rondel, Taylor (eds) New perspectives in beta blockade. Ciba, Horsham, pp 293-306
Taylor SH, Silke B, Lee PS, Hilal A (1982a) Haemodynamic dose-response effects of intravenous beta-blocking drugs with different ancillary properties in patients with coronary heart disease. Eur Heart J 3: 564-569
Taylor SH, Silke B, Ebbutt A, Sutton GC, Prout BJ, Burley DM (1982b) A long-term prevention study with oxprenolol in coronary heart disease. N Engl J Med 307 (21): 1294-1301
Textor SC, Fouad FM, Brevo EL, Tarazi RC, Vidt DG, Gifford RW (1982) Re-distribution of cardiac output to the kidneys during oral nadolol administration. N Engl J Med 307: 601-604
Tibblin G, Ablad B (1969) Anti-hypertensive therapy with alprenolol, a beta-adrenergic receptor antagonist. Acta Med Scand 186: 451-457
Trust PM, Rosei EA, Brown JJ, Fraser R, Lever AF, Morton JJ, Robertson JIS (1976) Effect on blood pressure, angiotensin II and aldosterone concentrations during treatment of severe hypertension with intravenous labetalol: comparison with propranolol. Br J Clin Pharmacol 3: 799-803
Tsukiyama H, Otsuka K, Higuma K (1982) Effects of beta-adrenoceptor antagonists on central haemodynamics in essential hypertension. Br J Clin Pharmacol 13: 269S-278S
Tuckman J, Martin R, Hodler J (1972) Hypertoniebehandlung mit hohen Dosen von oxprenolol, allein oder in Kombination mit dem vasodilator Dihydralazine. Helv Med Acta 36: 243-244
Tuckman J, Messerli F, Hodler J (1973) Treatment of hypertension with large doses of the beta-adrenergic blocking drug oxprenolol alone and in combination with the vasodilator dihydralazine. Clin Sci Mol Med 45: 159s-161s
Turi ZG, Braunwald E (1983) The use of beta-blockers myocardial infarction. JAMA 249: 12-16
Ulrych M, Frohlich ED, Dustan HP, Page IH (1968) Immediate haemodynamic effects of beta-adrenergic blockade with propranolol in normotensive and hypertensive man. Circulation 37: 411-416
Van Herwaarden CLA, Binkhorst RA, Fennis JFM, Van't Laar A (1979) Effects of propranolol and methprolol on haemodynamic and respiratory indices and on perceived exertion during exercise in hypertensive patients. Br Heart J 41: 99-105
Van Rooijen GJM, Boer P, Dorhout Mees EJ, Geyskes GG (1979) Effects of atenolol and propranolol when added to long-term antihypertensive diuretic therapy. Clin Pharmacol Ther 26: 420-427

Velasco M, Vizcarrondo H, Urbina-Quintana A, Hernandez-Pieretti O (1982) A comparative study between pindolol and nadolol on systemic and cardiac hemodynamics in hypertensive patients. Curr Ther Res 32 (5): 663-668
Vestal RE, Wood AJJ, Shand DG (1979) Reduced beta-adrenoceptor sensitivity in the elderly. Clin Pharm Ther 26 (2): 181-185
Veterans Administration Cooperative Study Group on Anti-Hypertensive Agents. (1977) Multiclinic controlled trial of bethanidine and guanethidine in severe hypertension. Circulation 55: 519-525
Veterans Administration Cooperative Study Group (1981) Oxprenolol vs propranolol: a randomized, double-blind, multiclinic trial in hypertensive patients taking hydrochlorothiazide. Hypertension 3: 250-256
Von Mollendorff E, Huschka C, Schroter E, Abshagen U (1981) BM 12343, a novel compound with vasodilating and beta-adrenoceptor blocking activities. Clin Sci 61: 477s-479s
Waal-Manning HJ (1966) Hypotensive action of propranolol. Clin Pharmacol Ther 7: 588-598
Waal-Manning HJ (1970) Comparative studies on the hypotensive effects of beta-adrenergic receptor blockade. Symposium on beta-adrenergic receptor blocking drugs. Ciba, Auckland, pp 64-72
Waal-Manning HJ (1976) The antihypertensive action of several beta-adrenoceptor blocking drugs. N Z Med J 83: 223-226
Waal-Manning HJ (1979) Can beta-blockers be used in diabetic patients? Drugs 17: 157-160
Waal-Manning HJ, Simpson FO (1974) Pindolol: a comparison with other anti-hypertensive drugs and a double-blind placebo trial. N Z Med J 80: 151-157
Waal-Manning HJ, Simpson FO (1982) Review of long-term treatment with labetalol. Br J Clin Pharmacol 13 [Suppl i]: 65S-73S
Webster J, Jeffers TA, Galloway DB, Petrie JC, Barker NP (1977) Atenolol, methyldopa and chlorthalidone in moderate hypertension. Br Med J 1: 76-78
Wikstrand J, Berglund G (1982) Anti-hypertensive treatment with beta-blockers in patients aged over 65. Br Med J 285: 850
Wilburn RL, Blaufuss A, Bennett CM (1975) Long-term treatment of severe hypertension with minoxidil, propranolol and furosemide. Circulation 52: 706-713
Wilcox RG, Hampton JR (1982) Comparison between atenolol and nadolol in essential hypertension at rest and on exercise. Br J Clin Pharmacol 13: 841-846
Wilcox RG, Mitchell JRA (1977) Contribution of atenolol, bendrofluazide and hydralazine to the management of severe hypertension. Br Med J 2: 547-550
Wilcox RG, Roland JM, Banks DC, Hampton JR, Mitchell JRA (1980) Randomised trial comparing propranolol with atenolol in immediate treatment of suspected myocardial infarction. Br Med J 281: 885-888
Wilhelmsen L, Wedel H, Tibblin G (1973) Multivariate analysis of risk factors for coronary heart disease. Circulation 48: 950-958
Wilkins MR, Kendall MJ (1984) Beta-adrenoceptor blocking drugs and the elderly. J R Coll Physicians Lond 18: 42-45
Williams LC, Murphy MJ, Parsons V (1979) Labetalol in severe and resistant hypertension. Br J Clin Pharmacol 8 [Suppl 2]: 143s-147s
Wilson M, Morgan G, Morgan T (1976) The effect on blood pressure beta-adrenoceptor blocking drugs administered once daily and their duration of action when therapy is ceased. Br J Clin Pharmacol 3: 857-861
Wilson C, Scott ME, Abdel-Mohsen A (1977) Atenolol and methyldopa in the treatment of hypertension. Postgrad Med J 53 [Suppl 3]: 123-127
Yusuf S, Ramsdale D, Peto R, Furse L, Bennett D, Bray C, Sleight P (1980) Early intravenous atenolol in suspected acute myocardial infarction. Lancet 2: 273-276
Zacest R, Gilmore E, Koch-Weser J (1972) Treatment of essential hypertension with combined vasodilation and beta-adrenergic blockade. N Engl J Med 286: 617-622
Zacharias FJ, Cowen KJ (1977) Comparison of propranolol and atenolol in hypertension. Postgrad Med J 53: 111-113
Zacharias FJ, Cowen KJ, Vickers J, Wall BG (1972) Propranolol in hypertension. A study of long-term therapy 1964-1970. Am Heart J 83: 755-761
Zacharias FJ, Cowen KJ, Cuthbertson PJR, Johnson TBW, Presst J, Thompson J, Vickers J, Simpson WT, Tuson R (1977) Atenolol in hypertension: a study of long-term therapy. Postgrad Med J 53 [Suppl 3]: 102-110

Discussion

Distler: There was some controversy as to the onset of the antihypertensive effect. Some authors claim that the antihypertensive onset is developed after just a few hours. Others state that it is obvious only after some days, still others after some weeks. What are your feelings on this?

Prichard: Right from the early days we were very well aware that in mild hypertension the onset was acute and the blood pressure was lowered. Many of the studies purporting to show that everything happens acutely did not in fact involve mild hypertension. But we certainly did observe evidence of a delayed effect in more severe grades of hypertension with propranolol. We examined the blood pressure fall in many patients, who were under observation in the clinic and compared it with that of patients who were receiving other drugs. We found no difference between the blood pressures at stabilization of dosage and 1 month after stabilization with bethanidine and methyldopa, whereas with propranolol we did see a further fall.

Middeke: I would like to ask you about the clinical significance of the so-called cardioprotection, especially as you had already mentioned it after the publication of the MRC trial and now the IPPPSH trial, comparing diuretics and beta blockers as first-line drugs. We have to face the fact that there was no cardioprotection. The incidence of mortality from cardiovascular diseases was equal in both the diuretic and the beta blocker groups in both trials. So, if we talk about cardioprotection in the primary treatment of essential hypertension, what do you think is the clinical significance now?

Prichard: Well, I think you have to look at this in three ways. One is the way you have just referred to, the final clinical pathway. Secondly there is the evidence from those patients at very high risk of infarction; and thirdly there is the experimental evidence. There is a lot of evidence from animal work in terms of reduction of infarct size, about the value of the prophylactic administration of beta receptor blockers in cutting down infarct size, and also shunting blood into ischemic zones to reduce myocardial blood flow. With high-risk patients; I think there is little doubt that those patients who have had a myocardial infraction get 20% or 25% protection in terms of infarction and mortality. In the IPPPSH study there was a trend in favour of oxprenolol in terms of reduction in mortality and infarction, and in the MRC trial in fact the patients had very mild hypertension, but if you dissect the results a little bit and look at those patients who were male non-smokers there was certainly a benefit in the propranolol group.

Koella: Among the side effects of beta blockers one always sees sleep disturbances listed, and usually there are two types of it. There are either REM sleep disturbances and/or slow-wave sleep disturbances. Now REM sleep disturbances, of course, can be easily explained by the beta blocking activity of the beta blockers. For many years we had difficulties in explaining the slow-wave sleep disturbances, until we started to find out through the work of Middlemiss that in fact some of the beta blockers also have a certain serotonin-receptor-blocking activity. That certainly gives us one chance to explain slow-wave sleep disturbances as side effects. However, the question I would like to ask is, shouldn't we start to consider also that the serotonin-blocking activity of some of the beta blockers may contribute to the peripheral effects on cardiovascular activity with these drugs?

Prichard: I think that is a very reasonable observation, and I think it could easily be true.

Göthert: May I comment on this very briefly. The serotonin receptor antagonist activity is related to a special type of 5HT receptor, namely the $5HT_1$ receptor, which may be present at the sympathetic nerve terminals. If you block this, you will decrease the inhibitory effect mediated by serotonin. But at present the physiologic importance of the presynaptic serotonin receptor on sympathetic nerves is not completely clear. In the central nervous system the situation is different, because there the $5HT_1$ receptor is the autoreceptor mediating autoinhibition.

Neyses: Two of the classical contraindications for beta blocker treatment are peripheral vascular disease and AV block. Now, very few cardiologists in the world would withhold beta blocker treatment for angina just because the patient has a marginal prolongation of the PQ time or because he has a walking distance of, let's say, 500 yards. The question then is, don't we have to give up those contra-indications in mild peripheral vascular disease and in marginal PQ time prolongation?

Prichard: Yes, I think we dealt with the PQ prolongation time and I agree that one would not regard that as a contraindication. Peripheral vascular disease, in fact the evidence in terms of Raynaud's phenomenon in patients with and without beta blockers, is very questionable when you look into it. There is no doubt, though, that there are some patients who are adversely affected, and one has to be careful. Generally speaking, I think this is a function of reduced cardiac output producing secondary peripheral vasoconstriction in response to the cardiac output, so we are going to see this with nonselective and cardioselective drugs. Possibly the only difference between these drugs might be some instances where you can say that the muscle blood flow is cut down by a nonselective drug. Probably with drugs with ISA activity you see less reduction in peripheral flow.

Cruickshank: I would just like to complement the remarks of Dr. Prichard on the MRC and IPPPSH studies concerning smoking. If you look at the incidence of coronary events and strokes in the placebo group, smoking doubled coronary events and also doubled stroke events, so undoubtedly smoking is a very wicked thing, certainly for doctors to be doing, and anybody who smokes should stop smoking. Now, when you look at the MRC and IPPPSH studies a little more closely, as the professor pointed out, about a third of men smoked. And the smoking totally inhibited and cancelled out the beneficial effect of propranolol and oxprenolol in coronary and stroke reduction. But if you look at the two-thirds of men who did not smoke, the reduction in coronary events was between 35% and 50%. So in the absence of smoking there is a very powerfull cardioprotective effect in hypertensives.

Effects of Antihypertensive Agents on Alpha and Beta Adrenoceptors*

A. DAUL, N. O'HARA, X. L. WANG, and O.-E. BRODDE

Universitätsklinikum Essen, Biochem. Forschungslabor der Medizinischen Klinik und Poliklinik, Abt. für Nieren- und Hochdruckkranke, Hufelandstr. 55, 4300 Essen 1, FRG

Introduction

Alterations in sympathetic activity might play an important role in inducing and/or maintaining elevated blood pressure in essential hypertension (De Champlain 1978; Folkow 1982; Weber and Drayer 1982). Because of the lack of a direct measurement of sympathetic activity in man, plasma noradrenaline concentrations have been taken as an index of sympathetic activity. Although numerous comparative studies of plasma catecholamines in hypertensives and normotensive controls exist, it is still a matter of controversy whether plasma noradrenaline levels are increased in essential hypertension (for a recent review see Goldstein 1983).

Human lymphocytes possessing a homogeneous population of β_2-adrenoceptors excitatorily coupled to the adenylate cyclase system, and human platelets containing a homogeneous population of α_2-adrenoceptors inhibitorily coupled to the adenylate cyclase system, which mediate aggregation, are suitable models in which to study alterations in adrenoceptor function in man (Brodde et al. 1985a). During the last few years several groups have found higher numbers of β_2-adrenoceptors in circulating lymphocytes of patients with essential hypertension than in normotensive controls (Landmann et al. 1983; Middeke et al. 1984; Brodde et al. 1984, 1985b). In addition, there was a significant positive correlation between β_2-adrenoceptor density and mean arterial blood pressure of the patients (Middeke et al. 1984; Brodde et al. 1985b). Changes of α_2-adrenoceptors in platelets, however, are controversial: Kafka et al. (1979) using ^{3}H-dihydroergorcriptine as ligand, found an increased density in female, but not in male, patients with essential hypertension, while Boon et al. (1983) and Motulsky et al. (1983), using ^{3}H-yohimbine as ligand, found no differences in platelet α_2-adrenoceptor density between normotensives and patients with essential hypertension. On the other hand, we recently observed that in patients with essential hypertension α_2-adrenoceptor density in platelets was significantly higher than in controls (Brodde et al. 1985b).

The aim of the present study was to investigate whether antihypertensive therapy might affect the density and/or responsiveness of α- and β-adrenoceptors in circulating blood cells of patients with essential hypertension and of healthy controls.

* This work was supported by the Landesamt für Forschung Nordrhein-Westfalen and the SANDOZ-Stiftung für Therapeutische Forschung.

New Aspects in Hypertension: Adrenoceptors
M. Middeke and H. Holzgreve (Eds.)
Springer-Verlag Berlin Heidelberg New York 1986

For this purpose we determined the effects of nifedipine, hydergine, and clonidine on α_2-adrenoceptor density in platelets (assessed by ^{3}H-yohimbine binding) and on β_2-adrenoceptor density in lymphocytes [assessed by (−)-^{125}iodocyanopindolol (ICYP) binding] of essential hypertension patients. In addition, we investigated the effects of β-adrenoceptor antagonists with and without intrinsic sympathomimetic activity (ISA) on β_2-adrenoceptor density in lymphocytes of healthy volunteers.

Methods

Lymphocyte β_2-adrenoceptor density was determined using ICYP binding, and lymphocyte cyclic AMP responses to isoprenaline stimulation and platelet α_2-adrenoceptor density using ^{3}H-yohimbine binding, as recently described (Brodde et al. 1985b). Plasma catecholamine concentrations were determined by an HPLC method using an electrochemical detection. The experimental data given in text and figures are means ± SEM of N experiments in each case. The maximal number of binding sites (B_{max}) and the equilibrium dissociation constants (K_D) for ICYP and ^{3}H-yohimbine were calculated from plots according to Scatchard (1949). Mean arterial blood pressure (MAP) was calculated by the equation $MAP = 2 \times P_{diast} + P_{syst})/3$. Linear regression analysis of the data was performed by the least-squares method. The significance of differences was estimated by Student's *t*-test. A *P*-value smaller than 0.05 was considered to be significant.

Results and Discussion

Effects of Nifedipine and Hydergine on Lymphocyte β_2- and Platelet α_2-Adrenoceptor Density in Patients with Essential Hypertension

To study whether the increases in α- and β-adrenoceptor density in the circulating blood cells of patients with essential hypertension (Brodde et al. 1985b) might be *directly* related to the elevated blood pressure levels, we investigated the effects of antihypertensive treatment with nifedipine and hydergine on platelet α_2- and lymphocyte β_2-adrenoceptor density in 18 male patients with essential hypertension [age: 50.4 ± 2.3 (32–60) years; blood pressure: 175.4 ± 2.8/102.6 ± 1.2 mmHg]. Therapy with nifedipine (2 × 20 mg/day) for 4 weeks led to a significant reduction in blood pressure from 180.1 ± 5.4/104 ± 1.3 to 154 ± 2/90 ± 3 mmHg (Fig. 1); concomitantly plasma noradrenaline levels increased from 378 ± 57 pg/ml to 658 ± 71 pg/ml (N = 9), while platelet α_2-adrenoceptor density decreased by approximately 30% (Fig. 2). Administration of hydergine (co-dergocrine, 2 × 2 mg/day) for 4 weeks reduced blood pressure from 169.8 ± 2.0/101.2 ± 1.0 mmHg to 151.4 ± 4.6/90.3 ± 3.5 mmHg (Fig. 1). Plasma noradrenaline levels were significantly reduced from 482 ± 58 to 327 ± 42 pg/ml (N = 9). Platelet α_2-adrenoceptor density, however, was not significantly affected by the hydergine treatment, although it showed a tendency to increase (Fig. 2). These opposite effects of nifedipine and hydergine on platelet

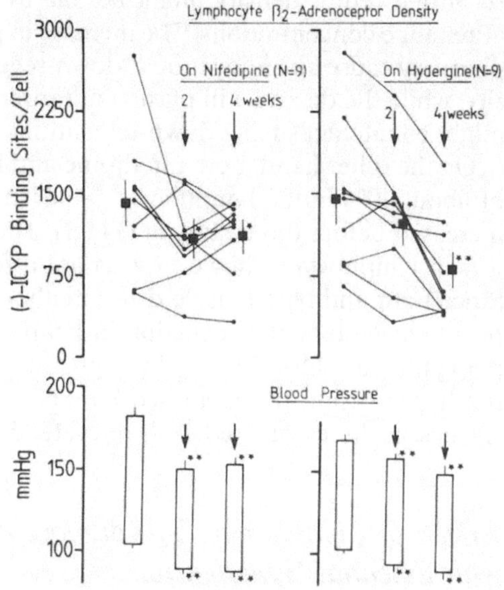

Fig. 1. Effects of nifedipine (2 × 20 mg/day) or hydergine (2 × 2 mg/day) on lymphocyte β_2-adrenoceptor density and blood pressure in 18 male patients with essential hypertension. *Ordinate (upper panel):* lymphocyte β_2-adrenoceptor density (determined by Scatchard analysis (1949) of ICYP binding) expressed as ICYP binding sites/cell; *lower panel:* blood pressure (mmHg)

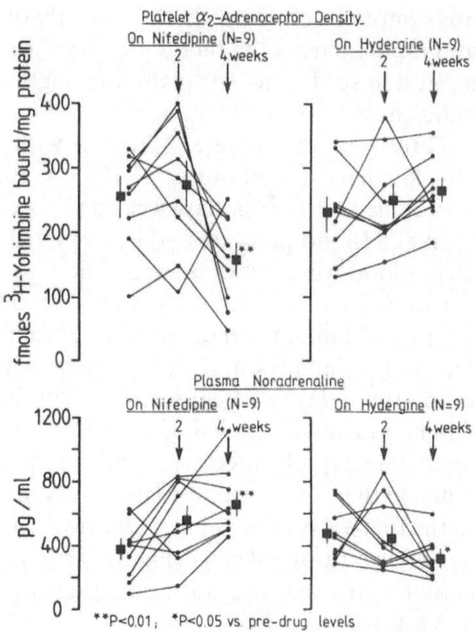

Fig. 2. Effects of nifedipine (2 × 20 mg/day) and hydergine (2 × 2 mg/day) on platelet α_2-adrenoceptor density and plasma noradrenaline levels in 18 male patients with essential hypertension. *Ordinate (upper panel):* platelet α_2-adrenoceptor density (determined by Scatchard analysis of ^{3}H-yohimbine binding) (fmol ^{3}H-yohimbine specifically bound/mg protein); *lower panel:* plasma noradrenaline levels (pg/ml)

α_2-adrenoceptor density might be due to the differential changes in plasma noradrenaline concentrations. The increase in plasma noradrenaline induced by nifedipine may cause an endogenous "down-regulation" of platelet α_2-adrenoceptor density, while the decrease in plasma noradrenaline following the hydergine treatment might counteract such a down-regulation.

On the other hand, both nifedipine and hydergine caused a significant reduction of about 40% in the lymphocyte β_2-adrenoceptor density, which was significantly increased before the treatment (Fig. 1). The affinity of ICYP for the β_2-adrenoceptors in lymphocytes, however, was not affected by the antihypertensive treatment. Since both antihypertensive drugs neither *directly* nor *indirectly* affect lymphocyte β_2-adrenoceptors, the reduction in lymphocyte β_2-adrenoceptor density accompanying the normalization of blood pressure lends credence to the idea that in essential hypertension the increased lymphocyte β_2-adrenoceptor density and responsiveness is directly linked to the elevated blood pressure.

Effects of Clonidine on α_2-Adrenoceptor Density in Patients with Essential Hypertension

By stimulating central α_2-adrenoceptors, clonidine depresses the sympathetic activity (Schmitt 1977; Kobinger 1978), and by stimulating peripheral presynaptic α_2-adrenoceptors it inhibits the release of endogenous noradrenaline (Starke 1977). Sudden withdrawal of clonidine produces a withdrawal syndrome with simultaneous symptoms of sympathetic overactivity such as unrest, perspiration, tachycardia, and rapid increases in blood pressure (for a review see Weber 1980). Thus, it was of interest to study whether clonidine might affect the number of α_2-adrenoceptors in platelets.

Three patients (1 male, 2 female) with mild essential hypertension (age: 42 ± 4 (36–46) years; blood pressure: $155 \pm 4/105 \pm 3.3$ mmHg) participated in this study. Clonidine (3×150 µg/day) was administered at 9, 15, and 21 h for 7 days (Brodde et al. 1982). Blood pressure and heart rate at supine rest were measured daily at 8 and 20 h. Blood was always taken at 9 h.

Clonidine decreased the patients' blood pressure from 155/105 mmHg to $125 \pm 10/85 \pm 11$ mmHg and the heart rate from 90 ± 8.3 to 72 ± 7 beats/min (Fig. 3). Plasma catecholamines and the number of platelet α_2-adrenoceptors had decreased even after 3 days of treatment and continued to decline during further treatment. After sudden withdrawal of clonidine, plasma catecholamines, blood pressure and heart rate rapidly increased and within 2–4 days reached values higher than or equal to their initial values. The α_2-adrenoceptor density, however, continued to fall in the first 3 days following withdrawal of clonidine, before returning to control values after a further 4 days (Fig. 3). The affinity of ^{3}H-yohimbine for the α_2-adrenoceptors, however, did not change during or after clonidine treatment (K_D values: 2–3 µ*M*).

Properties of α_2-adrenoceptors in human platelets determined by ^{3}H-yohimbine or ^{3}H-rauwolscine binding are very similar to those in other peripheral and/or central tissues (Eymer et al. 1982), including human cerebral cortex (Summers et al. 1983). Thus, changes in platelet α_2-adrenoceptor number can be taken as represen-

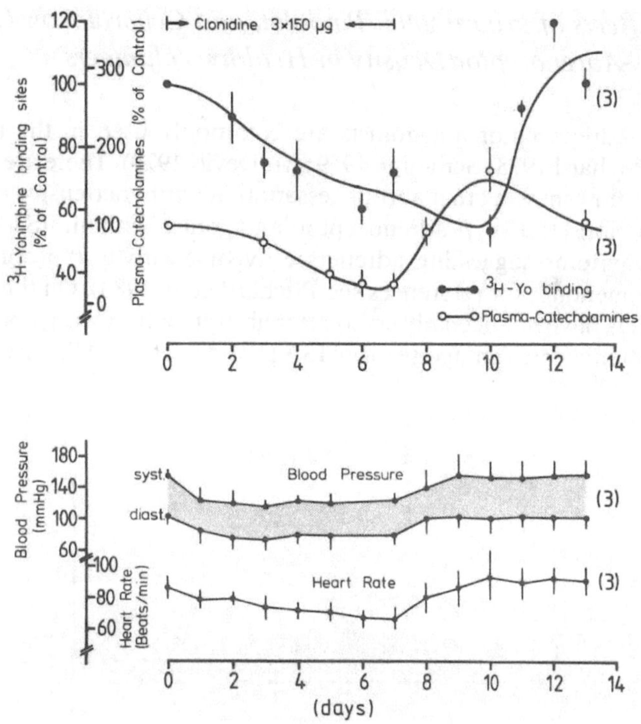

Fig. 3. Influence of clonidine treatment (3 × 150 μg/day for 7 days) on the number of α_2-adrenoceptors in platelet membranes, plasma catecholamine concentration, blood pressure and heart rate in hypertensive patients. ***Ordinate (upper panel):*** maximal number of ^{3}H-yohimbine binding sites (determined by Scatchard analysis) (●——●) as percentage of control (i.e. pretreatment) value: (^{3}H-yohimbine bound 158.1 ± 11.2 fmol/mg protein, N = 3; *left*); plasma catecholamine concentration (adrenaline + noradrenaline; O——O) as percentage of control [i.e., pretreatment value (0.55 ± 0.11 ng/ml); N = 3, *right*]; *lower panel:* blood pressure (mmHg) and heart rate (beats/min) N = 3. (From Brodde et al. 1982)

tative for changes of α-adrenoceptors in other tissues. From the present results, therefore, the following hypothesis can be proposed for the pathogenesis of the clonidine withdrawal syndrome: During treatment with clonidine the density of functional peripheral (presynaptic) and/or central α_2-adrenoceptors is reduced. Sudden withdrawal of clonidine results in an increased release of noradrenaline, as the release can no longer be regulated sufficiently as a result of the subsensitivity of α_2-adrenoceptors. Whether this effect is predominantly mediated peripherally or centrally cannot be decided from the present results. In this context it is worthwhile noting, however, that Engberg et al. (1982) found that following sudden withdrawal of clonidine in rats those central noradrenergic neurons which had a lower activity of α_2-adrenoceptors were overactive.

Effects of Propranolol, Pindolol, and Celiprolol on Lymphocyte β_2-Adrenoceptor Density in Healthy Volunteers

β-Adrenoceptor antagonists are commonly used in the therapy of hypertension (Prichard 1978; Scriabine 1979; McDevitt 1979). There are several reports in the literature showing that abrupt cessation of antihypertensive therapy with propranolol (a nonselective β-adrenoceptor antagonist without ISA) might lead to clinical symptoms suggesting adrenergic hypersensitivity ("propranolol withdrawal phenomenon"; for references see Prichard et al. 1983). On the other hand, rebound effects have not been observed after abrupt withdrawal of pindolol, a nonselective β-adrenoceptor antagonist *with* ISA (Walden et al. 1982; Szecsi et al. 1982). Obviously

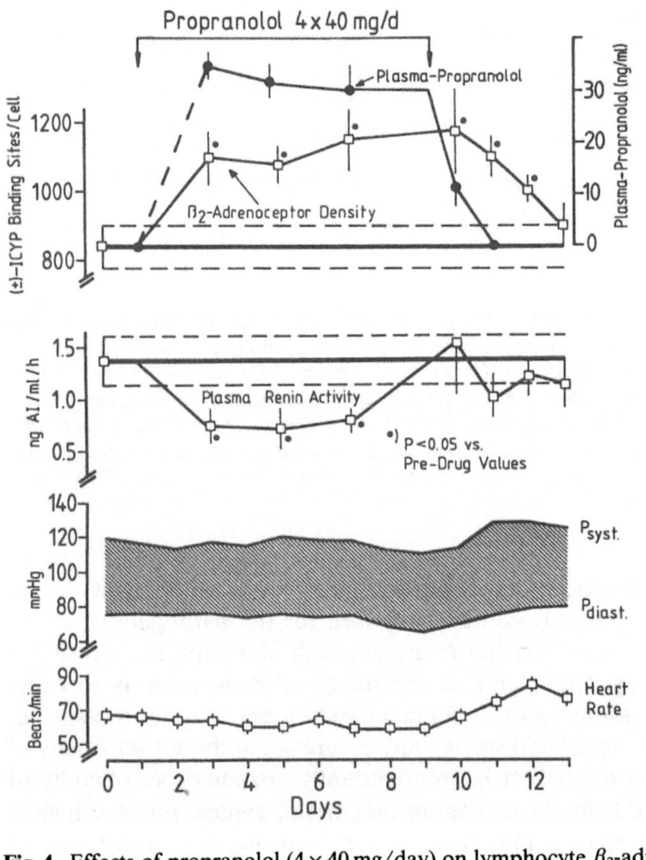

Fig. 4. Effects of propranolol (4 × 40 mg/day) on lymphocyte β_2-adrenoceptor density, plasma renin activity, blood pressure, and heart rate in six healthy male volunteers aged 27.0 ± 0.8 (24–30) years. *Ordinate* (top to bottom), *left:* β_2-adrenoceptor density in lymphocytes (determined by Scatchard analysis of ICYP binding) expressed as ICYP binding sites/cell; plasma renin activity (ng angiotensin I formed/ml/h); systolic and diastolic blood pressure (mmHg), and heart rate (beats/min); *right:* plasma propranolol levels (ng/ml). *Abscissa:* Days of study. Values plotted are means ± SEM from six experiments. *Horizontal lines* and *broken lines*, means ± SEM of predrug levels. *$p < 0.05$ vs predrug levels. (From Brodde et al. 1985c)

the ISA plays an important role in β-adrenoceptor antagonist-induced modulation of β-adrenoceptor density.

To test this hypothesis, the effects of the nonselective β-adrenoceptor antagonists propranolol (no ISA) and pindolol (strong ISA) and of the β_1-selective antagonist celiprolol *with* ISA on β_2-adrenoceptor density in lymphocytes (determined by ICYP binding) were investigated in normotensive young volunteers to gain further insights into the role of the ISA of β-adrenoceptor antagonists in modulating β-adrenoceptor density. A total of 22 healthy normotensive volunteers (16 male, 6 female) participated in the study after having given informed written consent. Propranolol (4 × 40 mg/day) was administered at 6, 12, 18, and 24 h, pindolol

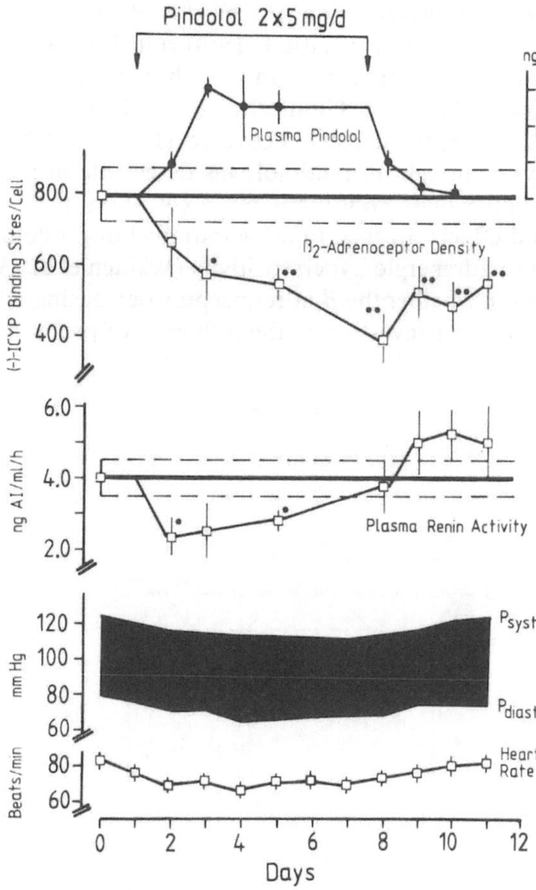

Fig. 5. Effects of pindolol (2 × 5 mg/day) on lymphocyte β_2-adrenoceptor density, plasma renin activity, blood pressure and heart rate in eight healthy male volunteers (4 male, 4 females, aged 24.5 ± 1.1 (20–28) years). *Ordinate* (top to bottom), *left:* β_2-adrenoceptor density in lymphocytes (determined by Scatchard analysis of ICYP binding) expressed as ICYP binding sites/cell; plasma renin activity (ng angiotensin I formed/ml/h); systolic and diastolic blood pressure (mmHg) and heart rate (beats/min); *right:* plasma pindolol levels (ng/ml). *Abscissa:* Days of study. Values plotted are means ± SEM from eight experiments. *Horizontal lines* and *broken lines,* means ± SEM of predrug levels. ** $P < 0.01$; * $P < 0.05$ vs predrug levels

(2 × 5 mg/day) at 7 and 19 h, and celiprolol (1 × 200 mg/day) at 19 h. β_2-Adrenoceptor density in lymphocytes was determined by ICYP binding (Brodde et al. 1985c; 1986).

Administration of propranolol (4 × 40 mg/day for 9 days) to healthy volunteers caused significant increases in lymphocyte β_2-adrenoceptor density, which amounted after 2 days to about 30%-35% (Fig. 4). A similar increase in lymphocyte β_2-adrenoceptor density in healthy volunteers following propranolol treatment has been also observed by Aarons et al. (1980) and Wood et al. (1982). After abrupt withdrawal of the drug β_2-adrenoceptor density declined slowly, remaining significantly elevated for 3-5 days, although 24 h after withdrawal no propranolol was detectable in plasma. Such a "supersensitivity" of β-adrenoceptors following the withdrawal of propranolol has been suggested to be the cause of the propranolol withdrawal phenomenon (Prichard et al. 1983). In contrast, administration of pindolol (2 × 5 mg/day) caused significant decreases in lymphocyte β_2-adrenoceptor density (Fig. 5), in accordance with recently reported data from Molinoff and Aarons (1983) and Giudicelli et al. (1984). After withdrawal of pindolol the β_2-adrenoceptor density recovered slowly, still being significantly reduced after 4 days, although no pindolol was detectable in plasma after 36 h. It is very likely that under these conditions rapid cessation of drug treatment will not induce rebound effects. In fact, rapid withdrawal of pindolol is not followed by any symptoms of adrenergic hypersensitivity (Walden et al. 1982; Szecsi et al. 1982).

To test whether the β-adrenoceptor-decreasing effect of pindolol is solely caused by its ISA we investigated the influence of propranolol on this pindolol effect. For

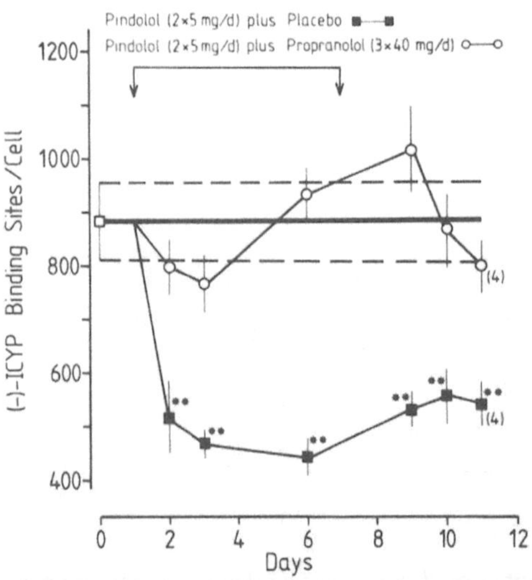

Fig. 6. Effects of pindolol (2 × 5 mg/day) *plus* placebo (■——■) or pindolol (2 × 5 mg/day) *plus* propranolol (3 × 40 mg/day; O——O) on lymphocyte β_2-adrenoceptor density in eight healthy male volunteers (aged 25.8 ± 1.6 (23-31) years). *Ordinate:* β_2-adrenoceptor density in lymphocytes (determined by Scatchard analysis of ICYP binding) expressed as ICYP binding sites/cell. *Abscissa:* Days of study. Values plotted are means ± SEM. Number of experiments in parentheses. *Horizontal line* and *broken lines*, means ± SEM of β_2-adrenoceptor density before treatment. ** $P <$ 0.01 vs predrug level. (From Brodde et al. 1986)

this purpose we conducted a double-blind test to determine the effects of simultaneous administration of pindolol (2 × 5 mg/day) *plus* placebo or pindolol *plus* propranolol (3 × 40 mg/day) on lymphocyte β_2-adrenoceptor density in eight healthy male volunteers. As shown in Fig. 6, propranolol completely abolished the pindol-induced decrease in lymphocyte β_2-adrenoceptor density, which suggests that in fact the ISA of pindolol is the cause of the lymphocyte β_2-adrenoceptor decreasing effect.

The β_1-selective antagonist celiprolol with ISA (= 0.32; 1 × 200 mg/day) produced effects comparable to those of pindolol: during treatment with celiprolol lymphocyte β_2-adrenoceptor density was significantly reduced (maximum decrease: 35%, Fig. 7). After withdrawal of celiprolol the β_2-adrenoceptor density re-

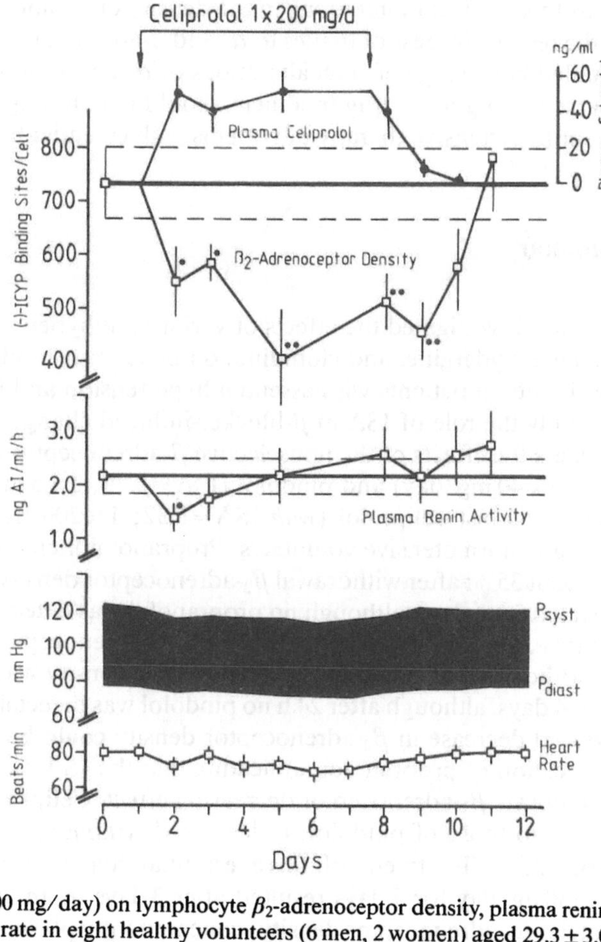

Fig. 7. Effects of celiprolol (1 × 200 mg/day) on lymphocyte β_2-adrenoceptor density, plasma renin activity, blood pressure and heart rate in eight healthy volunteers (6 men, 2 women) aged 29.3 ± 3.0 (20–46) years. *Ordinate* (top to bottom), *left:* β_2-adrenoceptor density in lymphocytes (determined by Scatchard analysis of ICYP binding) expressed as ICYP binding sites/cell; plasma renin activity (ng angiotensin I formed/ml/h); systolic and diastolic blood pressure (mmHg) and heart rate (beats/min); *right:* plasma celiprolol levels (ng/ml); *Abscissa:* Days of study. Values plotted are means ± SEM from eight experiments. *Horizontal lines* and *broken lines*, means ± SEM of predrug levels. ** $P < 0.01$; * $P < 0.05$ vs predrug levels. (From Brodde et al. 1986)

covered somewhat faster than after cessation of pindolol, reaching predrug levels after 3 days. The fact that the β_1-selective antagonist celiprolol decreases β-adrenoceptor density in lymphocytes, which contain exclusively β_2-adrenoceptors (Brodde et al. 1981) provides support for the idea that celiprolol might be an atypical β_1-selective antagonist which possesses β_2-agonistic activity in addition.

Conclusion

The present results clearly demonstrate that long-term administration of antihypertensive agents to patients with essential hypertension or to normotensive volunteers leads to significant alterations in the density of α- and β-adrenoceptors and hence in the responsiveness of tissues to α- and β-adrenergic stimulation or blockade. The detailed knowledge of such alterations of α- and β-adrenoceptors occurring in the course of long-term drug treatment should help to improve the individual efficacy of antihypertensive therapy of patients with essential hypertension.

Summary

We have investigated the effects of various antihypertensive agents (β-blockers, nifedipine, hydergine, and clonidine) on platelet α_2- and lymphocyte β_2-adrenoceptor density in patients with essential hypertension and in normotensive volunteers. To study the role of ISA in β-blocker-induced changes of β-adrenoceptor responsiveness the effects of the nonselective β-adrenoceptor antagonists propranolol (*no* ISA; 4×40 mg/day) and pindolol (ISA=0.39; 2×5 mg/day) and of the β_1-selective antagonist celiprolol (*with* ISA=0.32; 1×200 mg/day) were investigated in 22 young normotensive volunteers. Propranolol increased β_2-adrenoceptor density by about 35%; after withdrawal β_2-adrenoceptor density declined slowly, remaining elevated for 3 days, although no propranolol was detectable in plasma after 24 h. In contrast, pindolol (*with* ISA) decreased β_2-adrenoceptor density by about 50%; after withdrawal of pindolol β_2-adrenoceptor density was significantly reduced even after 4 days, although after 24 h no pindolol was detectable in plasma. The pindolol-induced decrease in β_2-adrenoceptor density could be prevented by simultaneous application of propranolol, indicating that the ISA of pindolol is the cause of the lymphocyte β_2-adrenoceptor decreasing effect. Celiprolol (*with* ISA) caused effects similar to those of pindolol: it decreased lymphocyte β_2-adrenoceptor density by about 35%. Treatment of three essential hypertension patients with clonidine 3×150 µg/day for 7 days resulted after 3 days in an about 30%–40% decrease of platelet α_2-adrenoceptor density; concomitantly plasma catecholamines were drastically reduced. After withdrawal of clonidine, plasma catecholamines increased rapidly, exceeding predrug levels after 2 days. α_2-Adrenoceptor density in contrast, increased slowly and did not reach predrug levels until 4–6 days after clonidine withdrawal. Treatment of nine male essential hypertension patients with nifedipine (2×20 mg/day, for 4 weeks) led to a significant reduction in blood pressure from

$180.1 \pm 5.4/104 \pm 1.3$ to $154 \pm 2/90 \pm 3$ mmHg ($P < 0.01$); concomitantly plasma noradrenaline levels increased from 378 ± 57 to 658 ± 71 pg/ml, while platelet α_2-adrenoceptor density decreased by approximately 35%. Administration of hydergine (2×2 mg/day for 4 weeks) reduced blood pressure from $169.8 \pm 2.0/101.2 \pm 10$ to $151.4 \pm 4.6/90.3 \pm 3.5$ mmHg ($N = 9$; $P < 0.01$); plasma noradrenaline was slightly reduced from 482 ± 58 to 327 ± 42 pg/ml. Platelet α_2-adrenoceptor density, however, was not significantly affected by treatment with hydergine, although it showed a tendency to increase. On the other hand, both nifedipine and hydergine caused a significant reduction ($\approx 30\%$–40%) in lymphocyte β_2-adrenoceptor density. These results demonstrate that long-term treatment of patients with essential hypertension with antihypertensive agents can alter density of α- and β-adrenoceptors and, by this, tissue responsiveness to α- and β-adrenergic stimulation or blockade. The detailed knowledge of such changes in α- and β-adrenoceptors over the course of long-term drug treatment should help to improve the individual efficacy of antihypertensive therapy in patients with essential hypertension.

References

Aarons RD, Nies AS, Gal J, Hegstrand LR, Molinoff PB (1980) Elevation of β-adrenergic receptor density in human lymphocytes after propranolol administration. J Clin Invest 65: 949–957

Boon NA, Elliot JM, Davies CL, Conway FJ, Grahame-Smith DG, Sleight P (1983) Platelet α-adrenoceptors in borderline and established essential hypertension. Clin Sci 65: 207–208

Brodde O-E, Engel G, Hoyer D, Bock KD, Weber F (1981) The β-adrenergic receptor in human lymphocytes: Subclassification by the use of a new radio-ligand, $(\pm)$-^{125}iodocyanopindolol. Life Sci 29: 2189–2198

Brodde O-E, Anlauf M, Graben N, Bock KD (1982) In vitro and in vivo down-regulation of human platelet α_2-adrenoceptors by clonidine. Eur J Clin Pharmacol 23: 403–409

Brodde O-E, Prywarra A, Daul A, Anlauf M, Bock KD (1984) Correlation between lymphocyte β_2-adrenoceptor density and mean arterial blood pressure: elevated β-adrenoceptors in essential hypertension. J Cardiovasc Pharmacol 6: 678–682

Brodde O-E, Daul A, O'Hara N, Khalifa AM (1985a) Properties of α- and β-adrenoceptors in circulating blood cells of patients with essential hypertension. J Cardiovasc Pharmacol 7 [Suppl 6]: S162–S167

Brodde O-E, Stuka N, Demuth V, Fesel R, Bergerhausen J, Daul A, Bock KD (1985b) Alpha- and beta-adrenoceptors in circulating blood cells of essential hypertensive patients: increased receptor density and responsiveness. Clin Exp Hypertens [A] 7: 1135–1150

Brodde O-E, Daul A, Stuka N, O'Hara N, Borchard U (1985c) Effects of β-adrenoceptor antagonist administration on β_2-adrenoceptor density in human lymphocytes. The role of the "intrinsic sympathomimetic activity". Naunyn Schmiedebergs Arch Pharmacol 328: 417–422

Brodde O-E, Schemuth R, Brinkmann M, Wang XXL, Daul A, Borchard U (1986) β-Adrenoceptor antagonists (non-selective as well as β_1-selective) with partial agonistic activity decrease β_2-adrenoceptor density in human lymphocytes. Evidence for a β_2-agonistic component of the partial agonistic activity. Naunyn-Schmiedebergs Arch Pharmacol (in press)

De Champlain J (1978) The contribution of the sympathetic nervous system to arterial hypertension. Can J Physiol Pharmacol 56: 341–353

Engberg G, Elam M, Svensson TH (1982) Clonidine withdrawal: activation of brain noradrenergic neurons with specifically reduced α_2-receptor sensitivity. Life Sci 30: 235–243

Eymer TH, Arroyo J, Prywarra A, Brodde O-E (1982) Properties of α_2-adrenoceptors in human platelets, guinea-pig kidney and calf cerebral cortex as evaluated by ^{3}H-yohimbine binding. Naunyn-Schmiedebergs Arch Pharmacol 321 [Suppl R]: 257

Folkow B (1982) Physiological aspects of primary hypertension. Physiol Rev 62: 347-504
Goldstein DS (1983) Plasma catecholamines and essential hypertension. An analytical review. Hypertension 5: 86-99
Giudicelli Y, Lacasa D, Agli B, Leneveu A (1984) Comparison of changes in the characteristics of β-adrenoceptors and responsiveness in human circulating lymphocytes during chronic and after chronic administration of pindolol and propranolol. Eur J Clin Pharmacol 26: 7-12
Kafka MS, Lake CR, Gullner H-G, Tallmann JF, Bartter FC, Fujita T (1979) Adrenergic receptor function is different in male and female patients with essential hypertension. Clin Exp Hypertens 1: 613-627
Kobinger W (1978) Central α-adrenergic systems as target for hypotensive drugs. Rev Physiol Biochem Pharmacol 81: 40-100
Landmann R, Bürgisser E, Bühler FR (1983) Human lymphocytes as a model for beta-adrenergic receptors in clinical investigation. J Recent Res 3: 71-88
McDevitt DG (1979) Adrenoceptor blocking drugs: clinical pharmacology and therapeutic use. Drugs 17: 267-288
Middeke M, Remien J, Holzgreve H (1984) The influence of sex, age, blood pressure and physical stress on β_2-adrenoceptor density in mononuclear cells. J Hypertens 2: 261-264
Molinoff PB, Aarons RD (1983) Effects of drugs on β-adrenergic receptors on human lymphocytes. J Cardiovasc Pharmacol 5 [Suppl 1]: S63-S67
Motulsky HJ, O'Connor DT, Insel PA (1983) Platelet α_2-adrenergic receptors in treated and untreated essential hypertension. Clin Sci 64: 265-272
Prichard BNC (1978) Beta-adrenergic receptor blockade in hypertension, past, present and future. Br J Clin Pharmacol 5: 379-399
Prichard BNC, Tomlinson B, Walden RJ, Bhattacharjee P (1983) The β-adrenergic blockade withdrawal phenomenon. J Cardiovasc Pharmacol 5 [Suppl 1]: S56-S62
Scatchard G (1949) The attraction of proteins for small molecules and ions. Ann N Y Acad Sci 51: 660-672
Schmitt H (1977) The pharmacology of clonidine and related products. In: Gross F (ed) Antihypertensive drugs. Handbook of Experimental Pharmacology, vol 39. Springer-Verlag, Berlin Heidelberg New York, pp 299-396
Scriabine A (1979) β-Adrenoceptor blocking drugs in hypertension. Annu Rev Pharmacol Toxicol 19: 269-284
Starke K (1977) Regulation of noradrenaline release by presynaptic receptor systems. Rev Physiol Biochem Pharmacol 77: 1-124
Summers RJ, Barnett DB, Nahorski SR (1983) The characteristics of adrenoceptors in homogenates of human cerebral cortex labelled by ^{3}H-rauwolscine. Life Sci 33: 1105-1112
Szecsi E, Kohlschütter S, Schiess W, Lang E (1982) Abrupt withdrawal of pindolol or metoprolol after chronic therapy. Br J Clin Pharmacol 13 [Suppl 2]: 353S-357S
Walden RJ, Bhattacharjee P, Tomlinson B, Cashin J, Graham BR, Prichard BNC (1982) The effect of intrinsic sympathomimetic activity on β-receptor responsiveness after β-adrenoceptor blockade withdrawal. Br J Clin Pharmacol 13 [Suppl 2]: 359S-364S
Weber MA (1980) Discontinuation syndrome following cessation of treatment with clonidine and other antihypertensive agents. J Cardiovasc Pharmacol 2 [Suppl I]: S73-S89
Weber MA, Drayer JIM (1982) The sympathetic nervous system in primary hypertension. Miner Electrolyte Metab 7: 57-66
Wood AJJ, Feldman R, Nadeau J (1982) Physiological regulation of beta-receptors in man. Clin Exp Hypertension [A] 4: 807-817

Discussion

Göthert: I noticed today that you showed in your in vitro experiments that the number of beta$_2$ adrenoceptors decreases under the influence of norepinephrine. Yesterday Dr. Brodde showed us that in the presence of in vivo elevated epinephrine concentrations the number of adrenoceptors apparently increases. Could you explain this discrepancy for me?

Daul: Yesterday the question was whether epinephrine really does regulate the beta$_2$ receptors, and there is probably a difference according as whether this process takes place in vivo, where other factors may contribute to the increase in beta$_2$ receptor density, or the process is investigated in vitro.

Göthert: I would say no, because in vitro you have better means of control. You can begin at very low concentrations, as we discussed yesterday, and of course you can also manipulate the system better at relatively high concentrations than is possible in vivo. You therefore have to find some condition under which an influence can really be exerted.

Brodde: I can't add much to that. When you infuse epinephrine in humans, you get a 100% increase in the beta receptor density. This persists for 2 hours. Then you discontinue the infusion, and after another 2 hours the receptors are low again and are destroyed. If you do the same thing in vitro, regardless of whether you use intact cells or membrane fractions, the receptor count drops immediately. When you incubate in vitro with agonists, the receptor density drops; in vivo with an agonist - regardless of whether you do it physiologically or with exercise, as discussed yesterday - it rises. When you infuse norepinephrine nothing happens to the beta$_2$ receptors. This means that unknown factors must be at work in vivo, which are not present in the in vitro system. That's why different regulation phenomena are found in vitro and in vivo.

Göthert: Thank you, that is clear and I find it convincing insofar as other factors, such as the corticoids, may also be present in vivo. Naturally we could try to simulate that in vitro as well, but I don't think we can say much more about it at the moment.

Heinz: I have a question regarding your nifedipine study. We conducted a similar study, but then combined it. We found no basal norepinephrine changes; only under ergometric stress were there changes. How large was your collective and what hypertensives were studied? Had they been treated previously?

Daul: No, they had not been treated previously. They were a total of 18 hypertensive patients, 9 of whom received Hydergine and 9 nifedipine.

Krawitz: Another question concerning your nifedipine study. Did you also investigate whether this preparation affected beta receptor binding in control subjects?

Daul: We have not yet done that.

Krawietz: The question is whether metabolites of nifedipine are involved.

Brodde: Dr. Philipp has conducted some experiments with nifedipine, alpha receptors, and catecholamines in healthy subjects and found that even in the short term the alpha receptors decrease under the influence of nifedipine. That's the study that was performed with healthy subjects.

Daul: These were acute studies with 20 mg sublingually.

Lemmer: A stupid question, perhaps. Dr. Prichard had said that the ISA is $beta_2$-related. Could you perhaps give some insight into how the ISA and blockade operate at the molecular level?

Daul: I can't tell you how they operate at the molecular level. The fact that the positive chronotropic effect of celiprolol is mediated by $beta_1$ receptors in the rat atrium and, on the other hand, that celiprolol, like pindolol, is able to reduce the $beta_2$ receptors indicate that the ISA is not subselective.

Kolloch: After 4 weeks you observed a further increase in the plasma catecholamine concentrations under the influence of nifedipine. Had you increased the dose, or how do you explain this rise? The second question I want to aks is: Did you find a correlation with the heart rate, since an acceleration of heart rate occurred in these patients?

Daul: We did not observe this, and after 2 weeks there was already a tendency for the plasma catecholamines to rise. After 4 weeks this rise was pronounced. This may be due to counterregulation of the vasodilatory effect.

Kolloch: You know that, in contrast to other reports in the literature, in which this increase in the plasma catecholamine levels was not observed ...

Daul: To return to the working group headed by Professor Distler, Dr. Philipp also found a tendency for the levels to rise, which only became significant during bicycle ergometric exercise. But there was at least a tendency for the plasma catecholamine levels to rise.

Kolloch: What was the mean age of these patients? Were they young?

Daul: No, they were elderly patients ranging in age from 32 to 60 years.

Kolloch: One last question: I'd be interested to know why you chose Hydergine for your investigations.

Brodde: We wanted a substance that was known or reported to reduce the plasma catecholamine levels by a mechanism not involving the alpha adrenoceptors. And the current hypothesis relating to Hydergine is that it reduces blood pressure by stimulating presynaptic $dopamine_2$ receptors, thus resulting in a reduction of the catecholamines.

But I'd like to make a serious comment with regard to the ISA. Dr. Pritchard mentioned earlier that the ISA is $beta_2$-related. I'd like to say a word of caution about making such global statements. I'd also like to explain why. Dr. Borchert showed us this ISA phenomenon in the rat heart and, as he said yesterday, it is clearly $beta_1$-related. Secondly, human lymphocytes are clearly a $beta_2$ model. After all, when $beta_1$ blockers without ISA, such as atenolol or bisoprolol, are given nothing happens; they don't react. If an ISA blocker reduces the receptor number of lymphocytes and all unselective agents change it, then lymphocytes must have a $beta_2$ system. The rat heart has a $beta_1$ system. It seems as if the ISA is unselective. But it goes on: although it is thought to have a $beta_2$ ISA, an ISA blocker is not able to stimulate the cAMP level in the lymphocytes, which an ISA blocker would have to do if it were $beta_2$-oriented. It gets worse: celiprolol, which according to the company and according to our own findings, has a $beta_2$ ISA, is not able to relax the human saphenous vein via $beta_2$ receptors. What I mean to say is that one should be very cautious, and Dr. Lemmer's question was more than justified. Essentially we still do not know, 30 years after the term ISA was coined, what it really means in molecular terms or in terms of subtype.

Göthert: One more question regarding this ISA problem, perhaps for the clinicians. In view of these findings would it be sensible to discontinue a beta blocker, to switch from, let's say, propranolol to a beta blocker with ISA, and only then discontinue therapy?

Krawietz: With regard to this ISA problem, or the problem of acute myocardial infarction - that's what you ultimately mean after discontinuation of beta blockers - I must say that Dr. Lichtlen expressed it very nicely when he said that he has performed acute coronary angiography in so-and-so many thousand patients, the last beta blocker dose usually being given on the eve of the angiographic examination, and he has never observed an acute myocardial infarction.

Mode of Action of Beta Blockers in Hypertension

J. M. Cruickshank
ICI plc Pharmaceuticals Division, Mereside, Alderly Park, Macclesfield, Cheshire Sk10 4TG
England

It should be stated quite clearly at the outset that the mechanism of action of beta blockers in lowering blood pressure (BP) is unknown. It is quite likely that several mechanisms exist and that one type might predominate under certain circumstances. All beta blockers will not necessarily lower BP in the same way - for example, under basal conditions propranolol does not lower peripheral resistance, but lowers cardiac output and BP (in responders): in contrast, under basal conditions pindolol lowers peripheral resistance, has little or no effect on cardiac output, but lowers BP to about the same degree as propranolol.

Several hypotheses exist as to the mode of action of beta blockers in lowering BP.

Central Nervous System

There have been observations in animals that suggest that beta-blocking drugs act centrally. When given intra-arterially, into either the carotid or the vertebral vessels in the anesthetised dog, propranolol produces a fall in BP of more rapid onset than when administered via the femoral artery [118]. Offerhaus and Van Zwieten [93] (1974) found that the non-beta-blocking dextroisomers of alprenolol and propranolol were as effective as the racemic mixtures when injected into the vertebral arteries of the chloralose anesthetized cat. This hypotensive effect of dextro and racemic mixtures alike was abolished by prior reserpinization [65]. The relevance of these observations is doubtful since the dextroisomer has no antihypertensive effect in man. The administration of several beta receptor antagonists (propranolol, alprenolol, pindolol, practolol, atenolol, sotalol, and oxprenolol) into the cerebral ventricle of conscious normotensive cats has been shown to produce a transient rise followed by a fall in BP, while the dextroisomers of propranolol and alprenolol showed only the initial pressor response [25] with no hypotensive effect. Intraventricular propranolol in doses giving levels in the brains of conscious rabbits comparable to those following intravenous infusion of 1.0 to 2.0 $mg kg^{-1} h^{-1}$ for 1-2 h also gave a fall of BP [90], and Reid et al. [106] have produced similar results. The former investigators also demonstrated brain penetration by propranolol in man. However, while *dl*-propranolol and bupranolol lowered the BP when injected into the cisterna magna of anesthetized dogs with neurogenic hypertension, other beta-adrenergic antagonist drugs, or *d*-propranolol, failed to result in a lowering of BP [86].

New Aspects in Hypertension: Adrenoceptors
M. Middeke and H. Holzgreve (Eds.)
Springer-Verlag Berlin Heidelberg New York 1986

Garvey and Ram [50] observed that oral or subcutaneous propranolol and pindolol given for 14 days lowered BP and heart rate in conscious hypertensive and normotensive rats. Propranolol was found to be concentrated particularly in the hippocampus, while pindolol was concentrated in the cerebral interventricular septum. Sotalol, however, failed to reduce BP, and significant concentrations were not found in the central nervous system. Sufficient amounts of all three drugs were given to produce persistent peripheral beta-adrenergic blockade. Direct injection of propranolol into the hippocampus, and pindolol into the septum, produced maximal effects on the BP and heart rate in chloralose anesthetised cats and dogs, with less effect being seen at other brain sites [51]. These procedures also produced reductions in efferent sympathetic and increases in parasympathetic nerve activity, while the injection of sotalol at various brain sites did not result in a fall in BP. Racemic propranolol given intravenously to the conscious rabbit gave a significant fall of BP and splanchnic efferent nerve activity after 2 h, whereas the dextroisomer did not [75]. However, in further experiments also in conscious rabbits, practolol did not reduce sympathetic nerve activity, but rather when pressures fell after larger doses, there was a rise in sympathetic nerve activity [30]. Other experiments in cats showed that racemic propranolol, dextroisomer propranolol, and pindolol were more effective in producing a fall in BP when given into the lateral ventricle than intravenously. The decline in BP was associated with a decrease in sympathetic nerve activity following sciatic nerve stimulation, whereas sotalol had no such effect [66].

The majority of beta adrenoceptor blocking drugs administered systemically penetrate the central nervous system and concentrations rapidly achieve a steady state. In cats, for example, there was no evidence of accumulation in the cerebrospinal fluid following 2 weeks' administration of alprenolol as compared with acute administration [93]. Other experiments in cats using equivalent hypotensive doses of metoprolol and atenolol have revealed a concentration up to ninefold higher of metoprolol in the brain compared with that of the lipid-insoluble atenolol [136]. These results have been confirmed in man, where brain concentration of the lipophilic beta blockers propranolol, oxprenolol, and metoprolol were 10–20 times higher than hydrophilic atenolol after chronic oral administration [91].

Thus, although some beta receptor-blocking drugs can influence central sympathetic activity, it is unlikely that this is the explanation for their antihypertensive action in man. However, it is not possible to rule out completely a central mechanism for beta blocker antihypertensive action, as even low brain levels of beta blocker such as occur with beta blockers like atenolol, sotalol, and nadolol, may be biologically active. There is also the possibility that beta blocker concentration in the cerebrospinal fluid (CSF) may be important; because the beta receptor resides on the outside of the cell membrane even hydrophilic agents like atenolol [91] would have ready access to it.

Inhibition of Sympathetic Nervous Activity

Adrenaline at low concentrations causes hypertension in the rat [80]; during beta blockade no such effect was observed. Elevated plasma adrenaline concentrations in patients with essential hypertension have been reported [1, 31, 47, 84, 114], possibly due to intermittent increased stimulation of the adrenal medulla by such factors as stress and anxiety [10]. It has been postulated that the development of hypertension occurs through increased adrenaline secretion from the adrenal medulla leading to stimulation of prejunctional beta receptors and consequent release of noradrenaline [79, 119, 120, 149] which effects vasoconstriction through stimulation of postjunctional alpha$_1$ receptors [10]. Figure 1 illustrates pre- and postjunctional alpha and beta receptors [130]. Many investigators have found evidence of higher levels of noradrenaline release in hypertension [7, 28, 31, 37, 42, 60, 96], though not all agree [63, 69, 112, 128]. Louis et al. [77] have shown a direct relationship between plasma noradrenaline concentration and DBP in patients with essential hypertension under basal conditions, and others have confirmed this [7]. Tuck et al. [132] have shown that in both normals and essential hypertensive circadian changes in BP relate to changes in both plasma renin activity and noradrenaline concentration, though levels were higher in the hypertensive group throughout 24 h, particularly during sleep.

There is evidence for a significant correlation between the magnitude of increase in plasma noradrenaline concentration during exercise and the subsequent decrease in mean arterial BP induced by the beta blocker atenolol [29]. Patients with low renin hypertension, who respond poorly to beta blockers, have a low plasma

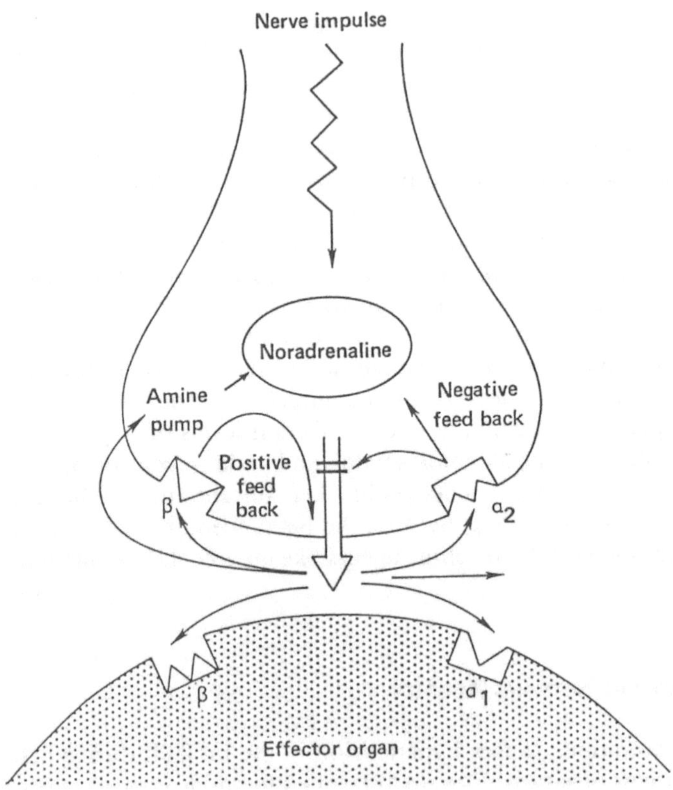

Fig. 1. Adrenergic nerve terminal: pre- and postjunctional alpha and beta receptors [130]

noradrenaline concentration and also a poor noradrenaline response to postural change [40]. On the other hand, hypertensives who have a high plasma renin activity (PRA) and respond well to beta blockade also have high plasma noradrenaline levels, which may be the cause of the increased PRA [41]. There is thus evidence to suggest that the degree of background sympathetic activity determines to what degree BP will fall with beta blockade [23, 29, 43], though not all agree [11]. Myers and De Champlain [89] showed that hypertensive patients with a high plasma noradrenaline concentration in the supine position responded well to atenolol with falls of 30/20 mmHg, compared with falls of 9/11 mmHg in those with lower noradrenaline concentration. It has been suggested that beta blockers lower BP by blocking prejunctional beta receptors and thus decreasing noradrenaline release from the nerve terminal resulting in a diminution of $alpha_1$-induced vasoconstriction [72].

If blockade of the prejunctional beta receptor and the resultant decrease in noradrenaline release is an important factor in the mechanism of lowering BP in the presence of beta-blockers, then evidence of decreased sympathetic activity should be present. However, beta-blockers tend to increase plasma catecholamine levels during exercise. At rest, beta blockers without ISA show a marked tendency to increase plasma noradrenaline concentration. Man in't Veld and Schalekamp [82] reviewed the literature and showed that beta blockers with no, or very little, ISA increased resting plasma noradrenaline levels by a mean of 30% in contrast to pindolol, which in seven studies lowered resting plasma noradrenaline by a mean of 33% (Fig. 2; [82]). Of particular interest is information indicating that plasma noradrenaline levels are reduced by pindolol only in responders, with levels remaining the same, or even raised, in nonresponders [148]. Buhler et al. [14] showed the same for propranolol, and others showed that propranolol lowered plasma noradrenaline, particularly if it was initially raised [135] alongside high PRA [16]. However, it must be remembered that plasma noradrenaline concentration is a reflection of both noradrenaline production and clearance. Clearance of plasma noradrenaline appears to be reduced during beta blockade [24, 44, 61]. Noradrenaline is cleared from the circulation mainly by the liver and lung, so that beta blockers without ISA, which lower cardiac output markedly [123] and reduce splanchnic-hepatic blood flow [24], will accordingly diminish noradrenaline clearance. Such effects will be magnified by exercise. By contrast, pindolol, which has little effect on cardiac output and splanchnic and hepatic blood flow at rest, will not reduce plasma noradrenaline clearance, and so the possible prejunctional effects on noradrenaline release become apparent. The fall in plasma noradrenaline did not correlate with the decrease in BP, however [7].

It has been suggested that the prejunctional beta receptor is of the $beta_2$ variety [56, 104]. Thus, if the blocking of this receptor is important in explaining how beta blockers lower BP, it might be expected that a $beta_1$-selective beta blocker such as atenolol would be relatively ineffective in lowering BP. This is clearly not the case, as atenolol is at least as effective as nonselective beta blockers in lowering BP. This, then, suggests that either the prejunctional beta receptor is of the $beta_1$, or mixed, variety or else adrenaline release from the adrenal medulla is decreased by the $beta_1$-blocking mechanisms. Vincent et al. [138] showed that isoprenaline-induced increases in plasma noradrenaline in man were blocked completely by propranolol, but only somewhat modified by cardioselective atenolol (Fig. 3 [138]) pointing pri-

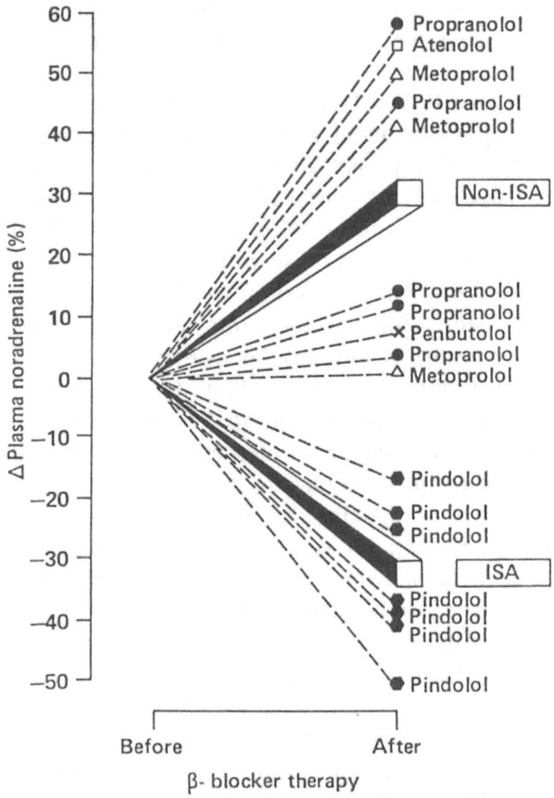

Fig. 2. Effect of beta blockade on plasma noradrenaline concentration in hypertensive patients [82]. Percentage change from baseline of plasma noradrenaline concentration in hypertensive patients during rest in supine position. Seventeen studies were included. Where beta blockers without ISA were investigated plasma noradrenaline increased by a mean of 30%. The seven studies with pindolol resulted in a mean decrease of 33% in plasma noradrenaline concentration

marily to a $beta_2$ mechanism possibly in the prejunctional area, though central actions could not be definitely ruled out. In contrast, the increase in noradrenaline, and adrenaline, with extreme exercise was greater with propranolol than with atenolol, with a resultant lower BP with the latter agent [83]. De Leeuw et al. [27] showed that even at rest, noradrenaline plasma concentration tended to be lower than pretreatment levels with atenolol but not with propranolol. Both propranolol [101] and atenolol are associated with increased plasma adrenaline levels during exercise, the latter somewhat less so [83], as is metoprolol [146]. Information on the effect of beta blockers on adrenaline clearance is required. Resting levels of plasma adrenaline have been shown to be unaffected by beta blockers [130], but during pleasant psychic stress plasma adrenaline did not rise with pindolol though it did with propranolol and metoprolol. In contrast, Dominiak and Grobecker [31] showed that pindolol significantly reduced resting, as well as "stress" adrenaline plasma levels. Buhler et al. [14] (1977) showed that in hypertensives, plasma adrenaline and noradrenaline tended to fall in responders to beta blockade compared with nonresponders. Com-

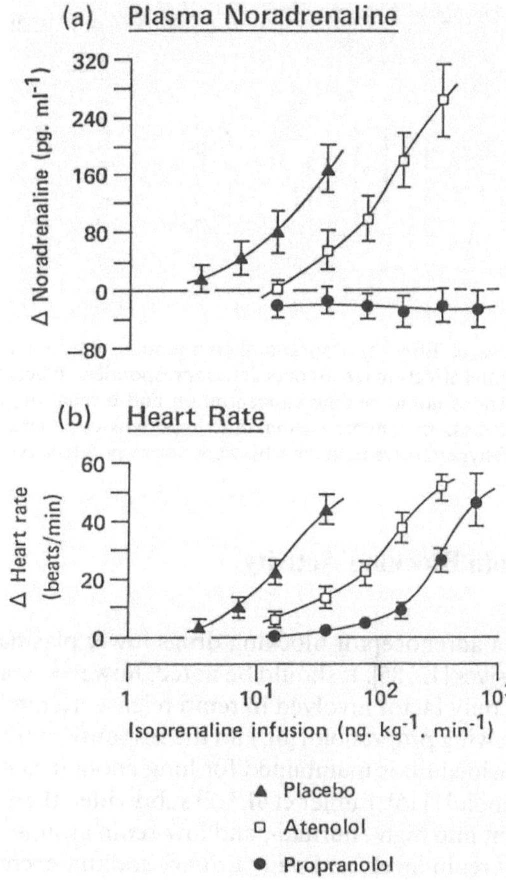

Fig. 3 a, b. Effect of isoprenaline infusion on **a** plasma noradrenaline concentration and **b** heart rate: Differential responses in the presence of atenolol and propranolol [138]. Mean (±SEM) change in **a** plasma noradrenaline and **b** heart rate in ten borderline hypertension patients during isoprenaline infusion in the supine position. Infusions were given before active therapy, after 7 days of oral atenolol (100 mg once a day) and after 7 days of oral propranolol (80 mg four times a day)

plementary to these observations are those of De Leeuw and Birkenhager [26], who showed that in nonresponders, but not responders, there was a significant secretion of noradrenaline from the kidneys (Fig. 4 [26]).

Others have shown that stress-induced (oral surgery) increases in plasma adrenaline are prevented by pindolol but not metoprolol [8]. The increase in plasma adrenaline associated with insulin-induced hypoglycemia is the same in the presence of placebo and pindolol, but greater with metoprolol and propranolol [110].

There is thus some evidence to suggest that beta blockers (at least pindolol) might lower BP by decreasing adrenaline release from the adrenal medulla and thus reducing prejunctional $beta_2$ receptor stimulation and the consequent noradrenaline release leading to a diminution of $alpha_1$-mediated vasoconstriction. However, more information is required in this area in order to substantiate such a hypothesis.

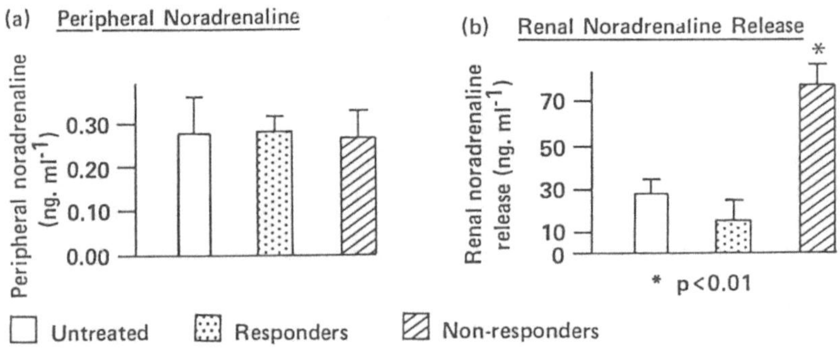

Fig. 4 a, b. Effect of propranolol on **a** venous noradrenaline and **b** renal noradrenaline release. Differential effects in responders and nonresponders to beta blockade [26]. Mean (± SEM) **a** peripheral venous noradrenaline concentration and **b** renal noradrenaline release in 15 patients with untreated essential hypertension, in 15 hypertensive patients who were responsive to propranolol, and in 10 hypertensive patients who were nonresponders to propranolol (maximum 480 mg/day)

Renin Blocking Activity

Beta adrenoceptor blocking drugs lower plasma renin in normals [147] and hypertensives [12, 85]. It should be noted, however, that beta-adrenergic stimulation is not the only factor involved in renin release. Renin levels rise after diuretics in patients receiving propranolol [6], and the response of the renin angiotensin system to tilting, provided tilt is maintained for long enough, is not abolished by metoprolol or propranolol [115]. Buhler et al. [12] subdivided their hypertensive patients prior to treatment into high-, normal-, and low-renin groups according to their ambulant peripheral renin levels and daily urinary sodium excretion (Fig. 5; [12]). The three groups were similar in age and severity of hypertension; up to 540 mg propranolol daily was used. The 12 patients with high renin showed the greatest falls of pressure, while the 14 patients with a low renin level showed only a very small effect. The 23 patients with normal renin levels had intermediate falls in BP. In additional, there was a good overall correlation between the fall in BP and PRA. Drayer et al. [33] also found slightly greater decreases in renin levels from propranolol in patients who showed a good response to BP, but falls in aldosterone levels were far greater in responders than in nonresponders. Propranolol, oxprenolol, LL21945, and the cardioselective agents atenolol and metoprolol were studied in a further series of 137 patients [13], and the results of Buhler et al. [12] were confirmed. Likewise, after treatment with alprenolol, falls in DBP correlated with reduction in plasma renin [17]. Fournier et al. [46] found a greater fall in BP when PRA was normal (as opposed to low) in patients treated with acebutolol, although initial PRA did not overall correlate with the fall in BP.

A study of Hollifield et al. [62] revealed a dissociation between the effect of low and high dosage of propranolol. They found that 160 mg propranolol a day caused a significant fall of BP in high-renin ($n = 13$, average 129 mmHg mean pressure to 114 mmHg) and normal-renin patients ($n = 18$, 131 mmHg to 119 mmHg); low-renin ($n = 9$) patients showed no change in pressure. Overall there was a positive

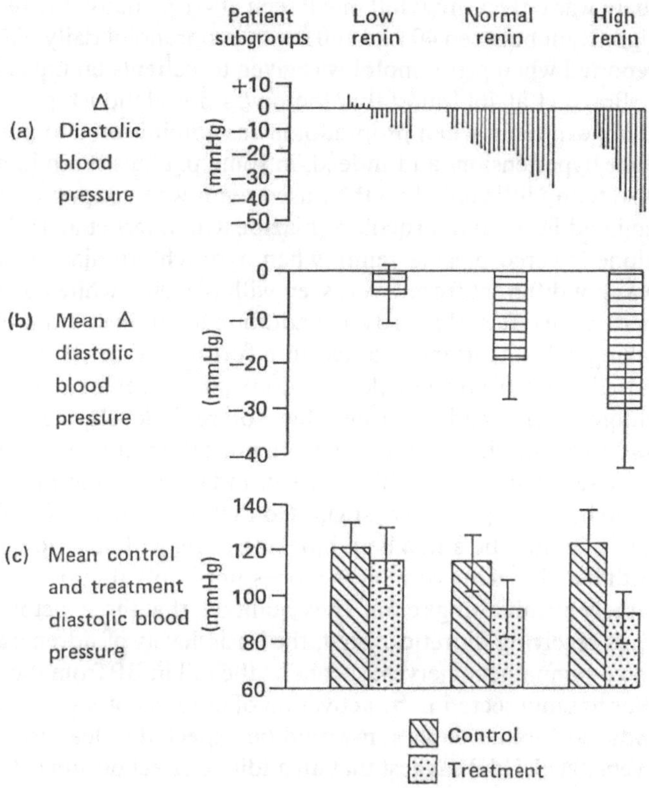

Fig. 5. Renin status and antihypertensive responsiveness to beta-blockade [12]. Changes in diastolic blood pressure after treatment with propranolol according to renin status classified prior to treatment. Results from 49 studies; mean ± SD *a* absolute changes in diastolic blood pressure in individual studies; *b* mean change in diastolic blood pressure; *c* mean control and treatment diastolic blood pressure

correlation between fall in renin and fall of BP. However, at higher doses of propranolol, 320–960 mg, there was a fall in BP in high- and low-renin patients independent of the effect on renin levels.

There is, however, considerable evidence that questions the importance of the renin effect in the antihypertensive action of beta-adrenergic blocking drugs. Many investigators have not found a relationship between pretreatment levels of plasma renin and the fall in BP following alprenolol [97], oxprenolol [59], propranolol [6, 15, 52, 58, 73, 87, 92, 121, 152]; practolol [39], pindolol [3, 70, 87]; sotalol [137]; timolol [113]; or metoprolol [53, 57]. Equal falls in BP with low-, normal-, and high-renin patients were seen by Morgan et al. [87].

Relatively small doses of propranolol which suppress plasma renin levels have little effect on BP [73, 85, 152]. Leonetti et al. [73] observed that a low dose of 40 mg propranolol daily produced almost maximal suppression of supine and frusemide-stimulated renin levels, and 60% of the fall in standing renin levels: a further fall in standing renin levels up to 160 mg of propranolol daily was significant. However, there was only a small fall in BP seen at 40 mg daily; the reduction in DBP was only significant between 40 and 160 mg of propranolol daily. There were similar findings reported when propranolol was given to patients taking chlorthalidone [88].

Bravo et al. [6] found that there was no relationship between the fall in BP and change in renin when propranolol was administered to patients taking diuretics for their hypertension, and indeed, in some patients renin increased. Gavras et al. [52] also found little effect on the raised renin when oxprenolol or propranolol was given in addition to hydrochlorothiazide. Chalmers et al. [18] found that while timolol alone lowered plasma renin, when hydrochlorothiazide was added, plasma renin was not different from levels seen with placebo, while there was an additive antihypertensive effect. Similarly, the additional administration of propranolol to patients taking chlorthalidone resulted in a further fall of BP and a partial reversal of the raised renin from the chlorthalidone [88]. Likewise, while metoprolol and hydrochlorothiazide had opposite effects on renin levels, the antihypertensive effect was additive, and the renin levels were not different from control [145]. Similar results were seen with the combined use of indapamide and pindolol [19].

Weber et al. [144] have suggested that the higher renin observed with a combination of a diuretic and a beta-blocking drug, with an additional fall in BP compared with beta blocking drug alone, does not imply that beta blocking drugs do not act largely by inhibiting renin. They point out that three factors can sustain renin in patients receiving diuretics: First, the basic levels of adrenergic stimuli, including the renal sympathetic nerves; secondly, the fall in BP from the diuretic would be a stimulus to renin secretion by activation of baroreceptor pathways; and thirdly, diuretic-induced sodium depletion would be expected to lead to increased renin secretion. Weber et al. [144] suggest that an additive effect occurs with diuretics, as beta blocking drugs will inhibit renin release from the first two mechanisms.

There is further evidence for the dissociation of effects on renin and BP: while intravenous propranolol lowers plasma renin, BP may not necessarily be reduced [5, 87]. It could be argued, however, that the fall in BP, although delayed, was secondary to an antirenin effect. Stokes et al. [121] found that while propranolol lowered plasma renin, substitution of pindolol for propranolol in nine patients for 48 h allowed plasma renin to reach control levels, although the hypotensive effect remained. Similarly, Stumpe et al. [122] noted that both pindolol and propranolol produced a similar fall in BP in patients with both borderline and established hypertension, but the fall in renin was greater with propranolol. Falls in BP and renin correlated with propranolol but not with pindolol. Man in't Veld and Schalekamp [82] illustrate clearly that beta blockers with no ISA markedly lower PRA, while pindolol has little effect (Fig. 6; [82]), and importantly, that vascular resistance and PRA are inversely correlated during long-term beta-blocker therapy. Likewise, Amery et al. [2] found that when they altered treatment from propranolol (480 mg) to atenolol (600 mg), the plasma renin concentrations rose and were no longer significantly different from placebo, but the hypotensive effect remained and indeed was improved somewhat. De Leeuw and Birkenhager [26] found that renin release from the kidney was suppressed to a greater extent in nonresponders by propranolol, and that in the nonresponders there was also a marked fall in cortical flow accompanied by increased release of noradrenaline.

Geyskes et al. [54] found saralasin infusion lowered the BP in a group of sodium-

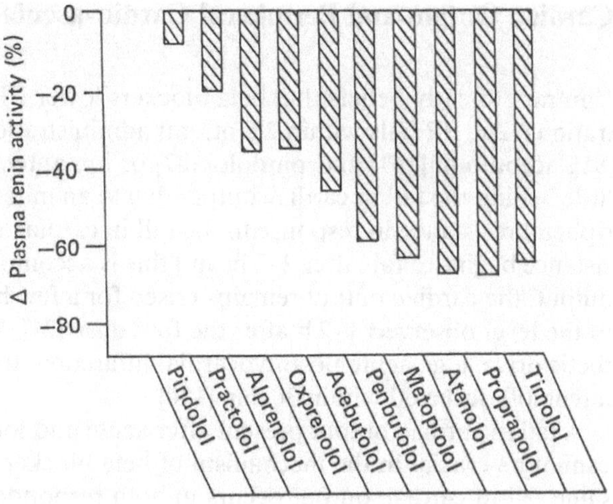

Fig. 6. Effect of intrinsic sympathomimetic activity on plasma renin activity [82]. Mean percentage change from baseline in plasma renin activity *(PRA)* during supine rest after long-term antihypertensive therapy with beta-blockers possessing different degrees of ISA. Beta blockers with high ISA are given from the *left*

depleted hypertensive patients in proportion to the renin levels, but there was much less effect after propranolol (80 mg q. d. s.) had been added to the low sodium diet. However Stumpe et al. [122] had four patients who showed a fall in BP with propranolol and a drop in renin levels. They found that the angiotensin antagonist saralasin failed to lower BP in these patients. Staessen et al. [116] found that the addition of propranolol to patients whose BP was resistant to the converting enzyme inhibitor captopril resulted in a significant fall in BP compared with placebo. On the other hand, others have failed to find any further fall of BP when propranolol was added to patients being treated with captopril [78].

It has been suggested that renin suppression may be important in lowering BP when beta-blocking agents are given to patients taking vasodilators, as they do reverse the rise in renin which results from the ingestion of vasodilators [98], or diuretics [151]. However, in patients taking alprenolol it was observed that the addition of hydralazine lowered BP without any significant change in renin levels [97].

In conclusion, while the fall in BP in some patients with high renin levels may be due largely to the antirenin activity of beta blocking drugs, the present evidence is still conflicting. Antirenin effect may be important when sodium depletion is present, e.g., diuretics. However, in general, inhibition of renin secretion from the kidney may contribute to the antihypertensive effect of beta blockers particularly at low dosage [62], but a primary role for this mechanism is unlikely. Initial renin status is possibly a useful predictor of response because it reflects sympathetic nervous activity [16, 32, 41, 122]. Van Baak et al. [134] consider that the antihypertensive mechanism of beta blockade is based upon a combination of cardiac beta receptor antagonism and a reduced intrarenal activity of the renin angiotensin system.

Cardiac Output and Peripheral Cardiovascular Mechanisms

Contrary to early beliefs that beta blockers lower BP only after long-term administration [126], BP falls within 2 h of oral administration of propranolol [21], atenolol [81], acebutolol [141] and pindolol [87] or i. v. antenolol [22]. The fall in BP lags a little behind the fall in cardiac output due to an initial compensatory increase in peripheral resistance in response to the fall in cardiac output. The total peripheral resistance begins to fall after 2-3 h, and this is accompanied by an increase in cardiac output: the cardiac output remains raised for a few hours before falling indefinitely to the level observed 1-2 h after the first dose [21]. In the presence of high sympathetic drive, e. g., acute postmyocardial infarction, the fall in BP to i. v. beta-blocker (atenolol) occurred within 30 min [150].

A fall in cardiac output present after acute and long-term beta blockade [58, 126] cannot be crucial in the mechanism of beta blocker antihypertensive action, as the same fall in cardiac output occurs in both responders and nonresponders [26, 45]. The differentiating factor in the responder and nonresponder is the raised compensatory (to decreased cardiac output) peripheral resistance which persists in the latter. The mechanism of the adaptive fall in peripheral resistance in responders is not understood, but must be of central importance to the antihypertensive action of beta blockers. Other differentiating points between responder and nonresponder are (a) a decreased velocity of left ventricular ejection and a slow rate of filling, i. e., altered wall relaxation or compliance in nonresponders [45]; and (b) marked reduction in cortical renal blood flow in nonresponders in contrast to responders, where there is no change [26].

There is little argument that the fall in BP with beta blockers correlates closely with the fall in peripheral resistance. With different beta blockers, however, the baseline peripheral resistance differs. Beta blockers with no ISA are associated initially with an increase in peripheral resistance arising from a compensatory vasoconstriction in response to a decreased cardiac output: this is followed within an hour or so by an adaptive fall in peripheral resistance back to, or perhaps slightly above, pretreatment values, with an accompanying fall in BP. Beta blockers like pindolol, with moderate to high ISA, cause little or no fall in cardiac output, and the fall in BP is associated with a fall in peripheral resistance to below pretreatment levels. These different hemodynamic profiles, however, are all associated with similar falls in BP, as has been well illustrated by Man in't Veld and Schalekamp [82] (Fig. 7) and by Hansson et al. [59] and Tsukiyama et al. [131].

It can therefore be concluded that although a fall in heart rate [22] and cardiac output may explain how beta blockers lower the BP of patients with labile hypertension and high output states [49], this is an inadequate explanation for the fall in BP in patients with classical essential hypertension. However, as Korner [67] concludes, the reduction in cardiac output is the major hemodynamic cause of the chronic reduction in BP. All beta blockers, with or without ISA, lower BP through lowering peripheral resistance, albeit from differing baselines. The mechanism for the fall in peripheral resistance is still unknown.

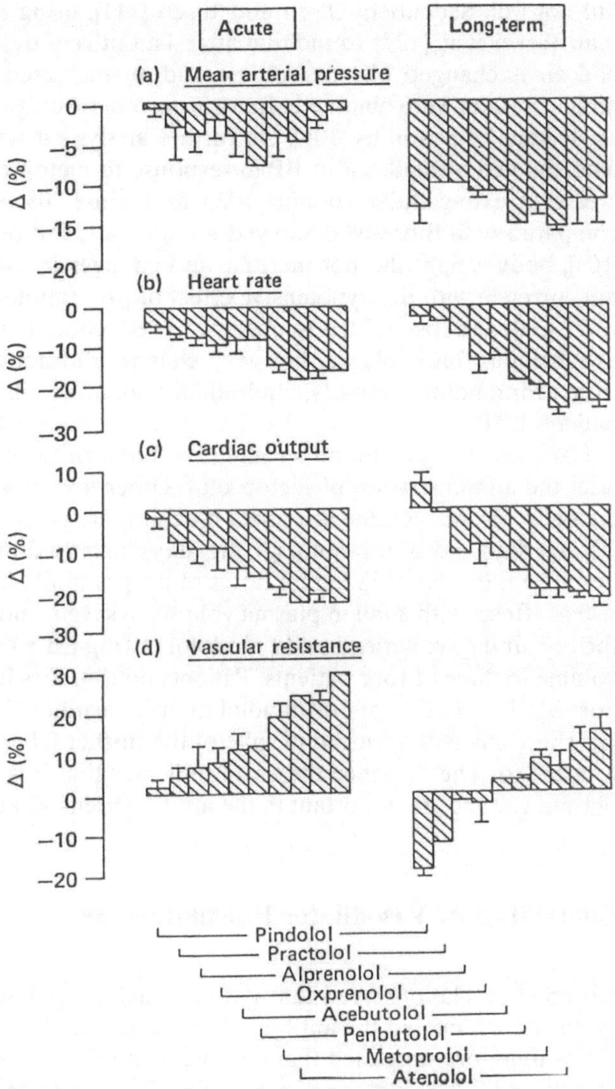

Fig. 7. Effect of intrinsic sympathomimetic activity on haemodynamic consequences of beta blockade [82]. Mean percentage change from baseline in supine resting patients after acute dosage or long-term antihypertensive therapy with beta-blockers possessing different degrees of ISA. Beta-blockers with a high degree of ISA are given from the *left*

Effect on Plasma Volume

Tarazi et al. [127] observed that propranolol reduced plasma volume in a series of 14 hypertensive patients, although this failed to correlate with the fall in BP. BP fell in some patients without a fall in plasma volume. Julius et al. [64] noted a fall in plasma volume after intravenous propranolol, but as others had shown before, BP did not fall. Sedenberg-Olsen and Ibsen [111], using higher doses of propranolol than Tarazi et al. [127], found that after 4 months of treatment hypertensive patients had an unchanged plasma volume and an increased extracellular fluid volume. Similar results were obtained after metoprolol (average dose 230 mg/day) given for an average of 5 months [105]. On further analysis it was found that those patients who showed a small fall in BP in response to metoprolol alone had a fivefold increase in extracellular volume, 1025 ml against 205 ml (statistically insignificant) compared with those who showed an adequate fall of BP. As in previous reports [103], body weight did not increase and changes in extracellular fluid volume did not correlate with the hypotensive effect of propranolol or other hypotensive drugs [107]. Leth and Ibsen [74] also observed a reduction in the ratio of plasma volume to extracellular fluid volume; however, changes did not correlate with the fall in BP from propranolol. Similarly, pindolol did not affect plasma volume in hypertensive patients [95].

Hansson et al. [57] found a small (5%) but significant increase of plasma volume after the administration of metoprolol. Other investigators have also found an increase in plasma volume after beta blocking drugs. Smaller doses of both pindolol (15 mg/day) and propranolol (30 mg/day) increased plasma volume after 1 month despite a fall in BP [55]. Larger doses of propranolol (40 mg t. d. s.) produced inconsistent effects with a fall in plasma volume in seven, and no change or an increase in the remaining six patients; and pindolol (10 mg t. d. s.) was found to reduce plasma volume in three of four patients. Patients on diuretics had a plasma volume 93% of normal; the addition of propranolol to their treatment increased it to 99% of normal [6]. These changes occurred in spite of the further fall of BP seen when propranolol was added. The evidence therefore indicates that it is improbable that changes in plasma volume are important in the antihypertensive action of beta blocking drugs.

Stimulation of Vasodilator Prostaglandins

Durao et al. [35] observed that indomethacin, a potent inhibitor of prostaglandin synthesis, attenuated the antihypertensive action of pindolol and propranolol, and it was therefore suggested that chronic beta receptor blockade might stimulate the formation of vasodilator prostaglandins. The antihypertensive effect of oxprenolol and atenolol is also blunted by indomethacin [108, 109]. This effect of indomethacin is not specific, as BP is raised to a similar degree in patients on propranolol or diuretics [76, 140], and there is a fall in urinary excretion products of prostaglandin metabolism when indomethacin is added to either propranolol or diuretics [140]. On the other hand, atenolol alone was found not to affect prostaglandin F_2 excretion [100]. Besides inhibition of prostaglandin synthesis, sodium retention from indomethacin [133] may be an alternative mechanism to explain its hypertensive effect and hence the effect in patients receiving beta-adrenergic blocking drugs; both possible actions may play a part. A less likely mechanism is a direct pressor effect [143].

Baroreceptor Resetting

The suggestion has been made [102, 103] that attenuation of pressor responses to various stimuli, by reducing the cardiac contribution, leads to the baroreceptors' generating their inhibitory impulses at lower levels of BP with a consequent fall in mean pressure. There is no reduction in baroreceptor responses to acute cardiovascular demands, such as posture. Generally, the heart is protected by β-blockade from responding to environmental stimuli; it amounts to a pharmacological "bed rest." When a hypertensive patient rests in bed, BP falls over a few days. There is a reduction of sensory input leading to a reduction of pressor events. This decline in environmentally induced stimulation means that the baroreceptors, being less stimulated, generate their impulses at a lower level of pressure. The BP falls while baroreceptor responses to acute physiological demand, e.g., posture, are still present. It was thus suggested that baroreceptor resetting is the primary mechanism, or at least a contributory factor, in the mode of action of beta adrenoceptor blocking drugs in hypertension. There seems little doubt that secondary resetting of the baroreceptors occurs after treatment with a variety of drugs in hypertension, because withdrawal of prolonged treatment not infrequently results in pressures remaining low for a variable period of time [94, 129].

If resetting of baroreceptors is primary in the mode of action of beta blocking drugs in hypertension, it does not necessarily mean that there is addition or alteration in actual receptor sensitivity. However, there is some work to suggest an increase in baroreceptor sensitivity. In dogs, chronic propranolol therapy blunted the pressor response to carotid occlusion [34], whereas short-term administration was without effect. If chronic propranolol administration enhanced baroreceptor sensitivity, then acute reduction in carotid sinus pressure (from carotid occlusion) should leave more inhibitory impulses remaining after occlusion. It is then possible that, with higher afferent inhibitory traffic, occlusion would result in a reduced rise in BP. Action potentials in aortic baroreceptor fibers have been recorded in anesthetized rabbits. It was found that the intravenous administration of propranolol, pindolol, and timolol all resulted in a fall in baroreceptor nerve acitivty, whereas this was not seen when a much larger fall in BP was induced by sodium nitroprusside [20, 48]. Angel-James and Bobik [4] also recorded action potentials in aortic baroreceptor fibers and reported an increase in activity in hypertensive rabbits treated with propranolol for 2 weeks, and even more in those treated for 15 weeks. The baroreceptor responses to pressor stimuli may be blunted in hypertension [9, 36, 71, 124]. The baroreceptor reflex is enhanced modestly by propranolol in normals [99] and in patients with borderline hypertension after intravenous propranolol, although sensitivity was not restored to that seen in control subjects [125]. These findings were confirmed with intravenous propranolol in borderline hypertensive subjects, both enhancing phenylephrine-induced bradycardia, and reducing the tachycardia from the increasing neck tissue pressure [139]. Watson et al. [142] found that acute oral administration of acebutolol, metoprolol, or propranolol only produced minor insignificant increases in baroreceptor sensitivity measured by phenylephrine-induced bradycardia, but the chronic administration of these drugs resulted in an increase in slope from 7.3 to 10.39 ms/mmHg ($P<0.005$). Moreover, while the increase in slope was significant for the nine patients under 40 years of age, the change in older patients ($n = 14$) was not significant. However, others have failed to find any significant increase in baroreceptor sensitivity in hypertensive patients treated with long-term timolol or acutely with propranolol [68, 113].

It must be concluded, then, that evidence does exist for beta blockers increasing baroreceptor reflex sensitivity, though there is not universal agreement on this matter. Such a mechanism could explain, at least in part, how beta blockers lower BP.

Beta Blockers and Calcium

Erne et al. [38] observed that in hypertensive patients there was a correlation between the free calcium concentration in platelets and both SBP and DBP. Antihypertensive therapy with calcium-entry blockers, beta blockers, and diuretics resulted in a fall in free calcium in the platelets, and this correlated with the fall in BP. It cannot be certain, however, that the changes in free calcium were not a result of, rather than a cause of, the fall in BP.

Summary

It is still not known how beta blockers lower BP. Various hypotheses have been put forward involving:

1. Action within the central nervous system (CNS)
2. Peripheral inhibition of sympathetic nervous activity
3. Inhibition of the extra- and intrarenal renin-angiotensin-aldosterone system
4. Decreasing heart rate and cardiac output
5. Diminishing plasma volume
6. Stimulation of vasodilator prostaglandins
7. Decreasing baroreceptor reflex sensitivity
8. A decrease in intracellular free calcium

It is quite possible that no one mechanism is at work. In patients whose hypertension is labile or associated with a hyperdynamic circulation, a decrease in heart rate and cardiac output is sufficient to explain the fall in BP. At times BP will be largely dependent on the renin-angiotensin-aldosterone system, e.g., in low sodium states such as might occur with diuretic therapy; under such circumstances inhibition of this system by a beta-blocker will result in a fall in BP. A beta-blocking action within the CNS cannot definitely be ruled out, but on balance it seems unlikely. Likewise, a decrease in baroreceptor reflex sensitivity may be relevant but has as yet not been proved to the satisfaction of everybody. The significance of the fall in platelet free calcium with beta blockers (as well as calcium channel blockers and diuretics) is still not understood. Perhaps the most attractive hypothesis involves beta blocker interference in the action of adrenaline upon the prejunctional beta receptor resulting in decreased noradrenaline release: however, more information on the effect of beta-blockers on adrenaline and noradrenaline release is required.

Whatever the mechanism, the end result is that in responders to beta blockers without ISA there is a chronic fall in cardiac output, and the fall in BP correlates with a fall in total peripheral resistance. Total peripheral resistance increases 1-2 h after the first dose of a beta blocker with no ISA and starts to fall 2-3 h after dosing. In the case of beta blockers with no ISA, the peripheral resistance adapts from a baseline higher than before treatment to a level at, or just above, pretreatment values: the fall in peripheral resistance associated with a beta blocker with moderate to high nonselective ISA, like pindolol, is from a baseline similar to pretreatment levels.

References

1. Amann FW, Bolli P, Kiowski W, Buhler FR (1981) Enhanced alpha-adrenoceptor mediated vasoconstriction in essential hypertension. Hypertension 3: I-119
2. Amery A, De Plaen JF, Fagard R, Lijnen P, Reybrouck T (1976) The relationship between beta-blockade, hyporeninaemic and hypotensive effect of two beta-blocking agents. Postgrad Med J 52 [Suppl 4]: 102-108
3. Anavekar SN, Louis JW, Morgan TO, Doyle AE, Johnston CI (1975) The relationship of plasma levels of pindolol in hypertensive patients to effect on blood pressure, plasma renin and plasma noradrenaline levels. Clin Exp Pharmacol Physiol 2: 203-212
4. Angell-James JE, Bobik A (1978) Modification of blood pressure and aortic baroreceptor activity in propranolol-treated hypertensive rabbits. J Physiol 278: 16P
5. Bravo EL, Tarazi RC, Dustan HP (1974) On the mechanism of suppressed plasma renin activity during beta-adrenergic blockade with propranolol. J Lab Clin Med 83: 119-128
6. Bravo EL, Tarazi RC, Dustan HP (1975) Beta-adrenergic blockade in diuretic treated patients with essential hypertension. N Engl J Med 292: 66-70
7. Brecht HM, Banthien F, Ernst W, Schoeppe W (1976) Increased plasma noradrenaline concentrations in essential hypertension and their decrease after long-term treatment with a beta-receptor blocking agent (prindolol). Clin Sci Mol Med 51: 485s-488s
8. Brisse B, Tetsch P, Jacobs W, Bender F (1982) Beta-adrenoceptor blockade in stress due to oral surgery. Br J Clin Pharmacol 13: 421S-427S
9. Bristow J, Honour AJ, Pickering GW, Sleight P, Smyth HS (1969) Diminished baroreflex sensitivity in high blood pressure. Circulation 39: 48-54
10. Brown MJ, Macquin I (1981) Is adrenaline the cause of essential hypertension? Lancet 2: 1079-1082
11. Bühler FR, Kiowski W (1980) Plasma catecholamines, renin, age and antihypertensive response of man to beta-blockers. In: Bevan JA, Godfraind T, Maxwell RA, Vanhoutte PM (eds), Vascular Neuroeffector Mechanisms, Raven Press, New York, 376-383
12. Bühler FR, Laragh JH, Baer L, Vaughan ED, Brunner HR (1972) Propranolol inhibition of renin secretion. A specific approach to diagnosis and treatment of renin dependent hypertensive diseases. N Engl J Med 287: 1209-1214
13. Bühler FR, Burkart F, Lutold BE, Kung M, Marbet G, Pfisterer M (1975) Antihypertensive beta-blocking action as related to renin and age: a pharmacologic tool to identify pathogenic mechanisms in essential hypertension. Am J Cardiol 36: 653-669
14. Bühler FR, Burkart F, Lutold BE, Bertel O, Pfisterer M (1977) Plasmakatecholamine und Hämodynamik im Verlauf der antihypertensiven Betablockade: verschiedene Muster bei Propranolol-Responders und Non-Responders. Schweiz Med Wochenschr 107: 1590-1591
15. Burris JF, Materson BJ, Freist ED (1983) Hydrochlorothiazide versus propranolol for monotherapy of hypertension. J Hypertension 1 [Suppl 2]: 329-331
16. Campese VM, Meyers MR, DeQuattro V (1977) Sympathetic nerve hyperactivity in 'high' renin primary hypertension: effects of propranolol. Clin Res 25 (2): 88a (Abstract)
17. Castenfors J, Johnsson H, Oro L (1973) Effect of alprenolol on blood pressure and plasma renin activity in hypertensive patients. Acta Med Scand 193: 189-195

18. Chalmers J, Horvath J, Tiller D, Bune A (1976) Effects of timolol and hydrochlorothiazide on blood pressure and plasma renin activity. Double-blind factorial trial. Lancet 2: 328-331
19. Chalmers J, Wing LMH, Grygiel JJ, West MJ, Graham JR, Bune AJ (1982) Effects of once-daily indapamide and pindolol on blood pressure, plasma aldosterone concentration and plasma renin activity in a general practice setting. Eur J Clin Pharmacol 22: 191-196
20. Chevalier-Cholat AM, Friggi A, Torresani J (1978) Action of beta-adrenoceptor blocking agents on haemodynamic variables and on baroreceptor and postganglionic sympathetic activities in rabbits. Biomedica 28: 67-72
21. Colfer HT, Cottier C, Sanchez R, Julius S (1984) Role of cardiac factors in the initial hypotensive action by beta-adrenoreceptor blocking agents. Hypertension 6: 145-151
22. Conway J (1983) Hypotensive mechanisms of beta-blockade. Eur Heart J 4 [Suppl D]: 43-50
23. Cousineau D, De Champlain J, Lapointee L (1978) Increased circulating catecholamines and cardiac functions in an important subgroup of essential hypertensive patients. Fifth scientific meeting of the inernational society of hypertension, Paris (Abstract)
24. Cryer PE, Rizza RA, Haymond MW, Gerich JE (1980) Epinephrine and norepinephrine are cleared through beta-adrenergic, but not alpha-adrenergic, mechanisms in man. Metab Clin Exp 29 [Suppl 1]: 1114-1118
25. Day MD, Roach AG (1974) Cardiovascular effects of beta-adrenoceptor blocking agents after intracerebroventricular administration in conscious normotensive cats. Clin Exp Pharmacol Physiol 1: 333-339
26. De Leeuw PW, Birkenhager WH (1982) Renal response to propranolol treatment in hypertensive humans. Hypertension 4 (1): 125-131
27. De Leeuw PW, Van Soest GAW, Punt R, Birkenhager WH (1983) Differences between selective and non-selective beta-blockade. Drugs (Symposium on beta-blockers in the 1980's) 25 [Suppl 2]: 250
28. De Quattro V, Chan S (1972) Raised plasma catecholamines in some patients with essential hypertension. Lancet 1: 806-807
29. Distler A, Keim HJ, Cordes U, Philipp T, Wolff HP (1978) Sympathetic responsiveness and antihypertensive effect of beta-receptor blockade in essential hypertension. Am J Med 64: 446-451
30. Dollery CT, Lewis PJ (1976) Central hypotensive effect of propranolol. Postgrad Med J 52 [Suppl 4]: 116-120
31. Dominiak P, Grobecker H (1982) Elevated plasma catecholamines in young hypertensive and hyperkinetic patients: effect of pindolol. Br J Clin Pharmacol 13: 318S-390S
32. Drayer JIM, Weber MA (1982) Antihypertensive agents which inhibit sympathetic activity: potentially adverse effects of combination treatment. Am Heart J 104 (3): 660-664
33. Drayer JIM, Weber MA, Longworth DL, Laragh JH (1978) The possible importance of aldosterone as well as renin in the long-term antihypertensive action of propranolol. Am J Med 64: 187-192
34. Dunlop D, Shanks RG (1969) Inhibition of the carotid sinus reflex by the chronic administration of propranolol. Br J Pharmacol 36: 132-143
35. Durao V, Prata MM, Goncalves LM (1977) Modification of antihypertensive effect of beta-adrenoceptor blocking agents by inhibition of endogenous prostaglandin synthesis. Lancet 2: 1005-1007
36. Eckberg DL (1979) Carotid baroreflex function in young men with borderline blood pressure elevation. Circulation 59: 632
37. Engelman K, Portnoy B, Sjoerdsma A (1970) Plasma catecholamine concentrations in patients with essential hypertension. Circ Res 27 [Suppl 1]: 141-145
38. Erne P, Bolli P, Burgisser E, Buhler FR (1984) Correlation of platelet calcium with blood pressure. N Engl J Med 310: 1084-1088
39. Esler MD (1974) Effect of practolol on blood pressure and renin release in man. Clin Pharmacol Ther 15: 484-489
40. Esler M, Randall O, Bennett J, Zweifler A, Julius S, Rydelek P, Cohen E, DeQuattro V (1976a) Suppression of sympathetic nervous function in low-renin essential hypertension. Lancet 2: 115-118
41. Esler M, Julius S, Randall O, DeQuattro V, Zweifler A (1976b) High-renin essential hypertension: adrenergic cardiovascular correlates. Clin Sci Mol Med 51: 181s-184s

42. Esler M, Julius S, Zweifler A et al. (1977 a) Mild-high renin essential hypertension: neurogenic human hypertension? N Engl J Med 296: 405-411
43. Esler MD, Zweifler A, Randall O, DeQuattro V (1977b) Pathophysiologic and pharmacokinetic determinants of the antihypertensive response to propranolol. Clin Pharmacol Ther 22: 299-308
44. Esler MD, Jackman G, Leonard P, Skews H, Bobik A, Jennings G (1981) Effect of propranolol on noradrenaline kinetics in patients with essential hypertension. Br J Clin Pharmacol 12: 375-380
45. Fouad FM, Slominski MJ, Tarazi RC, Gallagher JH (1983) Alterations in left ventricular filling with beta-adrenergic blockade. Am J Cardiol 51 (1): 161-164
46. Fournier A, Hardin JM, Alexandre JM, Lombaert M, Ronco G, Bezoc JF, Desmet G, Quichaud J (1976) Antihypertensive effect of acebutolol: its relation to sympathetic nervous system responsiveness and to plasma renin and dopamine beta-hydroxylase activities. Clin Sci Mol Med 51: 477s-480s
47. Franco-Morselli R, Elghozi JL, Joly E, Di Giulio S, Meyer P (1977) Increased plasma adrenaline concentrations in benign essential hypertension. Br Med J 2: 1251-1254
48. Friggi A, Chevalier-Cholat AM, Torresani J (1977) Haemodynamic and baroreceptor responses to beta-adrenoceptor blocking agents in rabbits with cardiopulmonary bypass. Eur J Pharmacol 45: 295-300
49. Frohlich ED, Tarazi RC, Dustan HP, Page IH (1968) The paradox of beta-adrenergic blockade in hypertension. Circulation 37: 417-423
50. Garvey HL, Ram N (1975 a) Comparative antihypertensive effects and tissue distribution of beta-adrenergic blocking drugs. J Pharmacol Exp Ther 194: 220-233
51. Garvey HL, Ram N (1975 b) Centrally induced hypotensive effect of beta-adrenergic blocking drugs. Eur J Pharmacol 33: 283-294
52. Gavras I, Gavras H, Sullivan PC, Tifft CP, Chobanian AV, Brunner HR (1979) A comparative study of the effects of oxprenolol versus propranolol in essential hypertension. J Clin Pharmacol 19: 8-14
53. Genest J, Dornier A, Boucher R, Nowaczynski W, Rojo-Ortega JM, Kuchel O (1976) Beta-adrenergic blocking agents and renin spectrum. In: Scriabine A, Sweet CS (eds) New antihypertensive drugs. Spectrum, New York, pp 215-226
54. Geyskes GG, Boer P, Vos J, Dorhout Mees EJ (1976) Renin dependency of blood pressure. Analysis by angiotensin II antagonist P113 in hypertensive patients treated with salt depletion and propranolol. Lancet 1: 1049-1051
55. Gordon RD (1976) Effects of beta-adrenoceptor blocking drugs on plasma volume, renin and aldosterone as components of their antihypertensive action. Drugs 11 [Suppl 1]: 156-163
56. Guimaraes S, Brandao F, Paiva MQ (1978) A study of the adrenoceptor-mediated feedback mechanisms by using adrenaline as a false transmitter. Naunyn-Schmiedebergs Arch Pharmacol 305: 185
57. Hansson BG, Dymling JF, Hedeland H, Hulthen UL (1977) Long-term treatment of moderate hypertension with the $beta_1$-blocking agent metoprolol. Eur J Clin Pharmacol 11: 239-245
58. Hansson L (1973) Beta-adrenergic blockade in essential hypertension. Effects of propranolol on haemodynamic parameters and plasma renin activity. Acta Med Scand 55 [Suppl 1]: 1-40
59. Hansson L, Svensson A, Gudbrandsson T, Sivertsson R (1983) Treatment of hypertension with beta-blockers with and without intrinsic sympathomimetic activity. J Cardiovasc Pharmacol 5: S26-S29
60. Henquet JW, Kho T, Schols M, Thijssen H, Rahn KH (1981) The sympathetic nervous system and the renin-angiotensin system in borderline hypertension. Clin Sci 60: 25-31
61. Hjemdahl P, Pollare T, Gillberg M, Akerstedt T (1980) Concentration-effect relationships for infused catecholamines in man: influence of propranolol and metoprolol. Naunyn-Schmiedebergs Arch Pharmacol 313: R61
62. Hollifield JW, Sherman K, Vander Zwaag R, Shand DG (1976) Proposed mechanisms of propranolol's antihypertensive effect in essential hypertension. N Engl J Med 295 (2): 68-73
63. Jones DH, Hamilton CA, Reid JL (1979) Choice of control groups in the appraisal of sympathetic nervous activity in essential hypertension. Clin Sci 57: 339-344
64. Julius S, Pascual AV, Abbrecht PH, London R (1972) Effect of beta-adrenergic blockade on plasma volume in human subjects. Proc Soc Exp Biol Med 140: 982-985

65. Kelliher GJ, Buckley JP (1970) Central hypotensive activity of dl- and d-propranolol. J Pharm Sci 59: 1276-1280
66. Klevans LR, Kovacs JL, Kelly R (1976) Central effect of beta-adrenergic blocking agents on arterial blood pressure. J Pharmacol Exp Ther 196: 389-395
67. Korner PI (1984) Beta-blockers, autoregulation, and experimental design. Hypertension 6 (2): 140-144
68. Krediet RT, Dunning AJ (1979) Baroreflex sensitivity in hypertension during beta-adrenergic blockade. Br Heart J 41: 106-110
69. Lake CR, Ziegler MG, Coleman MD, Dopin IJ (1977) Age-adjusted plasma norepinephrine levels are similar in normotensive and hypertensive subjects. N Engl J Med 296: 208-209
70. Lancaster R, Goodwin TJ, Peart WS (1976) The effect of pindolol on plasma renin activity and blood pressure in hypertensive patients. Br J Clin Pharmacol 3: 453-460
71. Lancet (1979) Baroreceptors and high blood pressure. Lancet 1: 1277-1279
72. Langer SZ, Cavero I, Massingham R (1980) Recent developments in noradrenergic neurotransmission and its relevance to the mechanism of action of certain antihypertensive agents. Hypertension 2 (4): 372-382
73. Leonetti G, Mayer G, Morganti A, Terzoli L, Zanchetti A, Bianchetti G, Disalle E, Morselli PL, Chidsey CA (1975) Hypotensive and renin suppressing activities of propranolol in hypertensive patients. Clin Sci Mol Med 48: 491-499
74. Leth A, Ibsen H (1976) Changes in the ratio of plasma to interstitial fluid volume during long-term antihypertensive therapy. J Lab Clin Med 87: 781-791
75. Lewis PJ, Haeusler G (1975) Reduction in sympathetic nervous activity as a mechanism for hypotensive effect of propranolol. Nature 256: 440
76. Lopez-Ovejero JA, Weber MA, Drayer JIM, Sealey JE, Laragh JH (1978) Effects of indomethacin alone and during diuretic or beta-adrenoceptor blockade therapy on blood pressure and the renin system in essential hypertension. Clin Sci Mol Med 55: 203s-205s
77. Louis WJ, Brignell MJ, McNeil JJ, Christophidis N, Vajda FJE (1978) Labetalol in hypertension. Lancet 1: 452-453
78. MacGregor GA, Markandu ND, Banks RA, Bayliss J, Roulston JE, Jones JC (1982) Captopril in essential hypertension; contrasting effects of adding hydrochlorothiazide or propranolol. Br Med J 284: 693-696
79. Majewski H, McCulloch MW, Rand MJ, Story DF (1980) Adrenaline activation of prejunctional beta-adrenoceptors in guinea pig atria. Br J Pharmacol 71: 435-444
80. Majewski H, Tung LH, Rand MJ (1981) Adrenaline-induced hypertension in rats. J Cardiovasc Pharmacol 3: 179-85
81. Maling TJB, Ferrara A, Muclow JC, Reid JL, Hamilton CA, Dollery CT (1979) Blood pressure and plasma noradrenaline during single high-dose beta-adrenoceptor blockade. Eur J Clin Pharmacol 15: 375-379
82. Man in't Veld AJ, Schalekamp ADH (1983) Effects of 10 different beta-adrenoceptor antagonists on hemodynamics, plasma renin activity, and plasma norepinephrine in hypertension: the key role of vascular resistance changes in relation to partial agonist activity. J Cardiovasc Pharmacol 5: S-30-S-45
83. McLeod AA, Brown JE, Kitchell BB, Sedor FA, Kuhn DC, Williams RS, Shand DG (1984) Hemodynamic and metabolic responses to exercise after alpha$_1$-, beta$_1$-, and nonselective beta-adrenoceptor blockade in man. Am J Med 76: 97-100
84. Meier A, Weidmann P, Grimm M, Keusch G, Gluck Z, Minder I, Ziegler WH (1981) Pressor factors and cardiovascular pressor responsiveness in borderline hypertension. Hypertension 3: 367
85. Michelakis AM, McAllister RG (1972) The effect of chronic adrenergic receptor blockade on plasma renin activity in man. J Clin Endocrinol Metab 34: 386-394
86. Montastruc P, Montrastruc JL (1978) Effects cardiovasculaires centraux de l'isoprenaline et de quelque beta-bloquants adrenergiques chez le chien hypertendu. Rôle des recepteurs beta centraux. J Physiol (Paris) 74: 651-658
87. Morgan TO, Roberts R, Carney SL, Louis WJ, Doyle AE (1975) Beta-adrenergic receptor blocking drugs, hypertension and plasma renin. Br J Clin Pharmacol 2: 159-164
88. Morganti A, Pickering TG, Lopez-Ovejero JA, Laragh JH (1979) Contrasting effects of acute beta-blockade with propranolol on plasma catecholamines and renin in essential

hypertension: a possible basis for the delayed antihypertensive response. Am Heart J 98: 490-494

89. Myers MG, De Champlain J (1983) Adrenergic status and the antihypertensive effects of atenolol and hydrochlorothiazide. Clin Pharmacol Ther 33 (2): 230
90. Myers MG, Lewis PJ, Reid JL, Dollery CT (1975) Brain concentration of propranolol in relation to hypotensive effect in the rabbit with observations on brain propranolol levels in man. J Pharmacol Exp Ther 192: 327-335
91. Neil-Dwyer G, Bartlett J, McAinsh J, Cruickshank JM (1981) Beta-adrenoceptor blockers and the blood-brain barrier. Br J Clin Pharmacol 11: 549-553
92. Nielsen I, Steiness E, Hesse B (1978) Acute and long-term salt depletion and beta-blockade. Plasma renin activity response and its relation to blood pressure reduction in long-term treatment. Acta Med Scand 203: 415-418
93. Offerhaus L, Van Zwieten PA (1974) Comparative studies on central factors contributing to the hypotensive action of propranolol, alprenolol and their enantiomers. Cardiovasc Res 8: 488-495
94. Page IH, Dustan HP (1962) Persistence of normal blood pressure after discontinuing treatment in hypertensive patients. Circulation 25: 433-436
95. Parving HH, Gyntelberg E (1973) Albumin transcapillary escape rate and plasma volume during long-term beta-adrenergic blockade in essential hypertension. Scand J Clin Lab Invest 32: 105-110
96. Pedersen EB, Christensen WWJ (1975) Catecholamines in plasma and urine in patients with essential hypertension determined by double isotope derivative techniques. Acta Med Scand 198: 373-377
97. Pedersen EB, Kornerup HJ (1977) Plasma renin concentration in essential hypertension during beta-adrenergic blockade and vasodilator therapy. Eur J Clin Pharmacol 12: 93-96
98. Pettinger WA, Mitchell HC (1976) Additive effect of beta-adrenergic blockers in combination with vasodilators in lowering blood pressure. Aust NZ J Med 6 [Suppl 3]: 76-82
99. Pickering TG, Gribbin B, Sleight P (1972) Comparison of the reflex heart rate response to rising and falling arterial blood pressure in man. Cardiovasc Res 6: 277-283
100. Pitkajarvi T, Ylitalo P, Metsa-Ketela T, Vapaatalo H (1979) The effects of $beta_1$-blocking agent, atenolol, on blood pressure, plasma renin activity and prostaglandin F_2 excretion in patients with essential hypertension. Acta Med Scand 206: 107-113
101. Planz G, Planz R (1980) Influence of propranolol on catecholamine concentration in blood of normotensive man during physical exercise and dependence of the drug effect on dosage intervals. Arch Int Pharmacodyn Ther 245 [Suppl]: 58-66
102. Prichard BNC, Gillam PMS (1964) Use of propranolol in the treatment of hypertension. Br Med J 2: 725
103. Prichard BNC, Gillam PMS (1969) Treatment of hypertension with propranolol. Br Med J 1: 7-16
104. Rand MJ, Majewski H, McCulloch MW, Story DF (1979) An adrenaline-mediated positive feed-back loop in sympathetic transmission and its possible role in hypertension. In: Langer SZ, Starke K, Dubocovich ML (eds) Presynaptic receptors. Pergamon, Oxford, p 263
105. Rasmussen S, Rasmussen K (1979) Influence of metoprolol, alone and in combination with a thiazide diuretic, on blood pressure, plasma volume, extracellular volume and glomerular filtration rate in essential hypertension. Eur J Clin Pharmacol 15: 305-310
106. Reid JL, Lewis PJ, Myers MG, Dollery CT (1974) Cardiovascular effects of intracerebroventricular d-, l- and dl-propranolol in the conscious rabbit. J Pharmacol Exp Ther 188: 394-399
107. Ronnov-Jessen V, Hansen J (1969) Blood volume and exchangeable sodium during treatment of hypertension with guanethidine and hydrochlorothiazide. Acta Med Scand 186: 255-263
108. Salvetti A, Arzilli F, Pedrinelli R, Beggi P, Motolese M (1982) Interaction between oxprenolol and indomethacin in blood pressure in essential hypertensive patients. Eur J Clin Pharmacol 22: 197-201
109. Salvetti A, Pedrinelli R, Magagna A, Abdel-Haq B (1983) The influence of indomethacin on some pharmacological actions of atenolol. In: Dunn MJ, Patrono C, Cinotti GA (eds), Prostaglandins and the Kidney, Plenum Publishing Corporation, New York, pp 287-295
110. Schluter KJ, Aellig WH, Petersen KG, Rieband HC, Wehrli A, Kerp L (1982) The influence of

beta-adrenoceptor blocking drugs with and without intrinsic sympathomimetic activity on the hormonal responses to hypo- and hyperglycaemia. Br J Clin Pharmacol 13: 407S-417S
111. Sedenberg-Olsen P, Ibsen H (1972) Plasma volume and extracellular fluid volume during long-term treatment with propranolol in essential hypertension. Clin Sci 43: 165-170
112. Sever PS, Osikowska B, Birch M, Tunbridge RDG (1977) Plasma noradrenaline in essential hypertension. Lancet 1: 1078-1081
113. Simon G, Kiowski W, Julius S (1978) Antihypertensive and beta-adrenoceptor antagonist action of timolol. Clin Pharmacol Ther 23: 152-157
114. Skrabal F, Aubock J, Hortnagl H, Brucke T (1981) Plasma epinephrine and norepinephrine concentrations in primary and secondary human hypertension. Hypertension 3: 373
115. Sondoni S, Agabiti-Rosei F, Fraser R, Leckie BJ, Morton JJ, Cumming AMM, Sood BP, Robertson JLS (1982) Response of the renin-angiotensin-aldosterone system to upright tilting and to intravenous frusemide: effect of prior metoprolol and propranolol. Br J Clin Pharmacol 13: 341-350
116. Staessen J, Fagard R, Lijnen P, Verschueren LJ, Amery A (1980) Beta-blockade during captopril treatment for hypertension. N Engl J Med 303 (19): 1121-1122
117. Starke K (1977) Regulation of noradrenaline release by presynaptic receptor systems. Rev Physiol Biochem Pharmacol 77: 1-24
118. Stern S, Hoffman M, Braun K (1971) Cardiovascular responses to carotid and vertebral artery infusions of propranolol. Cardiovasc Res 5: 425-430
119. Stjarne L, Brundin J (1975) Dual adrenoceptor-mediated control of noradrenaline secretion from human vasoconstrictor nerves. Facilitation by beta-receptors and inhibition by alpha-receptors. Acta Physiol Scand 94: 139-141
120. Stjarne L, Brundin J (1976) Beta-adrenoceptors facilitating noradrenaline secretion from human vasoconstrictor nerves. Acta Physiol Scand 97: 88-93
121. Stokes GS, Weber MA, Thornell IR (1974) Beta-blockers and plasma renin activity in hypertension. Br Med J 1: 60-62
122. Stumpe KO, Kolloch R, Gramann W, Vetter H, Ressel C, Higuchi M, Krück F (1976) Renin, aldosterone and arterial pressure responses to acute beta-adrenergic receptor blockade in hypertensive patients. Klin Wochenschr 54: 775-782
123. Svendsen TL, Hartling OJ, Trap-Jensen J, McNair A, Bliddal J (1981) Adrenergic beta-receptor blockade: hemodynamic importance of intrinsic sympathomimetic activity at rest. Clin Pharmacol Ther 29 (6): 711-718
124. Takeshita A, Tanaka S, Kuroiwa A et al. (1975) Reduced baroreceptor sensitivity in borderline hypertension. Circulation 51: 738-742
125. Takeshita A, Tanaka S, Nakamura M (1978) Effects of propranolol on baroreflex sensitivity in borderline hypertension. Cardiovasc Res 12: 148-151
126. Tarazi RC, Dustan HP (1972) Beta-adrenergic blockade in hypertension. Am J Cardiol 29: 633-640
127. Tarazi RC, Frohlich ED, Dustan HP (1971) Plasma volume changes with long-term beta-adrenergic blockade. Am Heart J 82: 770-776
128. Taylor AA, Pool JL, Lake CR et al. (1978) Plasma norepinephrine concentrations - no differences among normal volunteers and low, high or normal renin hypertensive patients. Life Sci 22: 1499-1510
129. Thurn RH, Smith WM (1967) On resetting of 'barostats' in hypertensive patients. JAMA 201: 301-304
130. Trap-Jensen J, Carlsen JE, Hartling OJ, Svendsen TL, Tango M, Christensen NJ (1982) Beta-adrenoceptor blockade and psychic stress in man. A comparison of the acute effects of labetalol, metoprolol, pindolol and propranolol on plasma levels of adrenaline and noradrenaline. Br J Clin Pharmacol 13: 391S-395S
131. Tsukiyama H, Otsuka K, Higuma K (1982) Effects of beta-adrenoceptor antagonists on central haemodynamics in essential hypertension. Br J Clin Pharmacol 13: 269S-278S
132. Tuck ML, Stern N, Sowers JR (1985) Enhanced 24-hour norepinephrine and renin secretion in young patients with essential hypertension: relation with the Circadian pattern of arterial blood pressure. Am J Cardiol 55: 112-115
133. Usberti M, Mileti M, Maiorca R (1975) Effect dell'indomethacina sulla funzione renale (Abstract in English). Minerva Nefrol 22: 299-303

134. Van Baak MA, Struyker Boudier HAJ, Smits JFM (1985) Antihypertensive mechanisms of beta-adrenoceptor blockade: a review. Clin Exp Hypertens [A] A7 (1): 1-72
135. Vandenburg MJ, Holly JMP, Goodwin FJ, Sharman VL, Marsh FP (1983) The effect of captopril and propranolol on the responses to posture and isometric exercise in patients with essential hypertension. Eur J Clin Pharmacol 25: 721-728
136. Van Zwieten PA, Timmermans PB (1979) Comparison between the acute haemodynamic effects and brain penetration of atenolol and metoprolol. J Cardiovasc Pharmacol 1: 85-96
137. Verniory A, Staroukine M, Telerman M, Delwiche F (1974) Effect of sotalol on arterial pressure and renin-angiotensin system in hypertensive patients. In: Smart E (ed) Clinical advances in beta-blocking therapy. Sotalol. Excerpta Medica IV, Amsterdam, pp 36-45
138. Vincent HH, Man in't Veld AJ, Boomsma F, Wenting GJ, Schalekamp MADH (1982) Elevated plasma noradrenaline in response to beta-adrenoceptor stimulation in man. Br J Clin Pharmacol 13: 717-721
139. Volpe M, Trimarco B, Ricciardelli B, Vigorito C, De Luca N, Rengo F, Condorelli M (1982) The autonomic nervous tone abnormalities in the genesis of the impaired baroreflex responsiveness in borderline hypertensive patients. Clin Sci 62: 581-588
140. Watkins J, Abott EC, Hensby CN, Webster J, Dollery CT (1980) Attenuation of hypotensive effect of propranolol and thiazide diuretics by indomethacin. Br Med J 281: 702-705
141. Watson RDS, Littler WA (1979) Onset and duration of beta-adrenergic receptor blockade following single oral dose acebutolol hydrochloride (Sectral). Br J Clin Pharmacol 7: 557-561
142. Watson RDS, Stallard TJ, Littler WA (1979) Effects of beta-adrenoceptor antagonists on sinoaortic baroreflex sensitivity and blood pressure in hypertensive man. Clin Sci 57: 241-247
143. Watson RDS, Eriksson BM, Hamilton CA, Reid JL, Stallard TJ, Littler WA (1980) Effects of chronic beta-adrenoceptor antagonism on plasma catecholamines and blood pressure in hypertension. J Cardiovasc Pharmacol 2: 725-738
144. Weber MA, Drayer JI, Laragh JH (1977) Beta-blockade, renin and blood pressure. Lancet 1: 367-368
145. Weber MA, Priest RT, Brewer DD (1980) Importance of low diuretic dosage in the combination treatment of hypertension. Clin Pharmacol Ther 27 (2): 292-293
146. Wilcox RG, MacDonald IA, Bennett T, Brown AM (1982) Metabolic and haemodynamic responses to exercise in hypertension: effects of beta-adrenoceptor antagonists. Cardiovasc Res 16 (7): 380-381
147. Winer N, Chokshi DS, Yoon MS, Freedman AD (1969) Adrenergic receptor mediation of renin secretion. J Clin Endocrinol Metab 29: 1168-1175
148. Winer N, Carter CH, Eddy HE, Gustafson SJ, Boling DA (1978) Pindolol vs methyldopa: a double-blind evaluation of effects on blood pressure, norepinephrine and renin. Clin Res 26: 596a
149. Yamaguchi N, De Champlain J, Nadeau RL (1977) Regulation of norepinephrine release from cardiac sympathetic fibers in the dog by presynaptic alpha and beta receptors. Circ Res 41: 108-117
150. Yusuf S, Sleight P, Rossi P, Ramsdale D, Peto R, Furze L, Sterry H, Pearson M, Motwani R, Parish S, Gray R, Bennett D, Bray C (1983) Reduction in infarct size, arrhythmias and chest pain by early intravenous beta-blockade in suspected acute myocardial infarction. Circulation 67 [Suppl 1]: I-32-I-41
151. Zanchetti A, Leonetti G, Terzoli L, Sala C (1983) Beta-blockers and renin. Drugs (Symposium on beta-blockers in the 1980's) 25 [Suppl 2]: 58-63
152. Zweifler AJ, Esler M (1976) Dissociation of fall in blood pressure, renin activity and heart rate during propranolol therapy. Circulation 54 [Suppl 2]: 87

Discussion

Lemmer: You pointed out that ISA blockers such as pindolol reduce norepinephrine concentration, whereas propranolol and some others increase it. Could it be that the indol moiety in the molecule of pindolol plays an important role, for the findings are based chiefly on pindolol. Perhaps a certain serotoninergic interaction of pindolol is at work here?

Cruickshank: Yes, that is a very good point. It probably is not the case, I think, because other beta blockers with nonselective ISA do in fact have a similar effect on plasma norepinephrine, but they do not have an indol moiety within their molecule. It is a good suggestion, but I think it is probably not relevant.

Curtis-Prior: I would like to clarify a point right at the very beginning of your talk, when you suggested that beta blockade of $beta_1$ receptors was the key point in the antihypertensive effect of the blocking agents; you suggested it because *d*-propranolol did not have an antihypertensive effect. Does that mean that *d*-propranolol is a $beta_2$ blocker?

Cruickshank: No, sorry. There was a step left out in that logic. What I should have said at that time is that $beta_1$-selective agents such as metoprolol and atenolol have a similar effect, so that $beta_1$ blockade lowers blood pressure.

Curtis-Prior: Yes, but you still haven't answered my question. Does that mean that *d*-propranolol is a specific $beta_2$ blocker?

Cruickshank: It has little or no beta-blocking action at all.

Curtis Prior: That's what I thought. Thank you.

Brodde: There are controversial results in the literature on the effects of $beta_2$ antagonists or, let's say, on the $beta_2$ antagonist ICI 118551, on blood pressure. The Schalekamp group claims that it decreases blood pressure, while a Swedish group claims the opposite. Do you have experience with ICI? You emphasized, at least in your abstract, the presynaptic theory, and then you have to conclude that $beta_2$ antagonists must decrease blood pressure.

Cruickshank: That's a good question. There have been four or five studies looking at the effect of $beta_2$ blockers on blood pressure, and I think one or two have been published. The effect of the $beta_2$ blockers is not essentially to lower blood pressure. I think that the Dutch group is slightly out on a limb there, and the weight of evidence suggests, if anything, that there might be small increase in blood pressure, which could well be the increase in peripheral resistance that you would get under these circumstances. So, on balance, there seems to be no fall in blood pressure with the $beta_2$ blockers.

Göthert: One of your slides showed that there was an influence on the beta adrenoceptor blockers on norepinephrine release from the renal vascular bed. How was this measured? I think that it is very difficult to measure norepinephrine release in humans.

Cruickshank: This is the work of Birkenhäger and his group, and I don't know the details of that study. I can only presume that they must have had catheters placed locally.

Göthert: Even so you would only measure norepinephrine overflow, because I think you cannot measure release under in vivo conditions.

Cruickshank: I agree with you entirely.

Subject Index